T0259180

Pediatrics

Editors

PETER M. DIGERONIMO
JOÃO BRANDÃO

VETERINARY CLINICS OF NORTH AMERICA: EXOTIC ANIMAL PRACTICE

www.vetexotic.theclinics.com

Consulting Editor
JÖRG MAYER

May 2024 • Volume 27 • Number 2

ELSEVIER

1600 John F. Kennedy Boulevard • Suite 1800 • Philadelphia, Pennsylvania, 19103-2899
http://www.vetexotic.theclinics.com

VETERINARY CLINICS OF NORTH AMERICA: EXOTIC ANIMAL PRACTICE Volume 27, Number 2
May 2024 ISSN 1094-9194, ISBN-13: 978-0-443-12877-6

Editor: Stacy Eastman
Developmental Editor: Varun Gopal

Veterinary Clinics of North America: Exotic Animal Practice (ISSN 1094-9194) is published in January, May, and September by Elsevier, Inc., 360 Park Avenue South, New York, NY 10010-1710. Subscription prices are $311.00 per year for US individuals, $100.00 per year for US students and residents, $362.00 per year for Canadian individuals, $377.00 per year for international individuals, $100.00 per year Canadian students/residents, and $165.00 per year for international students/residents. For institutional access pricing please contact Customer Service via the contact information below. To receive student/resident rate, orders must be accompanied by name of affiliated institution, date of term, and the *signature* of program/residency coordinator on institution letterhead. Orders will be billed at individual rate until proof of status is received. Foreign air speed delivery is included in all *Clinics* subscription prices. All prices are subject to change without notice. **POSTMASTER:** Send address changes to *Veterinary Clinics of North America: Exotic Animal Practice*, Elsevier Health Sciences Division, Subscription Customer Service, 3251 Riverport Lane, Maryland Heights, MO 63043. **Customer Service: Telephone: 1-800-654-2452** (U.S. and Canada); **1-314-447-8871** (outside U.S. and Canada). **Fax: 1-314-447-8029. E-mail: journalscustomerservice-usa@elsevier.com (for print support); journalsonlinesupport-usa@elsevier.com (for online support).**

Reprints. For copies of 100 or more of articles in this publication, please contact the Commercial Reprints Department, Elsevier Inc., 360 Park Avenue South, New York, New York 10010-1710. Tel.: 212-633-3874; Fax: 212-633-3820; E-mail: reprints@elsevier.com.

Veterinary Clinics of North America: Exotic Animal Practice is covered in *MEDLINE/PubMed (Index Medicus)*.

Contributors

CONSULTING EDITOR

JÖRG MAYER, Dr med vet, MSc
Diplomate of the American Board of Veterinary Practitioners (Exotic Companion Mammals); Diplomate of the European College of Zoological Medicine (Small Mammals); Diplomate of the American College of Zoological Medicine; Associate Professor of Zoological Medicine, Department of Small Animal Medicine and Surgery, University of Georgia College of Veterinary Medicine, Athens, Georgia, USA

EDITORS

PETER M. DIGERONIMO, VMD, MSc
Diplomate of the American College of Zoological Medicine; Associate Veterinarian, Philadelphia Zoo, Associate Adjunct Professor of Zoological Medicine, School of Veterinary Medicine, University of Pennsylvania, Philadelphia, Pennsylvania, USA

JOÃO BRANDÃO, LMV, MS
Diplomate of the European College of Zoological Medicine (Avian); Diplomate of the American College of Zoological Medicine; Associate Professor, Zoological Medicine, Debbie and Wayne Bell Professorship in Veterinary Clinical Sciences, Department of Veterinary Clinical Sciences, College of Veterinary Medicine, Oklahoma State University, Stillwater, Oklahoma, USA

AUTHORS

AMANDA ARDENTE, DVM, PhD
Founder, Ardente Veterinary Nutrition LLC, Ocala, Florida, USA

TRINITA BARBOZA, DVM, DVSc
Diplomate of the American College of Zoological Medicine; Assistant Professor, Zoological Companion Animal Service, Department of Clinical Sciences, Cummings School of Veterinary Medicine, North Grafton, Massachusetts, USA

JON ROMANO, DVM
Assistant Professor, Exotics and Lab Animal Medicine, Department of Veterinary Clinical Sciences, Long Island University College of Veterinary Medicine, Brookville, New York, USA

ERNESTO DOMINGUEZ-VILLEGAS, DVM
Diplomate of the American College of Veterinary Preventive Medicine; CWR, Veterinarian, Southwest Virginia Wildlife Center, Roanoke, Virginia, USA

MARION R. DESMARCHELIER, DMV, MSc
Diplomate of the American College of Zoological Medicine; Diplomate of the European College of Zoological Medicine (Zoo Health Management); Diplomate of the American College of Veterinary Behaviorists; Associate Professor, Department of Clinical Sciences, Faculté de médecine vétérinaire, Université de Montréal, Québec, Canada

ABIGAIL DUVALL, DVM
Diplomate of the American Board of Veterinary Practitioners- Avian Practice; Associate Veterinarian, Exotic Vet Care, Mt Pleasant, South Carolina, USA

DAVID ESHAR, DVM, MBA
Diplomate of the American Board of Veterinary Practitioners (Exotic Companion Mammal); Diplomate of the European College of Zoological Medicine (Small Mammal and Zoo Health Management); Director of Animal Health, Wildlife Hospital of Israel, Zoological Center Ramat Gan, Ramat, Israel

MIKEL SABATER GONZÁLEZ, LV, MRCVS, CertZooMed
Diplomate of the European College of Zoological Medicine (Avian); Veterinary Specialist, Manor Vets Edgbaston, Birmingham, United Kingdom

MOLLY GLEESON, DVM
Diplomate of the American College of Zoological Medicine; Clinical Veterinarian, Department of Exotic Pets, PETS Referral Center, Berkeley, California, USA

MICHELE GOODMAN, VMD
Director of Animal Care, Elmwood Park Zoo, Norristown, Pennsylvania, USA

CHRISTINE T. HIGBIE, DVM
Diplomate of the American College of Zoological Medicine; Associate Veterinarian, The Philadelphia Zoo, Philadelphia, Pennsylvania, USA

DARIA HINKLE, DVM
Department of Surgical Sciences, School of Veterinary Medicine, University of Wisconsin-Madison, Madison, Wisconsin, USA

LA'TOYA V. LATNEY, DVM, CertAqV
Diplomate of the European College of Zoological Medicine (Zoo Health Management); Diplomate of the American Board of Veterinary Practitioners (Reptile/Amphibian); Senior Clinician, Avian and Exotic Medicine and Surgery, The Animal Medical Center, New York, New York, USA

JULIANNE E. McCREADY, DVM, DVSc
Diplomate of the American College of Zoological Medicine; Assistant Professor, Zoological Medicine Service, Department of Veterinary Clinical Sciences, College of Veterinary Medicine, Oklahoma State University, Stillwater, Oklahoma, USA

COLIN T. McDERMOTT, VMD
Diplomate of the American Board of Veterinary Practitioners (Reptile and Amphibian Practice); Certified Aquatic Veterinarian, Clinical Assistant Professor, Department of Veterinary Clinical Sciences, Jockey Club College of Veterinary Medicine and Life Sciences, City University of Hong Kong, Kowloon Tong, Hong Kong, China

SARAH OZAWA, DVM
Diplomate of the American College of Zoological Medicine; Assistant Professor, Department of Clinical Sciences, College of Veterinary Medicine, North Carolina State University, Raleigh, North Carolina, USA

REBECCA PACHECO, DVM
Assistant Professor of Avian, Exotic, and Zoological Medicine, Department of Clinical Sciences, College of Veterinary Medicine and Biomedical Sciences, Colorado State University, Fort Collins, Colorado, USA

MIRANDA J. SADAR, DVM
Diplomate of the American College of Zoological Medicine; Service Head and Assistant Professor of Avian, Exotic, and Zoological Medicine, Department of Clinical Sciences, College of Veterinary Medicine and Biomedical Sciences, Colorado State University, Fort Collins, Colorado, USA

NICOLAS SCHOONHEERE, DMV
Associate Veterinary, Centre Vétérinaire Exclusif NAC VTNac Hingeon, Hingeon, Belgium

RHIANNON L. SCHULTZ, MA
Consultant and Project Manager, Animal Welfare Expertise Ltd, Littleton Manner, Littleton, Winchester, United Kingdom

BARBARA TODDES, MS
Nutrition Program Director, Philadelphia Zoo, Philadelphia, Pennsylvania, USA

NICOLE R. WYRE, DVM
Diplomate of the American Board of Veterinary Practitioners (Avian Practice); American Board of Veterinary Practitioners (Exotic Companion Mammal), Certified Veterinary Acupuncture, Certified Traditional Chinese Veterinary Medicine Palliative and End-of-Life Practitioner; Head Veterinarian, Zodiac Pet & Exotic Hospital, Fortress Hill, Hong Kong

GRAHAM ZOLLER, DMV, IPSAV (Zoological Medicine)
Diplomate of the European College of Zoological Medicine (Avian); Exotic Pet Department - Centre Hospitalier Vétérinaire OnlyVet, Saint-Priest, France

Contents

Ferrets are bred to be pets, utilized for hunting, and as laboratory models. Despite the fact that ferrets in some areas of the world are neutered by the breeder before entering the pet trade, the importance of pediatric management should not be overlooked. Pregnant, whelping, and lactating jills should be closely monitored and kept in a quiet, stress-free environment. Hand-rearing baby kits is very challenging due to their requirement for ferret milk. Minimizing maternal stress and disease can prevent the need to hand rear kits. Infectious diseases in juvenile ferrets include canine distemper virus, rotavirus, coccidiosis, feline panleukopenia virus (experimental only), and Toxoplasma-like disease. All juvenile ferrets should be vaccinated against canine distemper and rabies. Congenital diseases are reported to affect the auditory, ocular, cardiovascular, urogenital, central nervous, and musculoskeletal systems. Early detection of these diseases is important to prevent the progression of curable diseases.

Rabbits encompass roles spanning from companion animals, wildlife species to laboratory animal models. Pediatric care of these species therefore may extend to various disciplines of veterinary medicine. Rabbits are born altricial but have a unique perinatal relationship between kit and doe with infrequent nursing. Nursing is immunologically protective to the kit and close contact with the doe allows for colonization of their gastrointestinal tract with bacterial flora. The most common diseases that pediatric rabbits are faced with are gastrointestinal in nature with orphaned and hand-reared rabbits at higher risk due to the aforementioned effects on their immune system.

This article reviews the development, hand-rearing, feeding, housing, and social behavior of common pet rodent species (rats, mice, hamsters, gerbils, guinea pigs, chinchillas, and degus). In addition, common gastrointestinal, respiratory, cardiovascular, dermatologic, musculoskeletal, neurologic, and ophthalmic disorders in pediatric pet rodents are reviewed. Preventative care and indications for spaying and neutering are discussed.

disorders, and to provide minimal management guidelines to attempt to achieve a free of infecto-contagious disease collection.

exist has been compiled by wildlife rehabilitators, commercial breeders, and/or exotic captive breeding programs, such as those that exist in zoologic facilities. In this article, we discuss natural history, feeding strategies, energy requirements, digestive physiology and diet digestibility, and key nutrients of concern as factors for determining an appropriate diet for pediatric exotic species.

VETERINARY CLINICS OF NORTH AMERICA: EXOTIC ANIMAL PRACTICE

SERIES OF RELATED INTEREST

Veterinary Clinics: Small Animal Practice
https://www.vetsmall.theclinics.com/
Advances in Small Animal Care
https://www.advancesinsmallanimalcare.com

THE CLINICS ARE NOW AVAILABLE ONLINE!
Access your subscription at:
www.theclinics.com

Preface

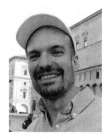
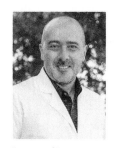

Peter M. DiGeronimo,
VMD, MSc, DACZM

João Brandão, LMV, MS,
DECZM (Avian), DACZM

Editors

Exotic animal practice has progressed substantially, mainly because of increased interest by veterinarians, but also because of the rise in popularity of these species. In order to support such growth, captive breeding is essential. Although much of the literature focuses on adult animals, pediatric medicine is relevant to exotic animal practice and is, in many aspects, different from the management of older animals. We are honored to organize this issue of *Veterinary Clinics of North America: Exotic Animal Practice* dedicated to pediatric medicine. This issue focuses on the management of several taxa during their development, birth, growth, and early age. Each article is organized to provide the reader with a general background on the husbandry, preventative care, and diseases specific to juveniles of each species and, when applicable, on the main considerations during incubation or pregnancy.

As editors, it is our privilege to introduce this comprehensive collection of knowledge and express our deepest gratitude to the exceptional authors who have made this resource possible. We are proud to have included clinicians from private practice, zoologic institutions, wildlife rehabilitation, and academia from countries around the globe. We believe that the veterinary profession benefits from greater representation of the diversity of our community and the fields in which we work. We are very grateful to the authors that have embarked with us on this endeavor and would like to thank each of them for the time and effort they devoted to writing each article.

Within this issue, you will find a wealth of information, practical insights, and clinical wisdom that illuminates the complexities associated with pediatric medicine across a diverse spectrum of nontraditional species. This issue covers some of the most common species of exotic companion animals, such as rabbits and ferrets, and also some other groups, including waterfowl and raptors, that may also be applicable to wildlife rehabilitation and zoo practice. Although our focus is on captive animals, we wanted to provide information that could also be useful for the management of native North American wildlife commonly presented to veterinarians. As very well stated by Dr Dominguez-Villegas, "Humans make very inadequate surrogate parents for wild

Vet Clin Exot Anim 27 (2024) xiii–xiv
https://doi.org/10.1016/j.cvex.2023.11.001
1094-9194/24/© 2023 Published by Elsevier Inc.

infants despite their ability to properly nourish them." Indeed, properly caring for juvenile wildlife requires much more than merely feeding them. We hope that this wildlife-specific article will be a useful resource for veterinarians presented with wild animals and will allow you to optimize the initial treatments you provide prior to transfer of the patient to a licensed wildlife rehabilitator.

Among mammals, marsupials have very unique reproductive characteristics, and for this reason, along with the increase in popularity of marsupials as pets, specific articles on macropods and sugar gliders have also been included. Along those lines, the unique reproductive strategies, physiologic needs, and diseases of birds and reptiles make these taxa deserving of special attention. We have included articles devoted to a diverse array of birds, including Anseriformes, Columbiformes, and psittacines, as well as an article reviewing considerations for the veterinary management of juvenile reptiles.

Caring for young animals requires special consideration of both their physical growth and their cognitive development. Articles specifically dedicated to nutrition and behavior provide valuable information to the reader on these aspects of pediatric medicine that are essential for the well-being of nontraditional species.

Last but not least, we would like to thank Dr Jörg Mayer, for the invitation to serve as guest editors, and the Elsevier staff, whose support was essential to finalize this work. We would like to specifically acknowledge Varun Gopal, Axell Ivan Jade Purificación, and Stacy Eastman for their investment in this publication.

We hope that this issue will become an invaluable resource for veterinarians, veterinary students, and all those who seek information on the management of pediatric patients. The information that has been compiled here will be essential to improve the management of nontraditional species.

Sincerely,

Peter M. DiGeronimo, VMD, MSc, DACZM
Philadelphia Zoo
Philadelphia, PA 19104, USA

School of Veterinary Medicine
University of Pennsylvania
Philadelphia, PA 19104, USA

João Brandão, LMV, MS, DECZM (Avian), DACZM
Department of Veterinary Clinical Sciences
College of Veterinary Medicine
Oklahoma State University
Stillwater, OK 74078, USA

E-mail addresses:
digeronimo.peter@phillyzoo.org (P.M. DiGeronimo)
jbrandao@okstate.edu (J. Brandão)

Ferret Pediatrics

Nicole R. Wyre, DVM, DABVP (Avian), DABVP (Exotic Companion Mammals), CVA, CTPEP

KEYWORDS

- Ferret • Pediatrics • Neonatal • Congenital diseases • Rotavirus
- Canine distemper virus

KEY POINTS

- Careful monitoring during whelping is important to ensure that the kits do not become tangled in the placenta and umbilical cords.
- Rotavirus and coccidiosis are common causes of diarrhea in kits that may require fluid therapy.
- Canine distemper is not always fatal in ferrets, especially if it is vaccine induced and appropriate treatment is started immediately.
- For immunity to develop, ferrets must receive at least 2 effective canine distemper vaccines after maternal antibodies have waned.
- Congenital diseases affect 3% to 4% of newborn kits and occur more frequently in jills that have had 0 to 2 pregnancies.

INTRODUCTION

Ferrets are common household pets as well as common laboratory animal models. In the Unites States, the majority of ferrets are spayed and neutered. Therefore, pediatric medicine may not be a common presentation to most veterinarians practicing in the United States, but this is not the case in the rest of the world where ferrets are intact and able to breed. Therefore, pediatric medicine is still an area that needs to be considered.

Gestation, Whelping, Neonatal Nutrition

Gestation in ferrets ranges from 39 to 43 days with primiparous jills usually whelping on day 41 and multiparous on day 42 (**Table 1**). It is very important to know the gestation length as kits that die *in utero* do so almost always after 43 days gestation.[1] Litter size can range from 1 to 18 kits, but jills are usually not able to nurse more than 11 kits at a time.[1] If there are multiple jills nursing at the same time, kits from large litters can be fostered to mothers with fewer kits. This fostering is most successful if the new kits are warm and fed a puppy milk replacer prior to placement.

Zodiac Pet & Exotic Hospital, Shop 102, 1/F, Victoria Centre, Fortress Hill, Hong Kong
E-mail address: wyredvm@gmail.com

Vet Clin Exot Anim 27 (2024) 155–170
https://doi.org/10.1016/j.cvex.2023.11.002
1094-9194/24/© 2023 Elsevier Inc. All rights reserved.

Table 1
Reproductive, neonatal, and pediatric data for domestic ferrets

Parameter	Value
Puberty female	7–12 mo (as early as 23 wk with photomanipulation)
Puberty male	8–12 mo (as early as 16 wk with photomanipulation)
Gestation	39–43 d *after day 43 of gestation, almost all kits will die in utero*
Litter size	8 kits (range, 1–18)
Weight at birth	10 g (range 6–12)
Weight at 5 day old	Double birth weight
Weight at 10 day old	Triple birth weight
Daily weight gain: 1st wk	2.5–30 gr/day
Daily weight gain: 2nd wk	4 gr/day
Daily weight gain: 3rd wk	6 gr/day
Deciduous teeth erupt	14 d
Permanent canine teeth erupt	47–52 d
Shed deciduous canine teeth	56–70 d
Ears open	32 d
Eyes open	34 d
Age to introduce moistened solid food	14–21 d
Weaning age	6–8 wk
Weight at weaning	300–350 g

Fox JG, Bell J, Broome R. Growth and reproduction. Biology and Diseases of the Ferret 2014:187 to 209.Jekl V, Hauptman K. Reproductive medicine in ferrets. Veterinary Clinics: Exotic Animal Practice 2017;20:629 to 663.Powers LV PD. Basic anatomy, physiology, and husbandry of ferrets In: Quesenbery KE OC, Mans C, Carpenter JW ed. Ferrets, Rabbits, and Rodents. 4 ed: Elsevier, 2020;1 to 12.

Careful monitoring during whelping is important. Pregnant jills should be housed separately in a quiet nest box. Approximately 5 kits are born per hour.[2,3] Kits can become entangled in the placenta and umbilical cords if they are born too rapidly or if there is improper bedding that can adhere to the umbilical cords. The cords should be trimmed to 1 cm in length as soon as possible. If the cord becomes tangled, sterile saline can be used to soften the cords to allow removal. The umbilical cord stumps should be disinfected with a 1% iodine solution to prevent ascending infection.[1] Kits should be kept at 18 to 21°C (65–70°F) in a nesting box that allows them to snuggle with their siblings without wandering off.[1] A heat lamp should be placed over half of the nesting box to allow them to select their ideal temperature. The bedding should be replaced frequently and should not contain any particulate matter. It is important to decrease the stress and handling of the jill to prevent her from hiding the kits or cannibalizing them. This is more frequently seen in primiparous jills.[2]

Ferret milk has a much higher fat content than cow's milk. Ferret milk contains 8% to 10% fat at parturition and 20% fat 3 weeks postpartum; therefore, jills should be fed a diet of 30% fat to help maintain their weight while nursing.[1] It is recommended to start feeding the kits a softened pelleted diet at 2 to 3 weeks old. This can help relieve the strain on the nursing jills. A pelleted diet can be mixed with warm water and a source of animal fat (ie, linoleic acid, fish oil, chicken fat). The mixture should contain at least 30% fat and 40% protein.[1] Kits should be weighed daily to ensure they are gaining adequate weight (see **Table 1**).

Fading kit syndrome can be seen if the mother is not able to properly care for the kit(s) due to poor milk production, mastitis, metritis, or other reasons. These kits need supplemental feeding or can be fostered to a healthy nursing jill. Completely hand-rearing kits is challenging as they require ferret milk for at least the first 10 days of life.[1] In a research setting, milk can be obtained from lactating jills but requires general anesthesia. If the dam is producing any milk at all, it is recommended that the kits stay with her and receive a puppy or kitten milk replacer every 4 hours. Kits older than 14 days of age can be fed canine or feline milk replacer from a plastic pipette or dropper. After 21 days of age, the ferrets can be fed a mixture of canned food and milk replacer. Solid food should be offered before their ears and eyes open (see **Table 1**). Another potential hand-rearing diet that can be given to ferrets 10 to 50 day old is a mixture of 80% cow's milk (4% fat) with either 20% chicken egg yolk or 20% strained beef liver.[1]

Infectious Diseases in Juvenile Ferrets

Canine distemper virus

Canine distemper virus (CDV) is an enveloped, nonsegmented RNA virus. It is transmitted via aerosol or direct contact with oral, respiratory, or ocular fluids and skin exudates containing the virus. It is fragile in the environment and requires close contact to spread. Unvaccinated ferrets of any age are susceptible to infection, but clinical disease is most commonly seen in 3-month to 6-month-old juvenile ferrets when they lose their protective maternal antibodies.[4] Subclinical infection can occur leading to disease outbreaks when these animals are introduced to unvaccinated ferrets.

CDV causes respiratory, dermatologic, and neurologic diseases. In naturally occurring infections, incubation is 11 to 56 days and the course of the disease is typically 14 to 36 days but has been reported to last as long as 7 weeks.[4,5] During the initial phase, the most common clinical signs are lethargy, oculonasal discharge, and diarrhea. Some ferrets may develop a fever during this phase, but it depends on the CDV strain.[4] During the mid-late phase, dermatologic signs occur and include severe pruritus with an erythematous papular rash that begins on the chin and spreads to the inguinal region. Hyperkeratosis of the nasal planum and foot pads can also occur. In the final stage of the disease, skin lesions progress and severe dyspnea can occur. Secondary bacterial pneumonia and skin infections can occur leading to sepsis and death. In neurotropic CDV strains, central nervous system (CNS) signs occur in the advanced stage of the disease and include hyperexcitability, muscle tremors, hypersalivation, paresis, myoclonus, convulsions, coma, and death.[4,5]

Hematology in ferrets with CDV can show varying degrees of leukopenia and nonregenerative anemia.[5,6] Pulmonary changes consistent with pneumonia can be seen on thoracic radiographs in the later stages of the disease.[6] CDV is diagnosed via reverse transcription polymerase chain reaction (RT-PCR) of conjunctiva swabs, respiratory secretions, or urine.[4] CDV titers are also available, but a single titer may be difficult to interpret if the ferret was previously vaccinated. Titers can be used to identify CDV in an outbreak and to diagnose recovery and clearance of the infection.[6]

Treatment is symptomatic focusing on supportive care and prevention of secondary bacterial infections. Broad-spectrum antibiotics given systemically are recommended to prevent secondary bacterial pneumonia and antibiotic eye drops are recommended to prevent bacterial conjunctivitis. Supportive care including supplemental feeding with a high fat, high protein liquid diet, and fluid therapy is important to prevent weight loss and dehydration secondary to decreased intake. When injected on the day of infection, intramuscular administration of vitamin A at a dose of 50,000 IU (15 mg) once daily for 2 doses improved recovery and decreased clinical signs in ferrets experimentally infected with CDV.[7] Oral vitamin C supplementation may be beneficial based on early studies of CDV in dogs, but this data have been subject to criticism.[4] Severe pruritus and painful skin lesions can be managed with antihistamines and opioids. Bronchodilators via nebulization may improve respiratory distress.[4,8]

Vaccination can be used as a treatment in the face of an outbreak. CDV vaccines are most effective when administered at a higher dose and within hours of exposure. The longer the interval between exposure and vaccination, the poorer the response. Vaccines are generally not an effective treatment if given greater than 48 hours post-infection but can still be used to prevent the spread of infection during an outbreak.[4,8]

The prognosis for naturally occurring CDV infection is poor with mortality rates as high as 100%.[4,5] This is not true for vaccine-induced CDV. Modified live vaccines (MLV) of canine and mink origin can produce disease in ferrets.[4] These vaccine-induced CDV cases are less fatal and may not be transmissible to unvaccinated ferrets.[4] The author successfully treated an 18-month-old male neutered ferret with vaccine-induced CDV after vaccination with a canine-origin MLV. The ferret was presented with extensive erythematous papules, hyperkeratosis of the front foot pads, periocular swelling, and an erythematous, pruritic rash on its chin (**Fig. 1**). The signs started 1-week after vaccination. Based on the clinical suspicion of CDV, it was started on oral amoxicillin-clavulanic acid and a 2% lignocaine topical anesthetic gel (Axcel Lignocaine 2% Sterile Gel, Kotra Pharma (M) Sdn Bhd, Malaysia) for its skin lesions. RT-PCR of conjunctival swabs and urine were both positive for CDV. The animal never developed respiratory disease or neurologic deficits, and recovered completely within 2 weeks.

A recent outbreak of vaccine-induced CDV in a large breeding facility in the United States also showed successful treatment of infected ferrets with survival rates of up

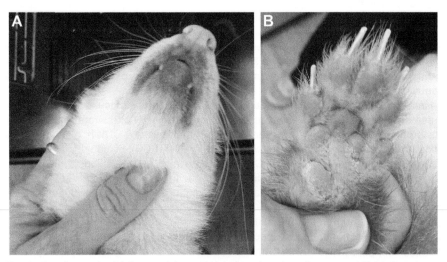

Fig. 1. An 18-month-old ferret with vaccine-induced canine distemper. (A) Erythematous, pruritic, papular rash on the chin, (B) Hyperkeratosis of the left front footpad.

to 80% to 85%.[9] Between September and December 2022, a large number of sick ferrets were developing CDV within days to weeks following vaccination with the Distemink vaccine (United Vaccines Inc, Fitchberg, WI, USA), a multivalent avian-origin vaccine. It was discovered that ferrets who were vaccinated at less than 9 to 10 weeks of age developed disease, whereas ferrets older than 10 weeks did not. Clinical signs included diarrhea, hyporexia, oculonasal discharge, open-mouthed breathing, dehydration, fever, and death within 48 to 72 hours. Ferrets were immediately treated and most had a positive response to treatment. Treatment included amoxicilin-clavulonate (12.5 mg/kg PO q 12 hr), vitamin A (50,000 IU or 15 g retinal palmitate IM or SC q 24 hr × 2 days), vitamin C (250 mg IV q 24 hr × 3 days), interferon (60–120 units SC q 24 hr), meloxicam (0.2 mg/kg PO q 24 hr), famotidine (2.5 mg/ferret SC q 24 hr), diphenhydramine (0.5–2 g/kg IM, IV, or PO q 8–12 hr), buprenorphine (0.01–0.5 mg/kg IM, SC q8-12 hr), vaccination (with either Purevax, Boehringer Ingelheim Animal Health, USA or Nobivac DPv, Merck, USA), nebulization with bronchodilators as needed, fluid therapy, and nutritional support.[9]

Prevention of CDV is achieved with proper vaccination and avoiding contact with potential carriers of the disease such as other ferrets and dogs (see below).

Rotavirus

Rotavirus group C is a nonenveloped RNA virus that causes diarrhea in juvenile ferrets and can cause mild infections in older ferrets.[4] It is transmitted via the fecal-oral route and possibly via the respiratory route. Viral particles are stable within feces and resistant to common disinfectants. Transmission in juvenile ferrets occurs primarily via contact with their infected mothers or a contaminated environment. Because it is stable in feces, the virus can remain for long periods of time on the contaminated fur of infected jills, making it difficult to eradicate. The morbidity is highest in primiparous jills (90%) and decreases by 10% to 20% with each gestation.

The disease is most commonly seen in ferrets 1 to 3 weeks of age but can occur in any juvenile ferret less than 2 month old. Clinical signs include yellow, watery diarrhea, dehydration, and even death. Physical examination findings include perianal fur staining, perineal erythema, and a distended abdomen due to gas and fluid-filled intestines.

Diagnosis is via RT-PCR on fecal samples or sections of small intestines. The commercial enzyme-linked immunosorbent assay (ELISA) kits for group A rotaviruses will not detect all ferret rotaviruses.

As with most viral infections, there is no targeted treatment for the virus itself. Treatment includes fluid resuscitation and prevention of secondary infection. Fluid therapy can be administered orally or parenterally. Antibiotics may improve recovery and decrease mortality rates. Support feeding is also indicated if the ferret is too sick to nurse or eat on their own. Immunoglobulin A (IgA) colostral antibodies can protect kits from rotaviral diarrhea but not from infection. Therefore, it is vital to try to encourage the kits to drink their mother's milk.

Proper environmental sanitation is vital to prevent rotavirus outbreaks. Chlorine solutions are the most effective at disinfecting the environment.

Coccidiosis

Eimeria furonis is common in ferret colonies and can cause diarrhea in weanling ferrets. Coccidia can be diagnosed with fecal floatation and treated with sulfa-based antibiotics or ponazuril.[10] Kits with severe diarrhea require fluid therapy and supplemental feeding to prevent dehydration. Treatment of the entire colony may be required.[1]

Feline panleukopenia virus

Feline panleukopenia virus (FPV) is a nonenveloped DNA parvovirus that has been shown to cause disease in ferret kits in an experimental setting. One-day and two-day-old kits that were inoculated intraperitoneally with a live FPV vaccine developed cerebellar ataxia at 6 to 7 weeks post-inoculation.[11] Their signs included ataxia, tremors, and loss of righting reflex. A post-mortem examination revealed cerebellar hypoplasia that was progressively more hypoplastic in kits inoculated at 2 days old. Three-day-old kits given the same intraperitoneal inoculation did not show clinical or pathologic changes. Pregnant ferrets were also inoculated intraperitoneally with the vaccine at varying intervals during gestation and neither the adults nor kits showed any adverse effects. Based on these findings, it is recommended to avoid housing neonatal ferrets with cats that may shed the FPV virus.[4] Cats with FPV-associated diarrhea can contaminate the environment which remains infectious for months and is resistant to physical and chemical decontamination.

Toxoplasma-like disease

A congenital Toxoplasma-like disease was implicated in the deaths of neonatal ferret kits on a single farm in New Zealand. Kits between 1 and 28 day old experienced a 36% mortality (270 deaths out of 750 kits) with no clinical signs prior to death.[12] Post-mortem changes showed Toxoplasma-like organisms in regions of multifocal necrosis of the liver, lungs, and heart. Parasitemia was suspected to have occurred in the pregnant females because the organisms were found in kits as young as 1-day-old. All adult ferrets on the farm had been anorexic 1 month prior to mating. It was suspected that this coincided with the period of initial infection and that the stress of pregnancy caused a relapse in these females resulting in parasitemia and subsequent transplacental infection of the kits.

Vaccination in Juvenile Ferrets

All juvenile ferrets should be vaccinated against CDV and rabies. A thorough discussion of these vaccine protocols and vaccine reactions was been recently published.[5]

Rabies

Several rabies vaccines have been approved for use in ferrets and are the only ones recommended to administer. The initial vaccine should be given at 12 weeks of age followed by annual boosters.[5]

Canine distemper

CDV vaccination is not as straightforward as the rabies vaccination. This is due to the difficulty of accessing the vaccine approved for use in ferrets, the risk of vaccine-induced CDV, and maternal antibodies that can interfere with vaccine effectiveness. A live canarypox vector recombinant vaccine (Purevax, Boehringer Ingelheim Animal Health, Atlanta, GA, USA) is licensed for use in ferrets and is the preferred vaccine. Due to its intermittent availability, many exotic companion mammal veterinarians have been using an attenuated live canine vaccine (Nobivac DPv, Merck, Upper Gwynedd, PA, USA).[5] Owners must be aware that this is not licensed for use in ferrets and contains both CDV and parvovirus.

Ferrets must receive at least 2 effective vaccines for immunity to develop. Maternal antibodies can be present in the kit for 6 to 14 weeks.[4] Kits from dams vaccinated with MLV had maternal antibodies below the limit of detection within 8 to 12 weeks and had to be at least 7 week old before attaining vaccine-induced immunity, whereas kits from unvaccinated dams attained vaccine-induced immunity at 8 days of age.[13] Kits should receive their first vaccine at 8 weeks of age. Because they may still have maternal antibodies at 8 weeks of age, it is recommended that they then receive boosters at 11 and 14 weeks of age.[5] After the recent outbreak of CDV from a major breeder in the United States, ferrets will now be released to retail pet stores at an older age (usually 12 week old) and should receive 2 vaccines at the breeding facility before reaching the retail pet stores (at 8–9 and 11–12 week old). With these ferrets, it is recommended that they are vaccinated again at 14 and 16 weeks of age.[9] Annual boosters are recommended, but some studies have shown that immunity may last longer.[5]

Congenital Diseases

Congenital anomalies are reported to affect 3% to 4% of newborn ferrets.[14] A higher frequency of congenital malformations was detected in females of low previous parity (ie, 0–2) than in those with 3 or more pregnancies.[15] There was no difference in the incidence based on maternal age or coat color.

Multiple congenital defects

Neural tube defects (NTD) have been reported in 5 stillborn ferret kits. In 1 case series,[16] an entire litter of 4 kits (3 stillborn and 1 that died minutes after delivery) was diagnosed with NTD. All 4 kits had varying degrees of iniencephaly with 2 having anencephaly (absence of cranial vault and cerebral hemispheres) and a third having anencephaly and an omphalocele (protrusion of the abdominal contents covered with peritoneum through the base of the umbilical cord). Of the 4 kits, 3 had palatoschisis (cleft palate), 2 had cheiloschisis (cleft lip), 1 had hydrocephalus, 1 had unilateral renal agenesis, and 1 had bilateral hydronephrosis. A previous litter sired by the same hob had resulted in similar birth defects, leading the author to conclude that this was a genetic condition. In humans, there is an increased risk of NTD after 1 child with NTD.[17] Another case report of NTD was a stillborn kit with spina bifida aperta.[18] The postmortem description did not discuss the kidneys. Congenitally defective kits with head defects and severe palatoschisis can cause dystocia and often several kits in affected litters have head deformities. This defect has been reported to be more common in jills with white markings on their head ("blaze").[1]

In ferrets, closure of the neural tube occurs from day 16 to 17 after fertilization.[16] Fetal insult during this time can include folic acid deficiency, gestational administration of salicylates, tetracycline, and sulfonamides.[16] In humans, folic acid supplementations can prevent NTD such as spina bifida by as much as 70%.[18] To avoid signs of deficiency, ferret kits < 13 weeks of age require a minimum of 0.5 mg of folate/kg of dry food.[18]

A less severe form of multiple congenital malformations was reported in a 2-month-old female ferret presenting with a malformed anus and the absence of both a tail and external genitalia.[19] Abdominal ultrasound and excretory urography revealed right kidney dysplasia. Iodinated contrast media injected into the anal orifice revealed the presence of a common chamber receiving the terminal segments of the colon, vagina, and urethra. The ferret was euthanized, and a post-mortem examination confirmed the presumptive diagnosis of congenital caudal spinal agenesis with anorectal and genitourinary malformation.

Auditory system

A 2014 study showed that congenital sensorineural deafness (CSD) in ferrets is strongly associated with a white patterned coat and premature graying.[20] In the study of 152 ferrets, 100% of the panda, American panda, and blaze ferrets were deaf (**Fig. 2**). Unilateral deafness was found in 7% of ferrets and bilateral deafness

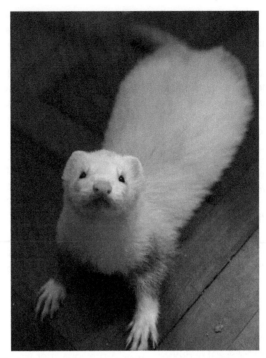

Fig. 2. Ferrets with white markings on their head, such as this American panda ferret, frequently have congenital sensorineural deafness. This 2-year-old male castrated ferret was deaf since adoption and startled easily but otherwise had a normal quality of life.

in 22% of ferrets. Deafness was suspected to be due to failure of migration/maturation, premature death, or dysfunction of neural crest melanocytes to the region of the stria vascularis of the cochlea. Interestingly, only 1 albino ferret was found to be deaf. This was suspected to be because albinism is a result of impaired expression of a pigment-producing gene, but they still have normal migration of melanocytes to the stria vascularis (the melanocytes are present, but clear rather than pigmented). Deaf ferrets in this study showed abnormal social interactions with other ferrets, biting tendencies, and louder than normal vocalizations. Based on this study, it is important to advise clients of ferrets with white patterned coats or premature graying ferrets that they could be deaf which can be associated with behavioral and training problems. If owners are considering breeding ferrets with these coat characteristics, brainstem auditory evoked response (BAER) testing should be performed to rule out CSD.

Congenital peripheral vestibular syndrome was diagnosed in a 3-month-old female intact ferret who had a left head tilt, circling to the left, vestibular ataxia, and positional strabismus that was noted at 3 weeks of age when it started ambulating.[21] MRI found a slight asymmetry in the morphology of the left labyrinth and cochlea. BAER testing was consistent with sensorineural deafness. The ferret accommodated with vestibular physiotherapy exercises and a liquid diet (due to difficulty in mastication).

External auditory canal atresia was diagnosed in a 6-month-old male ferret who had an absence of the opening of the left external acoustic meatus at the level of the conchal fossa since adoption.[22] A computed tomography (CT) scan with contrast showed a normal tympanic bulla but complete atresia of the left external auditory canal. No surgical intervention was needed as the animal showed no clinical signs attributed to the atresia.

Ocular system

Congenital dermoid cysts and persistent fetal intraocular vasculature (PFIV) have been described in juvenile ferrets. Dermoid cysts are a benign developmental anomaly due to the entrapment of ectodermal elements along the lines of embryonic closure and present with haired skin on the corneal surface of the eye.[23] PFIV is caused by the persistence of embryonal vascular vestiges within the eye that do not undergo normal involution during ocular development.[24] PFIV was found in 21/76 genetically related juvenile ferrets (5-week to 6-week-old) and 3/10 intact adult ferrets (parents of the juvenile ferrets) that had been bred for a research project. Slit lamp examination revealed diminutive vasculature with focal remnants of the posterior tunica vasculosa lentis, muscae volitantes, and an occluded hyaloid artery extending from the optic papilla to the anterior vitreous body. A hereditary basis for PFIV was speculated based on the histologic and clinical examination results in these closely related ferrets. Based on this study, ferrets intended for breeding should be screened with a slit lamp for the presence of PFIV.

Cardiovascular system

Congenital heart defects have been diagnosed in ferrets between 5 months and 6 years of age. Reported defects include an atrial septal defect, a ventricular septal defect, an atrioventricular (AV) canal defect, tetralogy of Fallot (TOF), and patent ductus arteriosus.[25] All congenital defects were diagnosed by echocardiogram.

The AV canal defect was diagnosed in a 4-year-old intact male ferret with hind leg weakness, ataxia, and hyporexia. Examination revealed a grade IV/VI systolic murmur and dyspnea. The animal was successfully managed with furosemide, spironolactone, enalapril, and diltiazem.[26]

The atrial septal defect was diagnosed in a 2-year-old, male castrated ferret that was presented with abdominal distention and muscle wasting despite a good appetite.[27] Physical examination revealed pale mucous membranes, prolonged capillary refill time, tachycardia (300 beats/min), and abdominal distention but no heart murmur or jugular vein distention. The ferret was euthanized. A post-mortem examination diagnosed decompensated right-sided heart failure due to an atrial septal defect and unrelated exudative peritonitis.

The ventricular septal defect was diagnosed in a 4-year-old male castrated ferret that was presented with a 1-year history of sporadic cough.[28] Physical examination revealed a right apical grade V/VI holosystolic murmur. The animal was managed with furosemide and benazepril for 2 months until it presented for respiratory distress which required thoracocentesis, an increase in furosemide, and initiation of pimobendan.

TOF has been diagnosed in 3 ferrets with various classifications (based on the classification of TOF in humans). One ferret was a 17-month-old male castrated ferret with mild exercise intolerance that had been diagnosed with a heart murmur at 12 weeks of age.[29] Physical examination revealed a right parasternal grade IV/VI systolic murmur and tachycardia. Atenolol was prescribed which resolved the tachycardia and exercise intolerance. The second ferret was a 6-year-old spayed female that was presented for routine examination.[30] Physical examination revealed a left basilar grade V/VI holosystolic murmur and tachycardia. In this case, the TOF was found to have bidirectional shunting which was suspected to be the reason the animal did not have clinical signs of disease even at 6 years of age. It was initially treated with ena-lapril and furosemide, but both were stopped due to side effects and difficulty medi-cating the patient. The animal died 5 months after diagnosis due to unrelated peritonitis and did not have clinical signs of heart disease prior to death. The third and most severely affected ferret was a 5-month-old intact male that was presented with lethargy, tachypnea, and exercise intolerance.[31] Physical examination found tachypnea, soft crackles, and cyanosis of the posterior body mucous membranes. A complete blood count revealed severe polycythemia. The patient was initially treated with phlebotomy and oxygen therapy but was euthanized due to continued respiratory distress. Necropsy confirmed extreme TOF and interstitial pneumonia caused by *Pneumocystis carinii.*

There is no information about the ferrets diagnosed with patent ductus arteriosus.[32]

Based on these case reports, any juvenile ferret with a cardiac murmur, exercise intolerance, and/or a chronic cough should receive an echocardiogram as most cases of congenital cardiac disease are able to be diagnosed with an echocardiogram and managed with medical therapy.

Musculoskeletal system

Several congenital abnormalities of the vertebral column have been documented in ferrets. A 2014 retrospective study of 172 ferrets found that there are 5 different formulas for the number of vertebrae.[33] All ferrets had 7 cervical vertebrae. The most common formulas had 14 thoracic vertebrae: C7/T14/L6/S3 (51.74%), C7/T14/L6/S4 (22.10%), and C7/T14/L7/S3 (6.98%) with the second formula being significantly more common in males than in females. The less common formulas contained 15 thoracic vertebrae and were C7/T15/L6/S3 (1.74%) and C7/T15/L6/S4 (0.56%).

This same study found congenital abnormalities in 16.86% of the ferrets and con-sisted of transitional vertebrae (89.7% of the abnormalities), block vertebrae (6.9%; 1 cervical and 1 lumbar), and wedge vertebrae (3.4%; thoracic).[33] Transitional verte-brae were found in the thoracolumbar region (50%), lumbosacral region (38%), or both regions (12%).[33] There was no information on clinical signs associated with the block vertebrae in the ferrets in Proks and colleagues,[33] but there has been 1 report of intervertebral disc protrusion and paraparesis in a ferret with T9-T10 block verte-brae.[34] This ferret, a 2-year-old spayed female, had a 4-month history of progressive paraparesis and urinary incontinence. A myelogram showed intervertebral disc herni-ations at T7-T8, T8-T9, and T10-T11. It was suspected that the block vertebrae caused extra loading on the adjacent vertebrae leading to degenerative changes allowing the disc herniation. Hemilaminectomy was performed. The ferret showed progressive improvement in its neurologic status 2 months after surgery.

Atlantoaxial subluxation secondary to congenital complex occipitoatlantoaxial mal-formation (OAAM) has been reported in 3 ferrets.[35,36] The first reported case was a 3-month-old male ferret with acute non-ambulatory tetraparesis and a right head tilt that began 10 days after adoption. Cervical radiographs showed that the atlas was fused to the occipital bone, the occipital condyles were absent, and the dens of the axis was incomplete and displaced. The ferret was euthanized due to a poor prognosis and a post-mortem myelogram showed mild compression of the spinal cord due to dorsal displacement of the hypoplastic dens.[35] The second case was an 18-month-old spayed female with chronic progressive ataxia and circling to the right since 3 months of age. The third case was a 5-month-old neutered male with acute onset tetraplegia and lethargy.[36] The 18-month-old female's cervical radiographs (lateral and ventro-dorsal extended) showed that the atlas was deformed and fused to the supraoccipital bone, the axis was deformed and fused to C3, and the dens was absent. The 5-month-old male's cervical radiographs (lateral flexed and rostro-caudal open-mouth) showed fusion of the atlas to the caudal skull, widening of the atlanto-axial (AA) space, dorsal subluxation of the body of the axis, and a present but small dens. CT scans of both ferrets confirmed what was seen on the radiographs, and an MRI in 1 ferret suggested chronic, dynamic spinal cord compression due to AA subluxation. Both ferrets were treated with a cervical brace and prednisolone. Unfortunately, both ferrets were eventually euthanized due to poor quality of life.

Based on these case reports, any juvenile ferret with tetraparesis, paraparesis, or ataxia should have spinal radiographs including the skull with a follow-up CT scan or myelogram. Ferrets with block vertebrae may develop intervertebral disc disease in adjacent vertebrae. Unfortunately, the prognosis is poor for ferrets diagnosed with OAAM.

Urinary system

Reported congenital defects of the urinary system include extramural ectopic ureters, circumcaval ureters, ureterovesicular stenosis, a vesicourachal diverticum, and suspected vestigial mesonephric or paramesonephric duct remnants on the dorsal aspect of the urinary bladder. Primary polycystic disease is suspected to be congenital.

Extramural ectopic ureters have been diagnosed in 2 ferrets. The first case of an extramural ectopic ureter was in a 6-month-old female spayed ferret with urinary incontinence and perineal/inguinal urine scald.[37] A left ectopic ureter was diagnosed via excretory urography. The patient was treated surgically with a left nephroureteroectomy. The patient's incontinence improved but was still present post-operatively. This was managed with phenylpropanolamine, although mild incontinence persisted. The second case was a 1-year-old intact female ferret that was also presented for incontinence and perineal urine scald. A left ectopic ureter was diagnosed via CT with contrast. This patient was also treated surgically with a left nephroureteroectomy. As with the first case, this patient's incontinence improved but was still present post-operatively. Based on these 2 cases, any juvenile female ferret with urinary incontinence should receive excretory urography (either radiographs or CT scan). Ultrasound was not helpful in the diagnosis of either case. Surgical treatment with nephroureteroectomy will improve, but not cure the incontinence.

Circumcaval ureter is caused by an anomaly in the development of the caudal vena cava in which a persistent right caudal cardinal vein leads to dorsal displacement and compression of the right ureter, resulting in hydroureter proximal to this compression. This congenital anomaly has been diagnosed in 3 ferrets, all of them male.

The first case was a 5-year-old male neutered ferret that was presented obtunded with a history of anorexia.[38] Blood revealed azotemia and an ultrasound showed right renal hydronephrosis and right proximal hydroureter. Circumcaval ureter was suspected based on an excretory urogram that found medial displacement of the proximal right ureter at the region that was dilated. The patient died and a postmortem examination confirmed the diagnosis.

The second case was a 3-year-old male neutered ferret presenting with weight loss, diarrhea, and anorexia.[39] This patient did not have azotemia at presentation. An abdominal ultrasound and CT scan with intravenous urogram revealed right-sided hydronephrosis and right proximal hydroureter with the dilation ending near the caudal vena cava. The proximal dilated portion of the right ureter was displaced dorsomedial to the vena cava with the dilation ending at the middle segment of the ureter (type I circumcaval ureter). Fluid therapy was initiated but the urea slowly increased and the patient deteriorated. Surgical right uretero-vesical anastomosis was performed, but the patient had worsening hydroureter 48 hours post-operatively and a right ne-phrectomy was performed. The patient died post-operatively.

The third case was a 4-year-old intact male ferret with palpable right renomegaly noted on routine physical examination.[39] This patient did not have azotemia and his urine spe-cific gravity was 1.050 (reference interval 1.034–1.070).[39] Abdominal ultrasound and CT scan with intravenous urogram revealed right hydronephrosis and right proximal hydro-ureter. The proximal dilated portion of the right ureter was displaced dorsomedial to the vena cava with the dilation ending at the proximal third of the ureter (also a type I circum-caval ureter). This patient was treated surgically with right nephrectomy and ureter resection with no post-operative complications or azotemia. Based on these cases, type I circumcaval ureter should be suspected in ferrets with right proximal hydroureter and hydronephrosis. This diagnosis can be confirmed with excretory urography.

Bilateral congenital ureterovesical junction (UVJ) stenosis has been diagnosed in 1 ferret. This case was an 8-month-old neutered male ferret presented for routine exam-ination and abdominal ultrasound of the adrenal glands to discuss preventative treat-ment.[40] Abdominal ultrasound revealed bilateral hydronephrosis and bilateral hydroureter that ended in marked narrowing of the ureters at the UVJ. Serum biochemistry showed mild elevation in urea with normal creatinine and urinalysis was unremarkable. Intravenous excretory urography with negative contrast cystogra-phy revealed bilateral hydronephrosis and hydroureter secondary to stenosis at the UVJ. A retrograde positive cystography found right vesicoureteral reflux. A subcutane-ous ureteral bypass device was placed in the left kidney but had to be removed 3 months after placement due to obstruction and persistent urinary tract infections. At the time of device removal, a left ureteroneocystostomy was performed with no post-operative strictures. Therefore, a right ureteroneocystostomy was performed 1 month later. During the right ureteroneocystostomy, 6 struvite uroliths were removed from the urinary bladder. Post-operative abdominal ultrasound showed progressive reduction in the size of the right and left renal pelvis and ureters.

A vesicourachal diverticulum occurs when the proximal portion of the urachus (in utero canal connecting the umbilical cord to the bladder) does not close postpartum which results in a blind-ended sac at the bladder apex. This congenital anomaly has been reported in a 4-year-old neutered male ferret that was presented for vomiting, weakness, and hyporexia.[41] Abdominal radiographs and ultrasound revealed several mineralized calculi in the urinary bladder and the distal left ureter. The patient was not azotemic. Urinalysis showed trace proteinuria and hematuria. Cystostomy and left ureterotomy were recommended to remove the uroliths. During the procedure, a urine-filled vesicourachal diverticulum associated with a urachal ligament was found and removed. Mineral analysis of the calculi found them to be calcium oxalate. The ferret recovered well without recurrence of urolithiasis.

A case series described the presence of variable-sized cystic structures on the dorsal aspect of the urinary bladder in 6 ferrets (4 male, 2 female) between 2 and 8 years old.[42] The cystic structures were diagnosed on post-mortem examination. Three of the 4 male ferrets had a history of dysuria; 1 of the 2 female ferrets had vulvar swelling; and 3 (2 male, 1 female) of the 6 ferrets had alopecia. The youngest ferret (2-year-old, female) did not have any clinical signs. In all ferrets, the cysts were palpable on physical examination as caudal abdominal masses. On gross post-mortem examination, all 6 ferrets had sin-gle or multiple semispherical or bilobed fluctuant cystic structures of various sizes located on the dorsal aspects of the urinary bladder. Histologic examination of the adre-nal glands was performed in 5 of the 6 ferrets (including the asymptomatic 2-year-old fe-male) and was abnormal in all 5: 1 ferret was diagnosed with cortical cell hyperplasia and 4 with neoplasia. The cystic structures in 2 of the 4 male ferrets were suggestive of prostatic cysts, which are commonly seen in male ferrets with adrenal gland disease. The cystic structures in the other 4 ferrets were suspected to be vestigial mesonephric or paramesonephric duct remnants that did not resorb postnatally and became cystic/enlarged due to excess androgen secretion from the diseased adrenal glands.

Renal cysts are a common incidental finding in ferrets and are suspected to be congenital. Primary polycystic kidney disease and simple cysts were prevalent in a retrospective study looking at cystic renal disease in postmortem samples from 3 institutes.[43] Primary polycystic kidney disease was found in 26% of ferrets and simple cysts in 22% of ferrets. The cyst sizes in ferrets with primary polycystic disease ranged from 1 to 25 mm in size and from 1 to 7 mm in size with simple cysts. In contrast to the hereditary primary polycystic kidney disease in humans, most of the ferrets in this study had glomerulocystic kidney disease.

Genital system

Reported congenital defects of the genital system in ferrets include a recto-vaginal fistula, segmental atresia of the uterus, a recessed vulva, and cryptorchidism.

A recto-vaginal fistula was diagnosed in a 3-year-old spayed female ferret that had feces passing through her vulva, chronic vaginal discharge, and vaginitis since adoption.[44] Conscious physical examination was unremarkable other than inflammation and pain of the vulva. Sedated examination with a catheter revealed communication between the rectum and the vulva. A fistula was confirmed radiographically by instilling contrast into the rectum which filled the vagina via a small fistula near the anus. Surgical repair of the fistula was successful.

Segmental atresia of the uterus was diagnosed in a 2-year-old intact female ferret during a routine ovariohysterectomy.[45] Exploration of the uterus showed that the right uterine horn had partial atresia proximal to the uterine body. The remaining portion of the right uterine horn distal to the atresic section was dilated and fluid-filled. Histologic diagnosis was segmental atresia of the right uterine horn associated with hydrosalpinx and hydrometra. Blood was submitted for chromosomal analysis which ruled out a chromosome-related congenital anomaly.

A congenital vulvar defect was diagnosed in a 1-year-old intact female ferret that was presented with dysuria and recurrent cystitis.[46] Estrus-related vulvar swelling would cause signs of discomfort and the animal never became pregnant after several attempts at breeding. Physical examination showed a recessed vulva with excess furred skin surrounding and folding over the vulva. Surgical correction with episioplasty was curative and the ferret was successfully bred the next year.

Cryptorchidism was reported in 0.75% of 1597 male ferrets presented to a veterinary clinic for elective castration over a period of 3 years.[47] All ferrets were presented for castration from a single breeder and were between 6 and 8 weeks old. Unilateral cryptorchidism was diagnosed in 83% of the ferrets and bilateral cryptorchidism in 17%. In the unilateral cryptorchid cases, 80% were on the left side, 20% were on the right side; 50% were located in the abdomen, and 50% were located in the inguinal region. In male ferrets, the testes typically descend into the scrotum during fetal development but in some cases can be delayed for several months after birth.[1] Therefore, if a juvenile male ferret presents with cryptorchidism, delaying the procedure until they are several months old may increase the chance of the testes descending into the scrotum.

Early detection of congenital disease is paramount in juvenile ferrets so that treatment can be initiated as soon as possible. Examination at the time of presentation for rabies and CDV vaccination should include a thorough cardiac auscultation, examination of the external genitalia, and a neurologic examination. Ferrets with white patterns should also receive BAER testing.

CLINICS CARE POINTS

- Juvenile kits require ferret milk for at least the first 10 days of life because ferret milk is higher in fat than cow's milk. If ferret milk is not available, a mix of 80% cow's milk and 20% chicken egg yolk or strained beef liver can be fed.

- Successful treatment of ferrets with CDV includes supplemental feeding, fluid therapy, intramuscular vitamin A injections, parenteral antibiotics, and analgesia. Vaccination can be useful if given within 48 hours post-infection. This disease can be prevented with routine vaccination.

- Juvenile ferrets with severe diarrhea require supplemental feeding and fluid therapy. Differentials include coccidiosis and rotavirus. Coccidiosis can be diagnosed with a fecal floatation.

- Any juvenile ferret with a cardiac murmur, exercise intolerance, and/or a chronic cough should receive an echocardiogram as most cases of congenital cardiac disease are able to be diagnosed with an echocardiogram and managed with medical therapy.

- Any juvenile ferret with tetraparesis, paraparesis, or ataxia should have spinal radiographs including the skull with a follow-up CT scan or myelogram. It is important to note that there are 5 different formulas for the number of vertebrae in ferrets and that ferrets with block vertebrae may develop intervertebral disc disease in adjacent vertebrae.

DISCLOSURE

This author has nothing to disclose.

REFERENCES

1. Fox JG, Bell J, Broome R. Growth and reproduction. Biology and Diseases of the Ferret 2014:187-209.
2. Richardson JPD. Reproductive biology. In: Johnson-Delaney C, editor. Ferret medicine and surgery. Boca Raton, FL: CRC Press; 2016. p. 64-9.
3. Jekl V, Hauptman K. Reproductive medicine in ferrets. Veterinary Clinics: Exotic Animal Practice 2017;20:629-63.
4. Kiupel M. Viral diseases of ferrets. In: Fox JG, editor. Biology and diseases of the ferret. Ames, IA: John Wiley & Sons; 2014. p. 439-518.
5. Wade LL. Vaccination of ferrets for rabies and distemper. Veterinary Clinics: Exotic Animal Practice 2018;21:105-14.
6. Powers LVPD. Basic anatomy, physiology, and husbandry of ferrets. In: Quesenbery KEOC, Mans C, Carpenter JW, editors. Ferrets, Rabbits, and Rodents. 4th edition. Philadelphia, PA: Elsevier; 2020. p. 1-12.
7. Rodeheffer C, Von Messling V, Milot S, et al. Disease manifestations of canine distemper virus infection in ferrets are modulated by vitamin A status. The Journal of nutrition 2007;137:1916-22.
8. Johnson-Delaney C. Ferret medicine and surgery. Boca Raton, FL: CRC Press; 2016.
9. Johnson-Delaney C. Canine distemper outbreak in ferrets in North America. Boston, MA: ExoticsCon; 2023.
10. Sledge DG, Bolin SR, Lim A, et al. Outbreaks of severe enteric disease associated with Eimeria furonis infection in ferrets (Mustela putorius furo) of 3 densely populated groups. J Am Vet Med Assoc 2011;239:1584-8.

11. Duenwald J, Holland J, Gorham J, et al. Feline panleukopenia: Experimental cerebellar hypoplasia produced in neonatal ferrets with live virus vaccine. Res Vet Sci 1971;12:394–6.
12. Thornton R, Cook T. A congenital Toxoplasma-like disease in ferrets (Mustela putorius furo). N Z Vet J 1986;34:31–3.
13. von Messling V. The ferret in morbillivirus research. Biology and Diseases of the Ferret 2014;641–51.
14. Willis L, Barrow M. The ferret (Mustela putorius furo L.) as a laboratory animal. Lab Anim Sci 1971;21:712–6.
15. McLain D, Harper S, Roe D, et al. Congenital malformations and variations in reproductive performance in the ferret: effects of maternal age, color and parity. Lab Anim Sci 1985;35:251–5.
16. Williams B, Popek E, Hart R, et al. Iniencephaly and other neural tube defects in a litter of ferrets (Mustela putorius furo). Vet Path 1994;31:260–2.
17. Hall J, Friedman J, Kenna B, et al. Clinical, genetic, and epidemiological factors in neural tube defects. Am J Hum Genet 1988;43:827.
18. Golini L, Di Guardo G, Bonnafous L, et al. Pathology In Practice. J Am Vet Med Assoc 2009;234:1263–5.
19. d'Ovidio D, Melidone R, Rossi G, et al. Multiple congenital malformations in a ferret (Mustela Putorius Furo). J Exot Pet Med 2015;24:92–7.
20. Piazza S, Abitbol M, Gnirs K, et al. Prevalence of deafness and association with coat variations in client-owned ferrets. J Am Vet Med Assoc 2014;244:1047–52.
21. Moya A, Mínguez JJ, Martorell J, et al. Congenital peripheral vestibular syndrome in a domestic ferret (Mustela putorius furo). J Exot Pet Med 2014;23:287–93.
22. Bo P, Med Vet S, Alberti BM, et al. External auditory canal atresia (EACA) in a ferret (Mustela putorius furo). Veterinaria (Cremona) 2018;32:295–8.
23. Myrna KE, Di Girolamo N. Ocular examination and corneal surface disease in the ferret. Veterinary Clinics: Exotic Animal Practice 2019;22:27–33.
24. Lipsitz L, Ramsey DT, Render JA, et al. Persistent fetal intraocular vasculature in the European ferret (Mustela putorius): clinical and histological aspects. Vet Ophthalmol 2001;4:29–33.
25. van Zeeland YR, Schoemaker NJ. Ferret cardiology. Veterinary Clinics: Exotic Animal Practice 2022;25:541–62.
26. Agudelo CF, Jekl V, Hauptman K, et al. A case of a complete atrioventricular canal defect in a ferret. BMC Vet Res 2021;17:1–5.
27. van Schaik-Gerritsen KM, Schoemaker NJ, Kik MJ, et al. Atrial septal defect in a ferret (Mustela putorius furo). J Exot Pet Med 2013;22:70–5.
28. Di Girolamo N, Critelli M, Zeyen U, et al. Ventricular septal defect in a ferret (Mustela putorius furo). J Small Anim Pract 2012;53:549–53.
29. Williams JG, Graham JE, Laste NJ, et al. Tetralogy of Fallot in a young ferret (Mustela putorius furo). J Exot Pet Med 2011;20:232–6.
30. Laniesse D, Hébert J, Larrat S, et al. Tetralogy of Fallot in a 6-year-old albino ferret (Mustela putorius furo). Can Vet J 2014;55:456.
31. Dias S, Planellas M, Canturri A, et al. Extreme tetralogy of fallot with polycythemia in a ferret (Mustela putorius furo). Top Companion Anim Med 2017;32:80–5.
32. Wagner RA. Ferret cardiology. Veterinary Clinics: Exotic Animal Practice 2009;12:115–34.
33. Proks P, Stehlik L, Paninarova M, et al. Congenital abnormalities of the vertebral column in ferrets. Vet Radiol Ultrasound 2015;56:117–23.
34. Orlandi R, Mateo I. Intervertebral disc protrusion in a Ferret with triple thoracic block vertebrae. J Exot Pet Med 2013;22:396–9.

35. N DC, Barreiro JD, Espino L. What is your diagnosis? J Am Vet Med Assoc 2014; 245:631–3.
36. Jayson SL, Dennis R, Mateo I, et al. Atlantoaxial subluxation with complex occipitoatlantoaxial malformation in two domestic ferrets (Mustela putorius furo). Vet Rec Case Rep 2018;6:e000530.
37. MacNab TA, Newcomb BT, Ketz-Riley C, et al. Extramural ectopic ureter in a domestic ferret (Mustela putorius furo). J Exot Pet Med 2010;19:313–6.
38. Di Girolamo N, Carnimeo A, Nicoletti A, et al. Retrocaval ureter in a ferret. J Small Anim Pract 2015;56:355.
39. Bernhard C, Linsart A, Mentré V. Circumcaval ureter in two ferrets. J Exot Pet Med 2022;42:42–6.
40. Vilalta L, Dominguez E, Altuzarra R, et al. Imaging diagnosis—radiography and ultrasonography of bilateral congenital ureterovesical junction stenosis causing hydronephrosis and hydroureter in a ferret (Mustela putorius furo). Vet Radiol Ultrasound 2017;58:E31–6.
41. Cojean O, Combes A, Maitre P, et al. Surgical treatment of congenital vesicourachal diverticulum associated with ureteral and vesical calcium oxalate urolithiasis in a domestic ferret (Mustela putorius furo). J Exot Pet Med 2019;29:22–6.
42. Li X, Fox J, Erdman S, et al. Cystic urogenital anomalies in ferrets (Mustela putorius furo). Veterinary pathology 1996;33:150–8.
43. Jackson CN, Rogers AB, Maurer KJ, et al. Cystic renal disease in the domestic ferret. Comp Med 2008;58:161–7.
44. Schlax K, Quiévreux L, Mélin M, et al. A rectovaginal fistula in a ferret (Mustela putorius furo) with a normal anus: a case report. J Exot Pet Med 2020;35:20–2.
45. Batista-Arteaga M, Alamo D, Herráez P, et al. Segmental atresia of the uterus associated with hydrometra in a ferret. Vet Rec 2007;161:759.
46. Bielli M, Giordano Nardini DM. Surgical correction of a vulvar congenital defect in a female ferret. 1st International Conference on Avian Herpetological and Exotic Mammal Medicine, Wiesbaden (Germany) 2013;277-280.
47. Bodri MS. Theriogenology question of the month. J Am Vet Med Assoc 2000;217: 1465–6.

Rabbit Pediatrics

Sarah Ozawa, DVM, DACZM[a],*, Molly Gleeson, DVM, DACZM[b]

KEYWORDS

- Kit • *Oryctolagus cuniculus* • *Sylvilagus floridanus* • Neonate

KEY POINTS

- Despite their reproductive efficiency, many rabbit species are endangered, emphasizing the importance of pediatric rabbit care.
- Rabbits are born altricial, and understanding the normal behavior and milestones of the juvenile is important from laboratory, wildlife, and companion rabbit care.
- Orphaned preweaning neonatal rabbits may have a relatively high mortality rate. Provision of nutrition and husbandry that most closely match their natural environment is imperative.
- Gastrointestinal disorders are the most common and important conditions in juvenile rabbits, especially parasitic infection with *Eimeria* species. Newly weaned rabbits are most susceptible and show the highest mortality rates.
- Prevention should be a major focus of pediatric rabbit care to reduce morbidity and mortality, with different goals depending on the setting and herd size. This includes providing appropriate husbandry and high-quality diet at all stages, practicing appropriate hygiene and management with large herds, and performing preventative care assessments and vaccinations at appropriate times.

NATURAL HISTORY

Rabbits belong to the order Lagomorpha which contains two families: the Leporidae family consists of rabbits, hares, and jackrabbits and the Ochotonidae consists of pikas.[1] Leporidae contains more than 60 species of animals.[2] Rabbit species are diverse and have evolved to survive in a variety of environmental conditions.[2] Leporidae species are therefore able to inhabit all continents outside of Antarctica with habitats ranging from fields, woodlands, and deserts to swamps.[1]

The most common species kept in captivity globally is the domesticated European rabbit (*Oryctolagus cuniculus*) which will be the focus of this article. In addition to human companionship, this species serves roles in meat and fur production, education, and laboratory medicine.[2] Within the European rabbit species, there are numerous breeds or varieties described (https://arba.net/recognized-breeds/) with significant

[a] Department of Clinical Sciences, College of Veterinary Medicine, North Carolina State University, 1060 Williams Moore Drive, Raleigh, NC 27606, USA; [b] Department of Exotic Pets, PETS Referral Center, 1048 University Avenue, Berkeley, CA 94710, USA
* Corresponding author.
E-mail address: sozawa@ncsu.edu

Vet Clin Exot Anim 27 (2024) 171–191
https://doi.org/10.1016/j.cvex.2023.11.003

diversity in appearance. The New Zealand White breed of *O cuniculus* is one of the most commonly represented animals used in biomedical research and is an important model for a variety of translational human diseases.[3] The most common wild rabbit genus in North America is the cottontail (*Sylvilagus* spp).[4] There are 17 species of cottontails throughout the world with the most widely distributed being the Eastern cottontail (*Sylvilagus floridanus*).

Despite their reproductive fecundity, many rabbit species are considered threatened. As of 2018, approximately 25% of lagomorph species were considered vulnerable, threatened, or endangered according to the International Union for the Conservation of Nature (IUCN) Red List of Threatened Species.[5] Species of note from North America include the Appalachian cottontail (*Sylvilagus obscurus*) listed as near threatened and the robust cottontail (*Sylvilagus robustus*) listed as endangered. Other species that are not endangered serve crucial roles as prey for predators and may be major players in the ecosystem. Therefore, understanding the biology, behavior, and care of pediatric rabbits has importance from a species survival standpoint as well.

DOMESTICATION

The European rabbit likely originated in the Iberian Peninsula according to fossil records and evolved as two separate lineages.[6] Although the initial purpose of domestication was likely due to their utilization as meat and fur, rabbits have served a long-standing role as a companion species. According to genomic data, wild French and domestic rabbits likely diverged at least 12,000 years ago.[7] The timing of the domestication of the rabbit is unclear and the development of specific breeds occurred within the last 200 years.[8,9] In comparison to other species, the domestication of the rabbit may be considered relatively recent.[10] Although dog domestication was initiated 14,000 years ago, evidence suggests that rabbit domestication only began in the last 1500 years.[9,10] However, domestication takes years and is an evolutionary process.[7] Selective breeding has led to the loss of genetic diversity in our companion species compared with wild counterparts.[11] Domestication of rabbits and this purposeful breeding has also resulted in the vast number of rabbit breeds that now exist. Although domestication has resulted in rabbits that are more approachable and easily handled, behavioral similarities to their wild counterparts still exist and should be considered especially in times of stress such as parturition and the early postnatal period.

NATURAL BEHAVIOR

The European rabbit develops social groups both in captivity and in the wild. In the wild, *O cuniculus* groups consist of a dominant male, several females, and their young. Larger groups may also include subordinate males. These groups may contain up to 20 adults and reside in burrows.[10] In these wild populations, some level of aggression is assumed to be normal and may help maintain their hierarchy.[12] This hierarchy is established after 10 weeks of age, and aggressive behavior is uncommon in rabbits less than 12 weeks of age.[13] In captivity, these species are also considered gregarious. However, rabbit group dynamics may be tenuous, and pairing of rabbits is a delicate process. Studies evaluating rabbits in research settings have demonstrated conflicting results regarding the benefits of social housing.[14,15] However, many institutions recommend attempting to at minimum pair-house rabbits to increase normal behavioral traits of the species.[16]

Social behaviors of young meat rabbits were investigated in a single breeding colony. This study found that young rabbits were submissive to adults and aggression was rare.[13] Therefore, housing of postweaning rabbits with adults may be possible.

In fact, 50% of the daytime behavior included lying in contact with conspecifics and animals were uncommonly alone.[13] In addition, dams were not the preferred social partner outside of suckling attempts. In this study, adult female aggression toward young was more common than male aggression toward young. Young rabbits displayed adult behaviors by 90 days of life and sexual behavior was present by day 70 in males.[13] In contrast, Eastern cottontails tend to be a more solitary species. Although there is male-to-female interaction, this species does not form true social groups and rabbit interactions are mainly centered on copulation and mothers and offspring.[10] These species do not create extensive burrows but instead produces shallow burrows covered in fur and grass. The young are contained within the burrows and the females reside above them during nursing.[10]

The mating preference of rabbits differs likely due to distribution of rabbits and environmental influence. Most of the European rabbits are polygamous, but monogamous pairs and harems are also described.[17]

The domestic rabbit as well as wild rabbits displays profound circadian patterns. Rabbits are a crepuscular species, with the majority of activity and foraging occurring in the early mornings and the evening.[18] Some sources, however, describe rabbits as more nocturnal beings.[19] This normal circadian cycle needs to be considered when housing and interacting with pet rabbits and wildlife.

JUVENILE MILESTONES AND MATERNAL CARE

Rabbit neonates before weaning are often referred to as kits and mothers as does.

The gestation length in rabbits is relatively short, with an average of approximately 30 days.[20,21] Parturition is typically rapid and is expected to take less than 30 minutes.[8,20] In a study evaluating the normal parturition of 10 chinchilla rabbits, longer parturition times were significantly associated with the number of stillbirths.[20] However, there was overlap in parturition duration between healthy and stillborn litters. Litter sizes vary and range from 4 to 12 young.[21] Smaller rabbits may produce smaller litters than larger rabbits.

Rabbit kits are often delivered separated from the placenta and free of membranes.[20] Rabbits are altricial and obtain most passive immunity before birth through the placenta.[8] Although not the focus of this article, hares are born more precocial with their eyes open. Additional antibodies are present in the colostrum and absorbed in the neonate intestine.[22] In rabbits, diversification of antibody genes present within gut-associated lymphoid tissue depends on intestinal microbial flora and occurs at 4 to 8 weeks of age.[23]

Newborn rabbits use olfactory cues to recognize the dam.[24] There is a gland near the nipple that produces these pheromones. Nursing of rabbits occurs infrequently with an approximately 24-hour interval between feedings. During each feeding, a kit can drink up to 20% of its body weight.[8] However, other sources cite the volume of the rabbit stomach to be up to 100 mL/kg so individual drinking volumes may vary.[4] Each feeding lasts around 3 minutes and constitutes the main interaction of the dam and young during this period of time.[25] This infrequent nursing pattern is likely evolutionary, as the dam seeks to avoid attention of the nest from predators. However, this feeding pattern is often misinterpreted by rabbit owners or good Samaritans as maternal neglect. Inappropriate interference, especially in wild rabbits, during this time can be detrimental.

During the nursing period, the doe does not spend a significant amount of time grooming or insulating the young. The doe also does not stimulate the kit to urinate, unlike other mammals. Rabbits consume exclusively milk before day 10 and begin to eat small amounts of solid food by day 12 to 18.[8,26] This solid food intake becomes significant by day 20. However, the availability of milk may influence weaning as the ingestion of solid food and water will increase as milk intake decreases.[26] For the first week, the neonate gastrointestinal tract is relatively sterile opposed to other species such as pigs and rats. In addition, the neonate stomach pH is higher than in adults. Rabbit milk contains bacteriostatic properties within fatty acids that are broken down by gastric lipase.[26] This is not present in artificial milk substitutes. Over time, colonization of the rabbit gastrointestinal tract occurs due to ingestion of the doe's and their own cecotrophs. In addition, the bacterial flora transitions over time with alterations in diet with a shift in anaerobic bacteria and increase in cellulolytic flora.[26] Significant cecotrophy occurs in the pediatric rabbit once regular solid food is consumed at approximately 3 weeks of age. The dam often leaves the young by 24 days of age. At the time of weaning, the gastric pH drastically decreases from 4 to 6 to less than 2.[26] Additional approximations of milestones and reproductive data are present in **Table 1**.

HUSBANDRY

Overall, the European rabbit is a social creature and there is a preference toward housing with a suitable companion. This species, however, can be selective regarding companionship and rabbits that are not "bonded" may exhibit aggressive behavior. Although young rabbits less commonly demonstrate aggressive behavior, as males approach puberty this can occur, separation may be recommended.[13] Adequate resources are critical in group housing to minimize aggression; this includes appropriate numbers of feeds, water sources, and hiding locations.[27] The exception to group housing, however, includes intact rabbits for which reproduction is to be prevented and scenarios in which co-housed intact males exhibit aggression. In addition, the does should ideally be housed alone during the periparturient period to avoid stress and risk of injury to the kits. In a study that group-housed production rabbit does, they found high rates of aggression among females, injury to the does, competition for nest space and kit mortality.[28] In addition, if breeding and reproduction are the desired outcome, reproductive performance may be dampened in a group setting due to high rates of pseudopregnancy.[29] Semigroup housing has been suggested in production rabbits where smaller groups of does are group-housed from 18 days of lactation until weaning, whereas they are individually housed before this and may show promise, though litter health and weight may still be inferior to that of does housed individually.[30]

Table 1	
Approximate milestones of pediatric rabbits and reproductive data for does	
Reproductive and Neonatal Data	
Gestation	30–32 d
Parturition	30 min
Litter size	4–12 kits
Birth weight	40–70 g
Eyes open	7–10 d
Ears functional	7 d
Begin eating solid food	12–15 d
Weaned	24–35 d

Stressed does are prone to cannibalism of the young, especially in the first few days following parturition. In addition, mutilation or other injury to the kits may occur post-parturition and may be more common in inexperienced does. It is imperative to limit disruptions and additional stressors in the periparturient period for the safety of the doe and kits.[31] In addition, other female and male rabbit companions may cannibalize the young, and therefore, the removal of other rabbits during late pregnancy is recommended. Intact males may also attempt to rebreed does shortly after giving birth, and rabbits are fertile starting at day 1 postpartum.[32] Conception in the periparturient period is however uncommon before day 8.[21]

Neonate rabbits should ideally be housed with the doe until fully weaned. A study in New Zealand White rabbits compared stress-associated behaviors in rabbits reared with the dam compared with weaned rabbits that were reared without their dam. In this study, bar-biting as well as cortisol levels was higher in the group weaned without the dam.[33] In addition, housing rabbits with conspecifics may lead to better socialization with other rabbits later in life.[18] Early human interaction may be beneficial for companion rabbits and those rabbits that will have frequent human interaction. Rabbits that were handled by humans in the first week of life during the peri-nursing period (15 minutes before and 30 minutes after nursing) resulted in less human avoidance behavior than those that were not handled.[34]

Reproducing does should be provided with a nest box or nesting area within the enclosure. The nesting area should be large enough for the entire litter and the doe to comfortably reside. As kits are born hairless, they require contact with conspecifics and this nest to aid in thermoregulation. Rabbits raised with littermates had higher body temperatures and a higher probability of survival compared with newborn rabbits housed alone.[35] Nesting material should provide warmth and comfort without the risks of trauma from the material to the kits. In a study evaluating nesting material preferences in rabbits, there was a preference for fine fiber material and hay over wood shavings.[36] The does often pull hair from their dewlap to help make these nests. It is important to distinguish this is a normal periparturient behavior opposed to self-destructive behavior. Commercial nesting products made of paper, bamboo, or wood are available (eg, Carefresh, Healthy Pet, Ferndale, WA) or natural products such as straw or hay can be used. During the periparturient period, rabbits should ideally be housed indoors in a thermally controlled environment. In farmed rabbits, temperatures in the nesting location should be around 27 to 35°C (80.6–95°F) at birth and 30°C (86°F) at 14 days of age.[30,37,38] Other sources recommend a nest box temperature of 26.7 to 29.4°C (80–85°F) and decreasing to 21 to 23.9°C (70–75°F) by week 3 of age.[39] This may differ in companion scenarios where there is often steady temperature control within the home as well as differences in body composition and hair coat in different breeds. The optimum temperature zone for most adult rabbits however is lower, approximately 15 to 21°C (60–70°F), and rabbits are susceptible to heat stress.[8] Therefore, being able to provide a separate microenvironment for the newborn rabbits may be advantageous for them as well as the doe.

Does housed with newborn and pediatric rabbits should be provided with a platform or a second level. This allows the doe to have an area of escape from the newborns, increases space availability, and minimizes injury to the neonate from the doe. Flooring of this platform and the cage should be flat bottomed and easily cleaned. Wire platforms and cages should be avoided due to the risk of the development of pododermatitis. In addition, slippery bottomed surfaces can lead to instability of the neonate and abnormal development of ligaments resulting in splay leg. The substrate of an enclosure should mimic the natural environment in the wild, providing pliability for movement of the foot and grip for the nails. Some options may include straw, grass hay, carpet, towels, blankets, and paper bedding. The behavior of the individual rabbit should also be considered as some rabbits will ingest carpet or blankets. Ideally, more than one substrate will be included in an enclosure to allow for self-selection of ideal flooring. As rabbits are prey species, it is important to not only provide a nest for the babies but also burrows or hides for adequate protection and hiding during all pediatric stages.

HAND-REARING RABBITS

As previously stated, neonate rabbits are ideally housed with a lactating doe. However, there are circumstances where hand-reading may be required. Some examples include abandonment of the neonate by the doe, inappropriate nursing, and insufficient care by the doe. If kits are confirmed to be abandoned or gaining insufficient weight and there is concern for lack of adequate nutrition, hand-rearing may be recommended.

Raising neonatal rabbits can be challenging and has a relatively high mortality rate. A study that evaluated orphaned and juvenile Eastern cottontails from a single wildlife center found an overall mortality rate of 18.9% within 72 hours of admission.[40] Rabbits before weaning require bottle or tube feeding. An estimated weaning weight of Eastern cottontail rabbits is approximately 70 to 140 g. The weight of a New Zealand White rabbit however at 4 weeks of age is closer to 500 g.[41] Differences in weaning weight by species and breed should be considered. In the above study evaluating Eastern cottontails, weight alone was not a predictor of survival. However, rabbits of a lower weight class that were brought in as a singleton opposed to a group were less likely to survive.[40] Another method to determine weaning age in rabbits is based on gross appearance which is used at some wildlife centers. In general, rabbits are partially self-feeding when they have eyes and ears opened, guard hairs fully grown in (opposed to a sleek fur coat) and are standing in an upright position (Dr Renee Schott, Wildlife Rehabilitation Center of Minnesota, personal communication, 2023).

Rabbit milk typically contains 13% to 15% protein, 10% to 12% fat, and 2% carbohydrates; these concentrations change throughout lactation. This is higher in protein and fat than many other species. For example, cow and goat milk have only 3.3% and 2.9% protein and only 3.8% and 4.5% fat, respectively, and are therefore inappropriate substitutes for rabbit milk.[8,42] A variety of recommendations have been made regarding an appropriate milk replacer to feed rabbits with similar tables provided in other sources (**Table 2**).[21] However, most feeding formulations, labeled for rabbit feeding or not, do not replicate the composition of rabbit milk or take into account the change in composition of rabbit milk over time during nursing. A study that compared the use of a canine milk replacer (Esbilac puppy milk replacer, Peg-Ag, Hamshire, IL) to a rabbit specific milk replacer (Womboo rabbit milk replacer, Perfect Pets Inc, Redford, MI) in infant Eastern cottontail rabbits at a rehabilitation center found that rabbits were 1.89 times more likely to survive when fed the rabbit-specific formulation.[43] The energy content of the rabbit-specific diet was higher compared with the canine diet in this study. Another study compared the use of a feline-specific feeding formulation (1 part Petag Kitten Milk replacer to 1 part Fox Valley Ultraboost) to a wild rabbit and rodent feeding formulation (Fox Valley 32/40). Eastern cottontails and desert cottontails (*Sylvilagus audubonii*) that received the feline formulation had a higher survival rate.[44] Some recipes advocate for the addition of egg yolk to feeding formulations to increase the fat and protein levels.[39] However, given the risk of bacterial enteritis in neonatal rabbits, the risks may not outweigh the benefits of this addition. In addition, most milk replacers do not contain the natural

Table 2
Examples of rabbit milk replacers and neonate feeding formulations. The formulations are not listed in order of recommendations

Number	Feeding Formulation	Citation
1	1 part Esbilac powder + 2 parts water	Kosmal[43] 2021
2	180 g Womboo powder + 330 mL water	Kosmal[43] 2021
3	1 part PetAg Kitten Milk Replacer (KMR) + 1 part Fox Valley Ultraboost + 3 parts water	Paul et al,[44] 2014
4	1 part Fox Valley 32/40 + 2 parts water	Paul et al,[44] 2014
5	6 parts Esbilac + 4 parts multi-milk	Taylor[39] 2002
6	1 part Esbilac + 1 part multi-milk + 1.5 parts water	Taylor[39] 2002
7	2 parts KMR + 1 part multi-milk	Taylor[39] 2002
8	1 part Esbilac + 1/4 part heavy cream + 1 part water	Taylor[39] 2002
9	1 part Zoologic milk matric 30/52 + 1 part water	Chankuang et al[102] 2020

antimicrobial fatty acids present in natural rabbit milk. Synthetic fatty acids may be present in some rabbit specific formulation (Womboo rabbit milk replacer), however whether these have the same antimicrobial effect as natural fatty acids is unknown. Therefore, this may make hand-reared rabbits more susceptible to gastrointestinal infections, emphasizing the need for sanitation and biosecurity during feeding. It is possible to foster neonatal rabbits to another lactating doe as an alternative to hand-rearing if a doe is available and may be considered to avoid these concerns.[45]

Neonatal rabbits can be fed with a nipple placed over a syringe or by tube feeding. Tube feeding is most often performed using a small red rubber catheter and may decrease the risks of aspiration that occur with bottle feeding. When tube feeding, the tip of the red rubber catheter should be measured from the mouth to the last rib to reach the stomach appropriately. The catheter should be primed with the feeding formulation being used and gently lubricated. The rabbit should swallow on advancement of the red rubber catheter and tube feeding should be stopped if there is any risk or concern for aspiration or regurgitation. To calculate the rabbits' daily caloric needs, the resting energy requirement (RER) should be calculated. This equation for most mammals is $RER = K \times body\ weight\ (kg)^{0.75}$. For this equation, K being constant for rabbits is 70 and body weight should be recorded in kilograms. Following calculation of basal metabolic rate (BMR), appropriate energy factors are used to calculate the maintenance energy requirement (MER); $MER = RER \times energy\ factor$. In young rabbits, an energy factor of at least 2 is recommended for growth. The rabbit stomach is readily distensible and can hold as much as 100 to 125 mL/kg at each feeding. Even though rabbits in the wild are fed once a day, hand-reared neonates are often fed two to three times a day to decrease the risks of aspiration and gastric distension while still providing appropriate caloric intake. Rabbits should be weighed regularly during this period to ensure they are gaining weight. This increase in weight is species and breed-specific.

Young rabbits should be offered grass hay, greens, young rabbit pellets, and a small portion of alfalfa hay starting at day 12 to 18 and often readily wean. The provision of alfalfa hay and young rabbit pellets provides additional protein, calcium, and calories that are needed in growing rabbits, but not most adult rabbits. Orphaned rabbits may reach milestones slightly later compared with their unorphaned counterparts. Throughout the weaning process, solid food intake should gradually increase as milk intake decreases. As microbial colonization is critical in the rabbit, cecotrophs from a healthy adult are occasionally fed to weaning rabbits as a method of transfaunation when they are hand-reared.[8] The diet should be transitioned at approximately 6 months of age to an adult diet that eliminates alfalfa hay and prioritizes grass hay, greens, and a small amount of adult pellets.

As rabbits cannot thermoregulate well during the neonatal period, they should be housed in a warm environment such as an incubator with adequate nesting material. Despite the fact that female rabbits in the wild do not groom them, those raising newborn rabbits still recommend stimulating the young to urinate and defecate by rubbing the perineal region with a warm moistened cloth after feeding.[8]

DISEASES AND CONDITIONS OF PEDIATRIC RABBITS

There are many disease processes and conditions that can affect young rabbits, including congenital conditions, gastrointestinal conditions, infectious disease, environmental effects, and nutritional deficiencies. Causes of morbidity and death in neonatal rabbits are often related to maternal and hand-rearing factors, whereas those in weanling rabbits are most commonly related to disorders of the gastrointestinal system.

Congenital Conditions

Multiple inherited and congenital conditions have been reported in rabbits, most commonly in farmed and pet rabbits.[46,47] Three of the most important conditions are discussed. However, other conditions to be aware of include congenital diaphragmatic hernia, hypotrichosis, achondroplasia, paralytic tremors, epilepsy, cortical renal cysts, hypogonadism, hydrocephalus, and cleft palate.[46]

The most common inherited disease in the rabbit is mandibular prognathism, leading to primary incisor malocclusion or "cross bite."[48–50] An autosomal recessive gene (mp) causes differential growth of the skull bones, which results in a mandible that is relatively longer than the maxilla.[48,51] This is most commonly seen in brachycephalic breeds, including dwarf and lop-eared rabbits.[49,50] More recently, the condition has been referred to as maxillary brachygnathism[52,53] as it is more likely there is reduced skull and maxilla growth rather than mandibular elongation.[54] Research has demonstrated that cranial morphometry differs between wild and domestic rabbits with this condition likely being a lesser concern in wild species.[55] Incisor malocclusion first appears around 3 weeks of age but may not be observed by owners until 10 to 12 weeks of age when significant clinical crown elongation has occurred.[49,54] Initially, incisors occlude edge to edge resulting in blunting of the cutting edge of each tooth. Later, the mandibular incisors shift to become positioned rostral to the maxillary first incisors. As they grow, the mandibular incisors elongate toward the upper lip due to the lack of opposing occlusion. The maxillary first incisors curve backward into the oral cavity and can cause lesions if they contact the palate or buccal mucosa. If not addressed, this can lead to ulceration and abscessation.[49,50,54] Over time, primary incisor malocclusion can lead to acquired premolar and molar malocclusion as the rabbit is unable to close its mouth fully.[50] Once diagnosed, treatment involves reestablishing normal occlusion with frequent incisor trims or incisor extractions.[49,50]

Congenital cardiac abnormalities are uncommon in rabbits but have been reported. Multiple cases of naturally occurring ventricular septal defects have been diagnosed in various breeds.[56–60] One of the authors (MG) has personally managed a case of ventricular septal defect in a young Holland lop rabbit with secondary dilated cardiomyopathy that was still alive at the time of writing, over a year after starting treatment. In addition, two cases of atrial septal defects were recently reported.[61,62] Any young rabbit with a heart murmur should have an echocardiograph performed to evaluate for these conditions. Anecdotally, physiologic murmurs in young rabbits seem less common than in puppies. Unfortunately, eventual progression to congestive heart failure is common and the prognosis at that time is considered poor.

Abnormalities associated with the ophthalmic system have also been reported in pediatric rabbits. Microphthalmia, anophthalmia, and congenital glaucoma have been described.[46] In a retrospective study evaluating the cause of death of 325 European rabbits and hares in Northern Spain, congenital glaucoma was identified in four rabbits (1.49%) and was the only congenital disease seen.[47] Congenital glaucoma is more common in albino breeds as the genes for both traits are located on the same chromosome.[46] It has been reported that does with the gene may have small litter sizes and decreased neonatal survival rates.[47]

Gastrointestinal Conditions

Digestive disorders are the most common and important conditions affecting pediatric rabbits. There seems to be a seasonal pattern with increased cases in autumn and early winter, which may coincide with better environmental conditions for the transmission of parasites.[47] An immature immune system and developing gut microbial population combined with environmental factors including poor hygiene, inadequate management systems, overcrowding, and suboptimal prophylactic health care likely increase the risks of digestive disorders in weanling rabbits. Hand-rearing or inappropriate weaning can disrupt the process of microbial colonization and increase the risk of dysbiosis. **Table 3** reports these conditions and the ages at which they typically present.

Table 3
The most common gastrointestinal conditions affecting neonatal and weanling rabbits

Disease	Organism/Primary Cause	Age
Dysbiosis	Antibiotic induced Exposure to pathogens/toxins Stress glucocorticoids Dietary factors	During or after cecal microbiota colonization (2–4 weeks old).
Hepatic coccidiosis	E stiedae	<6 mo
Intestinal coccidiosis	Eimeria spp E perforans = most common E magna, E media, E irresidua also seen	<6 mo
Cryptosporidium	Cryptosporidium parvum	30–40 d
Enterotoxemia	C spiroforme	3–6 wk
Tyzzer's disease	C piliforme	6–8 wk
Primary bacterial enteritis	E coli Campylobacter spp Salmonella typhimurium Klebsiella pneumoniae Klebsiella oxytoca Pseudomonas aeruginosa	<16 wk
Proliferative enterocolitis	Lawsonia intracellularis	8–16 wk
Epizootic rabbit enteropathy	Unknown pathogenesis	5–14 wk
Viral diarrhea	Rabbit enteric coronavirus Rotavirus	3–10 wk <6 wk

Endoparasites

Coccidiosis, caused by organisms of the genus *Eimeria*, is the most common parasitic condition affecting the rabbit gastrointestinal tract.[63] It is a frequent cause of illness in rabbits less than 6 month old, with those ages 1 to 4 months old being most affected.[63,64] In studies, suckling rabbits younger than 19 day old are not susceptible, which is potentially due to an intestinal environment incompatible with the endogenous development of coccidial organisms.[65] Digestive enzymes in the duodenum are required to break down ingested oocysts and release sporozoites that infect intestinal epithelium, which may not be present before the shift in intestinal environment that occurs with weaning.[66] Clinical coccidiosis can lead to mortality and impaired growth, especially in large colonies.[63] Affected rabbits will show anorexia, depression, weight loss, roughened haircoat, diarrhea of varying severity, and dehydration.[47,67] Chronic, severe diarrhea can lead to secondary complications such as intussusception.[66] Transmission is due to ingestion of infective sporulated oocysts from feed, the environment, or fomites with oocysts known to be stable in the environment for long periods.[68] Two primary forms of coccidiosis can be seen in rabbits.

Eimeria stiedae is the only extra-gastrointestinal *Eimeria* species in rabbits.[69] It infects the liver causing hepatic coccidiosis, primarily in young rabbits.[47] After invading the intestinal mucosa, sporozoites of this species travel into bile duct epithelial cells where they proliferate.[70] Clinical signs and laboratory findings are associated with bile duct obstruction and hepatic dysfunction. Pathogenicity depends on the number of oocysts ingested, which is different from intestinal species.[71] Biochemical analysis may show abnormalities in hepatic parameters, whereas hematology may reveal leukocytosis, eosinophilia, and thrombocytopenia.[67] Ultrasonographically, the liver of infected patients was diffusely heterogenous with multiple poorly defined, hyperechoic regions, and dilated hepatic blood vessels and bile ducts.[72] One of the authors (MG) has also identified similar ultrasonographic findings in rabbits diagnosed with this condition. Presumptive diagnosis can be made based on identification of *Eimeria* oocysts in the bile or feces in combination with the aforementioned laboratory findings, but hepatic histopathology is required for definitive diagnosis.[73]

At least 14 species of *Eimeria* have been identified as causes of intestinal coccidiosis in rabbits.[63] The two most pathogenic species are *Eimeria intestinalis* and *Eimeria flavescens*, whereas moderately pathogenic species include *E irresidua, E magna,* and *E piriformis*. The least pathogenic species are *E perforans, E neoleporis,* and *E media*.[71] Pathogenicity seems to be connected to localization of the particular species within the intestines and damage to the crypts.[69] Each *Eimeria* species has a particular site and depth of infection within the intestinal tract.[66] Mixed infections of multiple *Eimeria* species are common as well as coinfections with bacterial organisms, especially *Escherichia coli*.[63,66] Clinical signs vary depending on the species of *Eimeria*, age of the rabbit, immune status, and parasite burden. Presumptive diagnosis can be made by identifying *E* oocysts in the feces and definitive diagnosis relies on stained impression smears or histopathology of the intestines.[63]

Treatment of coccidiosis in rabbits depends on the housing environment. Many commercial breeders and farms use coccidiostats, such as monensin or salinomycin, as feed additives to prevent or minimize infection in their herds.[63] However, increased resistance to these drugs has been seen and increasing dosages have resulted in fatalities from toxicity.[47,69] More natural preventative alternatives are being explored, including herbal extracts such as garlic oil, banana stem extract, neem, clove, antioxidants, and acidifiers.[63] An important part of prevention and treatment is appropriate hygiene and management practices to reduce the number of oocysts in the environment.[68,69] Multiple medical therapies have been investigated for treatment of coccidiosis. For larger groups of rabbits, drinking water medicated with toltrazuril (2.5–5 mg/kg once daily for 2 days, repeating after 5 days), amprolium (50 mg/kg for 5 days), and a combination of both drugs has been demonstrated to be effective at controlling natural intestinal coccidial infections in rabbits. Treated rabbits had reduced fecal oocyst counts, resolution of clinical signs, and improved feed consumption and body weight.[74,75] Other toltrazuril doses as well as sulfadimethoxine in drinking water are also effective for both intestinal and hepatic coccidiosis.[74,76,77] A retrospective study from the Colorado Wild Rabbit Foundation reported a significant reduction in mortality ratio due to gastrointestinal disease from 29% to 7% when more aggressive treatment and prophylaxis of coccidiosis in young cottontail rabbits was implemented.[78] In 2020, all young cottontail rabbits were treated prophylactically with toltrazuril (25 mg/kg orally once daily for 2 days on, 5 days off) and those with clinical signs of gastrointestinal disease were treated more aggressively (25 mg/kg orally once daily for up to 5 days) until signs resolved.[78] For individual pet rabbits, primary treatment with sulfonamides is most recommended.[69] Options include sulfadimethoxine at 15 mg/kg orally twice daily for 10 days and trimethoprim-sulfamethoxazole at 30 to 40 mg/kg orally twice daily for 10 days.[66,73] The use of ponazuril, an active metabolite of toltrazuril, at 20 to 50 mg/kg orally once daily for up to 30 days has also been used.[79] One of the authors (MG) has found that cases of hepatic coccidiosis often need to be treated for longer. Rabbits that recover are immune from future reinfection, but no cross-immunity exists between *Eimeria* species.[66]

Bacterial Enteritis

Primary bacterial enteritis due to infection with *E coli* is seen in neonates and newly weaned rabbits around 4 to 7 weeks of age.[80] It is often associated with stressors like weaning, transport, and potentially overcrowding and can be a major cause of losses in commercial rabbitries and laboratories.[66] Although small numbers of nonpathogenic *E coli* can be found normally in the rabbit gastrointestinal tract, overgrowth can occur with changes in cecal pH and transmission of pathogenic serovars occurs through oral ingestion of contaminated water or feed.[81,82] Pathogenic *E coli* leads to primary pathology in the ileum, cecum, and colon.[83] Enteropathogenic *E coli* is the most common serovar found in rabbits.[84,85] It causes atrophy of the villi in the ileum and proximal colon leading to malabsorption and diarrhea.[84] Enterohemorrhagic *E coli* (EHEC), which produces shiga toxins, results in hemorrhagic colitis and diarrhea.[86] Renal lesions including glomerulonephritis and glomerular thrombotic microangiopathy leading to acute renal failure have also been reported with EHEC.[86] In severe cases of colibacillosis, rabbits may develop intussusception and rectal prolapse.[73] Definitive diagnosis requires histopathology as culture is not serotype-specific but may aid in choice of antibiotic therapy. Treatment can be challenging. A study evaluating the use of enrofloxacin in weanling New Zealand White rabbits experimentally infected with *E coli* found reduced bacterial shedding and improved body weight in treated rabbits that was further improved when probiotics were administered before infection.[87]

Multiple pathogenic *Clostridium* species can affect pediatric rabbits, with *C perfringens*, *C piliforme*, *Clostridium spiroforme*, and *C difficile* being the most common.[88] Stress, administration of enteral clindamycin, and feeding high-carbohydrate, low-fiber diets have been associated with proliferation of these organisms.[66,89] Endotoxemia is most often caused by *C spiroforme* and its associated iota-like toxin, which multiplies rapidly and alters the cecal microbiota.[66,90] The highest mortality is seen in newly weaned kits that are 3 to 6 weeks of age. Clinical signs include anorexia, depression, hypothermia, abdominal pain, and watery diarrhea that can contain blood and mucus. Death may occur within 24 to 48 hours due to dehydration and toxemia.[66,88] Definitive diagnosis may require fecal culture in combination with isolation of the toxin. Pathologic lesions include severe enteritis and typhlitis with petechiation and hemorrhage within the cecum, appendix, and/or colon.[73,89] *Clostridium piliforme* is the cause of Tyzzer's disease, which also causes morbidity and mortality in weanling rabbits around 6 to 8 weeks of age.[66] Affected rabbits exhibit depression, watery diarrhea, and dehydration.[73,89] Pathologic lesions include multifocal hepatic necrosis and mucosal necrosis within the ileum, cecum, and colon.[89,91] It is common to see mixed infections with *Clostridium*, other pathogenic bacteria, rotavirus, and *Eimeria*.[47,88,91] The Colorado Wild Rabbit Foundation found a reduction in mortality due to clostridial enteritis in young cottontail rabbits when prophylactic treatment of coccidiosis was implemented.[78] Treatment of clostridial enteritis should include aggressive supportive care, medications to improve cecal and colonic motility, and antimicrobials. The antibiotic of choice for clostridial infections is metronidazole at 20 mg/kg twice daily either intravenously or orally, but the use of tetracyclines in water and oral chloramphenicol has also been successful.[66,73] The use of cholestyramine to bind bacterial toxins may be helpful if used early on, with a recommended dose of 0.5 g/kg or 2 g/20 mL water administered once daily via gavage.[73,79]

Viral Diarrhea

Rotavirus and rabbit enteric coronavirus (REC) cause diarrhea in rabbits, typically affecting larger colonies rather than individual pet rabbits. Neonatal rabbits are most susceptible, but transplacentally derived maternal antibodies to rotavirus can provide some level of protection until weaning.[66,73] REC has been implicated in outbreaks of diarrhea in weanling rabbits associated with very high morbidity and mortality (almost 100%).[73,92]

Other Gastrointestinal Disease

Epizootic rabbit enteropathy (ERE), also known as mucoid enteritis, is a major cause of morbidity and mortality in postweaning rabbits.[73] One retrospective study found a higher prevalence in female farmed rabbits, compared with pet or wild rabbits, and it was more common in the autumn and winter months.[47] Affected rabbits exhibit anorexia, lethargy, weight loss, mucoid yellowish diarrhea, and impaction of the cecum and colon from excessive mucus production.[47,73] Mortality rates of 35% to 95% have been reported with most rabbits dying within 1 to 3 days.[66] The true pathogenesis of the condition is still unclear; however, is it possibly related to changes in cecal pH and inadequate fiber content.[82,93] Prognosis is considered poor but treatment with antibiotics and general gastrointestinal support can be considered for pet rabbits.[66] Providing appropriate fiber to newly weaned rabbits may help reduce the chances of ERE.

Non-Gastrointestinal Infectious Diseases

Pasteurella multocida is both a commensal and opportunistic pathogen in rabbits as serogroups have variable pathogenicity.[94] It is most problematic in large colonies where sources of stress may be increased.[92,95] Respiratory disease in newly acquired young rabbits, especially from a pet store, is commonly related to *P multocida*.[92] Acute respiratory infections and septicemia can occur in pediatric rabbits, showing increasing prevalence with age. Treatment involves isolation of infected animals, increased hygiene, optimization of husbandry, and antibiotic therapy based on culture and sensitivity of respiratory samples.[92]

While not a common cause of morbidity in pediatric rabbits, rabbit hemorrhagic disease virus type 2 (RHDV2) has caused disease and mortality in kits as young as 15 to 20 day old and has been demonstrated to be more virulent than classical RHDV.[96] It may be a cause of mortality in young wild rabbits with peracute infection leading to rapid death.[47] *Encephalitozoon cuniculi* can cause phacoclastic uveitis in young rabbits due to intrauterine transmission of the organism into the lens before capsule formation.[97] Mortality in young rabbits due to meningoencephalitis and multifocal granulomatous interstitial nephritis from *E cuniculi* infection has also been reported.[47]

Environmental Conditions

As noted earlier, pediatric rabbits are sensitive to thermal stress and thus will succumb to heat stroke more readily than older rabbits. Clinical signs associated with heat stress can include reduced food intake, immune suppression, increased respiratory rate, prostration, hypoglycemia, seizures, and pulmonary edema.[95] Acute shock with renal and pulmonary compromise can lead to death especially during late spring and summer months.[47] Temperatures higher than 35°C (95°F) are often associated with this condition.[47,95] Pediatric rabbits should be housed in a controlled environment and protected from extremes in temperature fluctuation as much as possible.

Trauma to pediatric rabbits can occur in many forms, including predation, conspecific or maternal trauma, and inappropriate enclosures. Predation is likely a higher risk for rabbits housed outdoors and they should be kept in a secure enclosure, especially at night. Young rabbits encountered in the wild should not be uncovered or left exposed. However, indoor rabbits are also at risk of injury from other household pets like cats, dogs, and ferrets. Trauma from does and other members of the group is discussed earlier.

Conditions Associated with Orphaned or Hand-Reared Rabbits

Infant rabbits with poor maternal care that require hand-rearing are more likely to succumb to hypothermia, dehydration, hypoglycemia, aspiration pneumonia, and/or malnutrition as mentioned previously. Hypoglycemia is often encountered when recently or inappropriately weaned rabbits are obtained as new pets. Suboptimal diets can lead to malnutrition and hypoglycemia, causing these rabbits to present moribund, hypothermic, and potentially seizing. The investigators have experienced especially high numbers of these cases around Easter, when rabbits are often given as gifts. The assessment of blood glucose concentrations in rabbits should be done with a laboratory analyzer if available, but point of care assessment in critical patients can be performed using a human glucometer (eg, Accu-Chek, Roche Diabetes Care Inc, Indianapolis, IN) based on available studies.[98] Treatment involves intravenous dextrose supplementation, thermal support, nutritional support, and treatment of any secondary infections.

Nutritional Deficiencies

The nutritional deficiencies seen in juvenile rabbits are often due to deficiencies in the doe or inappropriate diet in the early stages of life but can also result when gastrointestinal diseases lead to poor absorption of nutrients. Hypovitaminosis A in young, growing rabbits can result in hydrocephalus from defective bone growth and stenosis of the cerebral aqueduct.[99] Deficiencies in vitamin E can lead to nutritional muscular dystrophy resulting in paresis or paralysis from degeneration and necrosis of skeletal muscle myofibers and may also develop myocardial dysfunction.[99,100] Effects on the skeletal system are also seen with manganese deficiency, which causes poor bone

Table 4
Vaccines available for rabbits in North America and the age at which they can first be administered

Vaccine	Type of Vaccine	Availability	Age	Protocol
Rabbit Hemorrhagic Disease				
Medgene[a]	Inactivated recombinant subunit vaccine against capsid protein of RHDV2	USA	7 wk	2 dose primary series, 21 d apart. No information on dosing interval yet.
Filavac VHD K C + V	Inactivated RHDV 1 + 2	France	10 wk	Primary dose, then booster annually
Eravac	Inactivated RHDV2 only	Spain	30 d	Primary dose, then booster annually
Nobivac Myxo-RHD PLUS	Trivalent Live recombinant vector vaccine for myxomatosis + RHDV1 + 2	United Kingdom	5 wk	Primary dose, then booster annually
P multocida				
BunnyVac	Killed *P multocida* bacterin	USA	6 wk	2 dose primary series, 30 d apart, then booster annually.

[a] The Medgene RHDV2 vaccine is not yet FDA-approved as of the writing of this article and has been granted emergency use authorization due to the introduction and spread of RHDV2 in the United States.

quality, and nutritional hyperparathyroidism from hypocalcemia and/or hypovitamino-sis D.[99] Hypomagnesemia can cause seizures and mimic other primary neurologic conditions.[100]

PREVENTATIVE CARE

As in adult rabbits, preventative care can help ensure the health of pediatric rabbits and reduce the risk of the aforementioned conditions in this article. It is important to reduce stress on neonatal and weaning rabbits, so the authors recommend waiting to perform a wellness visit until after rabbits have been fully weaned. The most efficient strategy is to perform a rabbit's first wellness examination in combination with a pri-mary vaccine series, which is typically after 5 weeks of age. If neonatal or weaning rab-bits show signs of illness they should be evaluated by a veterinarian sooner, with precautions taken to reduce stress, maintain appropriate environmental tempera-tures, and avoid any injury associated with handling. Following any necessary vacci-nation visits, young rabbits should be evaluated for a pre-neuter examination around 4 to 5 months of age, depending on breed and size. Female rabbits should ideally be spayed before 6 months of age, before the development of significant mesometrial fat stores. If breeding is desired then female can be spayed later, but it is recommen-ded no later than 3 years of age due to the high incidence of uterine adenocarcinoma. Male rabbits should be castrated between 4 and 7 months of age, around the time of sexual maturity, with smaller breeds maturing faster than larger breeds. However, the same neoplastic risk is not present in male rabbits, and some owners may elect to keep their male rabbits intact.

Examination of young rabbits should include a full physical examination with partic-ular attention paid to body condition, hydration, body temperature, cardiac ausculta-tion, abdominal palpation, evaluation of fecal quality and consistency, and oral examination. Fecal evaluation from individuals or pooled from a litter may be useful to evaluate for the presence of coccidia or other parasites, especially in farm or com-mercial settings. Bloodwork should be performed during pre-neuter evaluations to help formulate an appropriate anesthetic plan and evaluate for any unexpected anes-thetic risks.

Vaccination

Vaccine recommendations for rabbits depend on geographic location. For rabbits in North America, vaccination for RHDV2 is currently recommended in all rabbits living in the southwestern United States, including those housed indoors, and considered for those at high risk in other locations. A killed *P multocida* vaccine is available in the United States, which may reduce clinical disease associated with this pathogen.[8] It has been shown to be more effective when given subcutaneously rather than intra-nasally.[101] Vaccination for *P multocida* is not typically recommended for house rabbits but may be important for rabbitries. Although routinely used in Europe, a vaccine for myxomatosis is not currently available in the United States. **Table 4** lists the specific vaccines and their availability. When vaccinating rabbits intended for human con-sumption, an appropriate withdrawal time should be used after vaccination.

SUMMARY

Understanding the natural behavior and husbandry of periparturient and pediatric rab-bits is imperative to the provision of appropriate pediatric care. Mimicking the natural environment with provision of appropriate substrate, temperatures, maternal support, and diet may improve animal health in the post-natal period. Unfortunately, many causes of morbidity in neonatal rabbits are related to maternal and hand-rearing factors. Veterinary intervention in the early pediatric period is not always necessary unless poor indicators of health are identified. However, given the propensity of pediatric rabbits to develop certain diseases, such as gastrointestinal disease, careful monitoring is recommended, and medical care may be required for the previously mentioned disease processes. Further research is likely needed regarding therapeutic interventions and nutritional support in pediatric rabbits.

CLINICS CARE POINTS

- Neonatal rabbits are ideally raised by the doe with littermates until fully weaned. If not possible, the provision of adequate heat support, environmental factors, and nutrition is required.
- Rabbit milk has relatively high protein and fat compared with cow and goat milk. Therefore, using a milk replacer that most closely mimics the natural lactational milk of rabbits is recommended.
- Treatment of gastrointestinal conditions in weanling rabbits should include fluid therapy, thermal and nutritional support, use of antimicrobials to treat specific pathogens, and optimization of husbandry.
- Combining a first wellness examination with the primary rabbit hemorrhagic disease virus type 2 vaccine series may reduce stress associated with veterinary visits in young rabbits.

DISCLOSURE

The authors have nothing to disclose.

REFERENCES

1. Donnelly TM, Vella D. Basic Anatomy, Physiology, and Husbandry of Rabbits. In: Katherine Q, Christoph M, Connie O, et al, editors. Ferrets, rabbits, and rodents : clinical medicine and surgery. Philadelphia: Saunders; 2020. p. 131–49.
2. Fontanesi L, Di Palma F, Flicek P, et al. LaGomiCs—Lagomorph Genomics Consortium: An International Collaborative Effort for Sequencing the Genomes of an Entire Mammalian Order. J Hered 2016;107:295–308.
3. Fan J, Kitajima S, Watanabe T, et al. Rabbit models for the study of human atherosclerosis: from pathophysiological mechanisms to translational medicine. Pharmacol Therapeut 2015;146:104–19.
4. Tseng FS. Natural History and Medical Management of Lagomorphs. In: Hernandez SM, Barron H, Miller E, et al, editors. Medical management of wildlife species: a guide for practitioners. Hoboken, NJ: New Jersey Wiley; 2019. p. 185–96.
5. The IUCN red list of threatened species. Version 2022-2. 2022. Available at: www.iucnredlist.org. Accessed April 26, 2023.
6. Fontanesi L, Utzeri VJ, Ribani A. The evolution, domestication and world distribution of the European rabbit (Oryctolagus cuniculus). In: Fontanesi L, editor. The genetics and genomics of the rabbit. Wallingford: CAB International; 2021. p. 1–22.
7. Irving-Pease EK, Frantz LAF, Sykes N, et al. Rabbits and the Specious Origins of Domestication. Trends Ecol Evol 2018;33:149–52.

8. Smith MV. Rabbit Basic Science. In: Varga Smith M, editor. Textbook of rabbit medicine. 3rd edition. Philadelphia, PA: Elsevier Health Sciences; 2023.

9. Carneiro M, Afonso S, Geraldes A, et al. The Genetic Structure of Domestic Rabbits. Mol Biol Evol 2011;28:1801–16.

10. Somerville AD, Sugiyama N. Why were New World rabbits not domesticated? Animal Frontiers 2021;11:62–8.

11. Alves JM, Carneiro M, Afonso S, et al. Levels and patterns of genetic diversity and population structure in domestic rabbits. PLoS One 2015;10:e0144687.

12. DiVincenti L Jr, Rehrig AN. The social nature of European rabbits (Oryctolagus cuniculus). JAALAS 2016;55:729–36.

13. Lehmann M. Social behaviour in young domestic rabbits under semi-natural conditions. Appl Anim Behav Sci 1991;32:269–92.

14. Fuentes GC, Newgren J. Physiology and clinical pathology of laboratory New Zealand White rabbits housed individually and in groups. JAALAS 2008; 47:35–8.

15. Chu L-r, Garner JP, Mench JA. A behavioral comparison of New Zealand White rabbits (Oryctolagus cuniculus) housed individually or in pairs in conventional laboratory cages. Appl Anim Behav Sci 2004;85:121–39.

16. Thurston S, Burlingame L, Lester PA, et al. Methods of pairing and pair maintenance of New Zealand White rabbits (Oryctolagus cuniculus) via behavioral ethogram, monitoring, and interventions. JoVE 2018;e57267.

17. Cowan D, Bell D. Leporid social behaviour and social organization. Mamm Rev 1986;16:169–79.

18. Crowell-Davis S. Rabbit behavior. Veterinary Clinics of North America, Exotic Animal Practice, 24, 2021, Elsevier; Philadelphia, PA, 53–62.

19. Gunn D, Morton DB. Inventory of the behaviour of New Zealand White rabbits in laboratory cages. Appl Anim Behav Sci 1995;45:277–92.

20. Hudson R, Cruz Y, Lucio RA, et al. Temporal and Behavioral Patterning of Parturition in Rabbits and Rats. Physiol Behav 1999;66:599–604.

21. Donneley T, Vella D Ch. 11. Basic Anatomy, Physiology and Husbandry of Rabbits. In: Quesenberry K, Mans C, editors. Ferrets, rabbits, and rodents: clinical medicine and surgery. 4th edition. Philadelphia: Elsevier; 2020. p. 131–49.

22. Peri B, Rothberg R. Mucosal immunity and tolerance in neonatal rabbits. Recent Advances in Mucosal Immunology: Part A: Cellular Interactions 1987;739–50.

23. Lanning D, Zhu X, Zhai S-K, et al. Development of the antibody repertoire in rabbit: gut-associated lymphoid tissue, microbes, and selection. Immunol Rev 2000;175:214–28.

24. Luo M. Got milk? A pheromonal message for newborn rabbits. Bioessays 2004; 26:6–9.

25. González-Mariscal G, Caba M, Martínez-Gómez M, et al. Mothers and offspring: The rabbit as a model system in the study of mammalian maternal behavior and sibling interactions. Horm Behav 2016;77:30–41.

26. Gidenne T, Fortun-Lamothe L. Feeding strategy for young rabbits around weaning: a review of digestive capacity and nutritional needs. Anim Sci 2002;75: 169–84.

27. Clauss M, Hatt J-M. Evidence-Based Rabbit Housing and Nutrition. Veterinary Clinics of North America. Exotic Animal Practice 2017;20:871–84.

28. Szendrő Z, Mikó A, Odermatt M, et al. Comparison of performance and welfare of single-caged and group-housed rabbit does. Animal 2013;7:463–8.

29. Rommers JM, Boiti C, De Jong I, et al. Performance and behaviour of rabbit does in a group-housing system with natural mating or artificial insemination. Reprod Nutr Dev 2006;46:677–87.

30. Szendrő Z, Trocino A, Hoy S, et al. A review of recent research outcomes on the housing of farmed domestic rabbits: reproducing does. World Rabbit Sci 2019; 27:1–14.

31. Rashwan A, Marai I. Mortality in young rabbits: a review. World Rabbit Sci 2000; 8:111–24.

32. Lamb IC, Partridge GG, Fuller MF, et al. Fertility of the early postpartum, lactating domestic rabbit. Theriogenology 1988;30:75–82.

33. Gharib HS, Abdel-Fattah AF, Mohammed HA, et al. Weaning induces changes in behavior and stress indicators in young New Zealand rabbits. Journal of Advanced Veterinary and Animal Research 2018;5:166–72.

34. Pongrácz P, Altbäcker V. The effect of early handling is dependent upon the state of the rabbit (Oryctolagus cuniculus) pups around nursing. Dev Psychobiol 1999;35:241–51.

35. Bautista A, Drummond H, Martínez-Gómez M, et al. Thermal benefit of sibling presence in the newborn rabbit. Dev Psychobiol 2003;43:208–15.

36. Farkas TP, Szendrő Z, Matics Z, et al. Preference of rabbit does among different nest materials. World Rabbit Sci 2018;26:81–90.

37. Bautista A, Castelán F, Pérez-Roldán H, et al. Competition in newborn rabbits for thermally advantageous positions in the litter huddle is associated with individual differences in brown fat metabolism. Physiol Behav 2013;118:189–94.

38. Rödel H, Hudson R, Von Holst D. Optimal litter size for individual growth of European rabbit pups depends on their thermal environment. Oecologia 2008;155: 677–89.

39. Taylor K. Orphan Rabbits. In: Gage L, editor. Hand-rearing wild and domestic mammals. Ames, IA: Iowa State Press; 2002. p. 5–12.

40. Principati SL, Keller KA, Allender MC, et al. Prognostic indicators for survival of orphaned neonatal and juvenile eastern cottontail rabbits (Sylvilagus floridanus): 1,256 Cases (2012–17). J Wildl Dis 2020;56:523–9.

41. Masoud I, Shapiro F, Kent R, et al. A longitudinal study of the growth of the New Zealand white rabbit: Cumulative and biweekly incremental growth rates for body length, body weight, femoral length, and tibial length. J Orthop Res 1986; 4:221–31.

42. Petrescu-Mag V, Bud I, Gavriloaie C. The chemical composition of rabbit milk compared to the milk composition of other mammal species. Rabbit Genetics 2020;10:13–4.

43. Kosmal P. Survival of infant eastern cottontails (Sylvilagus floridanus) rehabilitated using a rabbit-specific and non-specific milk replacer: a retrospective study. J Wildl Rehabil 2021;41.

44. Paul G, Friend DG. Comparison of outcomes using two milk replacer formulas based on commercially available products in two species of infant cottontail rabbits. J Wildl Rehabil 2017;37.

45. Abecia L, Fondevila M, Balcells J, et al. The effect of lactating rabbit does on the development of the caecal microbial community in the pups they nurture. J Appl Microbiol 2007;103:557–64.

46. Botha M, Petrescu-Mag IV, Hettig A. Genetic disorders in domestic rabbits (Oryctolagus cuniculus). Rabbit Genetics 2014;4.

47. Espinosa J, Ferreras MC, Benavides J, et al. Causes of mortality and disease in rabbits and hares: a retrospective study. Animals 2020;10:158.

48. Lindsey JR, Fox RR. Inherited diseases and variations. In: Manning PJ, Ringler DH, Newcomer CE, editors. The biology of the laboratory rabbit. San Diego, CA: Academic Press; 1994. p. 293–319.
49. Lord B. Dental disease in the rabbit Part 2: Dental disease causes, clinical signs and diagnosis. UK Vet Companion Animal 2011;16:39–42.
50. Legendre LF. Malocclusions in guinea pigs, chinchillas and rabbits. Can Vet J 2002;43:385–90.
51. Fox R, Crary D. Mandibular Prognathism in the Rabbit: Genetic studies: Genetic studies. J Hered 1971;62:23–7.
52. Verstraete FJ, Osofsky A. Dentistry in pet rabbits. Compendium 2005;27: 671–84.
53. Proorocu M, Safirescu OC, Petrescu-Mag IV. Malocclusion in Oryctolagus cuniculus: causes, diagnosis, prevention, treatment. Rabbit Genetics 2022;12:9–14.
54. Jekl V, Redrobe S. Rabbit dental disease and calcium metabolism–the science behind divided opinions. J Small Anim Pract 2013;54:481–90.
55. Böhmer C, Böhmer E. Shape variation in the craniomandibular system and prevalence of dental problems in domestic rabbits: a case study in evolutionary veterinary science. Veterinary sciences 2017;4:5.
56. Voros K, Seehusen F, Hungerbuhler S, et al. Ventricular septal defect with aortic valve insufficiency in a New Zealand White rabbit. J Am Anim Hosp Assoc 2011; 47:e42–9.
57. Hildebrandt N, Leuser C, Miltz D, et al. Restrictive ventricular septal defect in a dwarf rabbit. Tierarztliche Praxis Ausgabe K, Kleintiere/Heimtiere 2016;44: 59–64.
58. Ozawa S, Guzman DS-M, Keel K, et al. Clinical and pathological findings in rabbits with cardiovascular disease: 59 cases (2001–2018). J Am Vet Med Assoc 2021;259:764–76.
59. Crary DD, Fox RR. Hereditary vestigial pulmonary arterial trunk and related defects in rabbits. J Hered 1975;66:50–5.
60. Kanemoto I, Chimura S. Congenital Heart Disease of the Rabbit I. A Case of Ventricular Septal Defect. Advances in Animal Electrocardiography 1983; 16:52–6.
61. Di Girolamo N, Palmieri C, Baron Toaldo M, et al. First Description of Partial Atrioventricular Septal Defect in a Rabbit. J Exot Pet Med 2018;27:5–9.
62. Nakata M, Miwa Y, Chambers JK, et al. Ostium secundum type of atrial septal defect in a rabbit. J Vet Med Sci 2018;80:1325–8.
63. El-Ghany WAA. Coccidiosis: a parasitic disease of significant importance in rabbits. World's Vet J (WVJ) 2020;10:499–507.
64. Varga I. Large-scale management systems and parasite populations: coccidia in rabbits. Vet Parasitol 1982;11:69–84.
65. Pakandl M, Hlásková L. The reproduction of Eimeria flavescens and Eimeria intestinalis in suckling rabbits. Parasitol Res 2007;101:1435–7.
66. Varga Smith M. Digestive disorders. In: Varga Smith M, editor. Textbook of rabbit medicine. 3rd edition. Poland: Elsevier; 2023. p. 156–91.
67. Jing J, Liu C, Zhu S-X, et al. Pathological and ultrastructural observations and liver function analysis of Eimeria stiedai-infected rabbits. Vet Parasitol 2016; 223:165–72.
68. Bangoura B, Daugschies A. Eimeria. In: Florin-Christensen M, editor. Parasitic protozoa of farm animals and pets. 2018. p. 55–101.
69. Pakandl M. Coccidia of rabbit: a review. Folia Parasitol 2013;56:153–66.

70. Kraus A, Weisenbroth S, Flatt R, et al. Biology and diseases of rabbits. In: Fox J, editor. Laboratory animal medicine. Orlando, FL: Academic Press; 1984. p. 240–70.

71. Coudert P, Licois D, Drouet-Viard F. Eimeria species and strains of the rabbits. In: Eckert RB J, Shirley MW, Coudert P, editors. Guidelines on techniques in coccidiosis research European Commission, Directorate-General XII. Luxembourg: Science, Research and Development Environment Research Programme; 1995. p. 52–73.

72. Hrženjak NM, Zadravec M, Švara T, et al. Hepatic coccidiosis in two pet rabbits. J Exot Pet Med 2021;36:53–6.

73. Oglesbee BL, Lord B. Gastrointestinal Diseases of Rabbits. In: Quesenberry KE, Orcutt CJ, Mans C, et al, editors. Ferrets, rabbits, and rodents. 4th Edition. Philadelphia: Elsevier; 2020. p. 174–87.

74. Redrobe S, Gakos G, Elliot S, et al. Comparison of toltrazuril and sulphadimethoxine in the treatment of intestinal coccidiosis in pet rabbits. Vet Rec 2010; 167:287–90.

75. El-Ghoneimy A, El-Shahawy I. Evaluation of amprolium and toltrazuril efficacy in controlling natural intestinal rabbit coccidiosis. Iran J Vet Res 2017;18:164.

76. Berdiyevich DR, Khudoiyberdi KA, Ilhomovna KM. Epizootology of eimeriosis (coccidiosis) of rabbits, treatment and preventive measures. Ann For Res 2022;65:602–7.

77. Singla L, Juyal P, Sandhu B. Pathology and therapy in naturally Eimeria stiedae-infected rabbits. J Protozool Res 2000;10:185–91.

78. Paul G, Friend D. Aggressive treatment of young cottontail rabbits (Sylvilagus spp.) for coccidiosis resulted in large reduction in gastrointestinal disease mortality from all causes. J Wildl Rehabil 2021;41:7.

79. Varga Smith M. Therapeutics. *Textbook of rabbit medicine.* 3rd edition. Poland: Elsevier; 2023. p. 100–37.

80. Boullier S, Milon A. Rabbit colibacillosis. In: Maertens L, editor. Recent advances in rabbit sciences. 2006. p. 171–9.

81. Davies RR, Davies JAR. Rabbit gastrointestinal physiology. Veterinary Clinics: Exotic Animal Practice 2003;6:139–53.

82. Lelkes L, Chang C-L. Microbial dysbiosis in rabbit mucoid enteropathy. Lab Anim Sci 1987;37:757–64.

83. Harkness J, Turner P, Van de Woude S, et al. Specific diseases and conditions. Biology and medicine of rabbits and rodents. 5th edition. Ames, IA: Wiley-Blackwell; 2010. p. 249–396.

84. Heczko U, Abe A, Finlay BB. In vivo interactions of rabbit enteropathogenic Escherichia coli O103 with its host: an electron microscopic and histopathologic study. Microb Infect 2000;2:5–16.

85. Swennes AG, Buckley EM, Parry NM, et al. Enzootic enteropathogenic Escherichia coli infection in laboratory rabbits. J Clin Microbiol 2012;50:2353–8.

86. García A, Marini RP, Feng Y, et al. A naturally occurring rabbit model of enterohemorrhagic Escherichia coli-induced disease. J Infect Dis 2002;186:1682–6.

87. Ismail A, Abdien H, Hamed D, et al. Prevalence of some Enteric Bacterial Infections Causing Rabbit Enteritis and Attempts to Control Rabbit Coli Enteritis with Phytobiotics. Zagazig Veterinary Journal 2017;45:91–101.

88. Khelfa D, Abd El-Ghany WA, Salem HM. Recent status of clostridial enteritis affecting early weaned rabbits in Egypt. Life Sci J 2012;9:2272–9.

89. Percy DH, Muckle CA, Hampson RJ, et al. The enteritis complex in domestic rabbits: a field study. Can Vet J 1993;34:95.

90. Borriello SP, Carman R. Association of iota-like toxin and Clostridium spiroforme with both spontaneous and antibiotic-associated diarrhea and colitis in rabbits. J Clin Microbiol 1983;17:414–8.

91. Peeters J, Geeroms R, Carman R, et al. Significance of Clostridium spiroforme in the enteritis-complex of commercial rabbits. Vet Microbiol 1986;12:25–31.

92. Varga Smith M. Infectious diseases of domestic rabbits. Textbook of rabbit medicine. 3rd edition. Poland: Elsevier; 2023. p. 264–335.

93. Jin DX, Zou HW, Liu SQ, et al. The underlying microbial mechanism of epizootic rabbit enteropathy triggered by a low fiber diet. Sci Rep 2018;8:1–15.

94. Percy D, Bhasin J, Rosendal S. Experimental pneumonia in rabbits inoculated with strains of Pasteurella multocida. Can J Vet Res 1986;50:36.

95. Varga Smith M. Cardiorespiratory disease. In: Varga Smith M, editor. Textbook of rabbit medicine. 3rd edition. Poland: Elsevier; 2023. p. 300–13.

96. Gleeson M, Petritz OA. Emerging infectious diseases of rabbits. Veterinary Clinics: Exotic Animal Practice 2020;23:249–61.

97. Ozkan O, Karagoz A, Kocak N. First molecular evidence of ocular transmission of Encephalitozoonosis during the intrauterine period in rabbits. Parasitol Int 2019;71:1–4.

98. Selleri P, Di Girolamo N, Novari G. Performance of two portable meters and a benchtop analyzer for blood glucose concentration measurement in rabbits. J Am Vet Med Assoc 2014;245:87–98.

99. Fisher PG, Künzel F, Rylander H. Neurologic and Musculoskeletal Diseases. In: Quesenberry KE, Orcutt CJ, Mans C, et al, editors. Ferrets, rabbits, and rodents. 4th Edition. Philadelphia: W.B. Saunders; 2020. p. 233–49.

100. Varga Smith M. Neurological and Locomotor Disorders. In: Varga Smith M, editor. Textbook of rabbit medicine. 3rd edition. Poland: Elsevier; 2023. p. 282–99.

101. Suckow MA, Haab RW, Miloscio LJ, et al. Field trial of a Pasteurella multocida extract vaccine in rabbits. JAALAS 2008;47:18–21.

102. Chankuang P, Linlawan A, Junda K, et al. Comparison of rabbit, kitten and mammal milk replacer efficiencies in early weaning rabbits. Animals 2020;10: 1087.

Rodent Pediatrics

Julianne E. McCready, DVM, DVSc, DACZM[a,*],
Trinita Barboza, DVM, DVSc, DACZM[b]

KEYWORDS

- Pediatrics • Rat • Mouse • Hamster • Gerbil • Guinea pig • Chinchilla • Degu

KEY POINTS

- Rats, mice, hamsters, and gerbils are born altricial and hairless while guinea pigs, chinchillas, and degus are precocial.
- Knowledge of the social behavior of different rodent species is important for appropriate management of breeding groups as well as for appropriate housing of animals following weaning.
- Tyzzer's disease (*Clostridium piliforme*) is a common problem in juvenile rodents of multiple species and proliferative ileitis (*Lawsonia intracellularis*) is a significant cause of morbidity and mortality in young hamsters.
- Heart murmurs of varying intensity are commonly found on routine examinations in chinchilla kits. Low grade murmurs are likely physiologic.
- Prophylactic ovariectomy is recommended in young female rats and guinea pigs to prevent reproductive problems (mammary and pituitary tumors in rats, ovarian cysts in guinea pigs) later in life.

INTRODUCTION

The Latin root for rodent is *rodere*, meaning "to gnaw," referring to the continuously-growing incisors of animals in this order.[1] The most common pet rodents are in the suborders Myomorpha and Hystricomorpha. Myomorpha includes Norway or brown rats (*Rattus norvegicus*), mice (*Mus musculus*), Mongolian gerbils (*Meriones unguiculatus*), and hamsters. The hamster species commonly kept as pets include the golden or Syrian hamster (*Mesocricetus auratus*); the winter white, Russian, Siberian, or Djungarian hamster (*Phodopus sungorus*); the Campbell's hamster (*Phodopus campbelli*); the Roborovski hamster (*Phodopus roborovskii*); and the Chinese hamster (*Cricetulus griseus*).[2,3] *P. campbelli* and *P. sungorus* are capable of interbreeding.[4] Other species, including the Armenian or gray hamster (*Cricetulus migratorius*) and the European

[a] Department of Veterinary Clinical Sciences, Zoological Medicine Service, College of Veterinary Medicine, Oklahoma State University, 2065 West Farm Road, Stillwater, OK, USA;
[b] Department of Clinical Sciences, Zoological Companion Animal Service, Cummings School of Veterinary Medicine, 200 Westboro Road, North Grafton, MA, USA
* Corresponding author.
E-mail address: julianne.mccready@okstate.edu

Vet Clin Exot Anim 27 (2024) 193–219
https://doi.org/10.1016/j.cvex.2023.11.004
1094-9194/24/© 2023 Elsevier Inc. All rights reserved.

hamster (*Cricetus cricetus*), have also been used in research.[5] Pets within Hystrico-morpha include guinea pigs (*Cavia porcellus*), long-tailed chinchillas (*Chinchilla lanigera*), and degus (*Octodon degus*).[1] Prairie dogs, squirrels, and chipmunks, which are within the suborder Sciuromorpha, are occasionally kept as pets.[6–8] This review will focus on the common pet rodent species and not discuss the rodent suborders of Sciuromorpha, Anomaluromorpha (springhares), and Castorimorpha (beavers and kangaroo rats), which are not commonly kept by private individuals.[1]

MILESTONES OF JUVENILE DEVELOPMENT

A summary of developmental milestones in different rodent species is presented in **Table 1**.

Rats

Gestation in rats is 21 to 23 days.[9] Rat pups are born virtually hairless and unable to hear or see (**Fig. 1**A, B).[10] They are able to vocalize immediately after birth, but hearing does not develop until approximately 9 days of age.[9] The haircoat is complete by day 7 to 10 (**Fig. 1**C, D).[9] Coat color changes may occur in the first weeks of life in juvenile rats with certain color patterns (**Fig. 2**). The eyelids open at 14 to 17 day old (**Fig. 1**E), but complete development of the eye does not occur until day 60.[9] Incisors appear at 6 to 8 days old, while molar eruption occurs between 16 and 34 days.[9] Antibody transfer via colostrum peaks at 14 days and is complete by 21 days.[9]

In male rat pups, the testicles descend into the scrotum at day 15.[9] Prior to this, sexing pups is more difficult but still possible. There is a larger anogenital distance in males and the penis can be distinguished from the urethral papilla of females.[9] Female rodents have separate vaginal and urethral openings, which makes sexing easier in rodents compared to rabbits.[4] In addition, nipples can be observed from day 10 and are only present in female rats and mice, not males.[10] Rat pups are weaned at 20 to 21 days (**Fig. 1**F); caution should be exercised with earlier weaning, as younger rats may still require their mother to stimulate them to urinate.[9] However, prolonged delaying of separation of males and females should be avoided due to the risk of unwanted pregnancies. Males should be separated from females by 5 weeks of age (**Fig. 1**G).[11] Males begin producing sperm at approximately day 45, but puberty is delayed until day 62 to 65.[9] Puberty generally occurs earlier in females than males; however, variable ages for female puberty have been reported, ranging from 40 to 72 days.[9] Female rats may begin to show signs of estrus before puberty.[9] Play fighting begins in young rats at around 5 weeks of age and lasts until 5 to 6 months of age.[12] Social maturity occurs at 5 to 6 months of age, and it is at this point that young male rats may establish dominance hierarchies.[12]

Mice

Gestation in mice is briefer than that in rats at 19 to 21 days.[13] The eyes of mouse pups are closed at birth and open at day 12 to 13.[13] Pups are typically nursed for 21 days, similar to rats.[13] Puberty occurs at 28 to 49 days of age.[13]

Hamsters

The gestation period is 15 to 18 days in Syrian hamsters. Similar to rats and mice, Syrian hamsters are born hairless with their eyes and ears closed.[5] In contrast to rats, incisors are present at birth.[5] Their ears open at day 5 and their eyes open at day 15.[5] Hair begins to grow on day 9.[5] They wean at approximately 21 to 28 days, similar to rats and mice.[5] Sexing is similar to that of rats and mice, with males having a larger

Table 1
Developmental milestones in companion rodent species[5,9,13,16–18,24,25,33,34,38]

Species	Altricial vs. Precocial	Gestation Period (Days)	Eyes Open (Age in Days)	Weaning Age (Age in Days)	Sexual Maturity (Age in Days)
Rat (*Rattus norvegicus*)	Altricial	21–23	14–17	20–21	40–72 (females), 62–65 (males)
Mouse (*Mus musculus*)	Altricial	19–21	12–13	21	28–49
Syrian hamster (*Mesocricetus auratus*)	Altricial	15–18	15	21–28	56–84 (females), 42–56 (males)
Chinese hamster (*Cricetulus griseus*)	Altricial	20.5	10–14	21–25	56–84
Russian and Campbell's hamsters (*Phodopus* spp.)	Altricial	18	10–14	21	42–56
Gerbil (*Meriones unguiculatus*)	Altricial	24–27	16–18	21	70–90 (females), 70–84 (males)
Guinea pig (*Cavia porcellus*)	Precocial	59–72	birth	21–28	60 d (females), 90 d (males)
Chinchilla (*Chinchilla lanigera*)	Precocial	105–118	birth	42–56	120–180 (females), 240–270 (males)
Degu (*Octodon degus*)	Precocial	87–93	birth	28–42	120–180

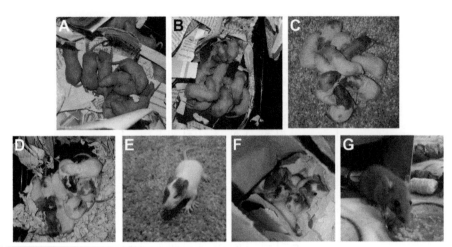

Fig. 1. Stages of development in rat (*Rattus norvegicus*) pups, with pups shown at 2 (*A*), 5 (*B*), 7 (*C*), 10 (*D*), 14 (*E*), 20 (*F*) days, and (*G*) 6 to 8 weeks of age. (*A*) Pups are born hairless and unable to see or hear. (*B*) At day 5, pups are still mostly hairless but their markings are visible. (*C*) The haircoat is visible on 7-day-old pups. (*D*) The haircoat is complete by day 10. (*E*) Pups open their eyes at day 14 to 17. (*F*) Rat pups at 20 days of age, showing complete haircoat and fully opened eyes. Pups are weaned at around this age. (*G*) Juvenile rat of approximately 6 to 8 weeks of age, the age at which they are typically adopted into new homes. Photographs A-F courtesy of Allison Dianis, DVM.

anogenital distance, a prominent scrotum, and no nipples.[5] Female hamsters begin to enter estrus at 6 to 8 weeks and can become pregnant at 8 weeks of age or earlier.[5] Pups are separated from their mother after 19 days of age.[5] Young females can be kept together until 40 to 50 day old, while male littermates can be kept together longer.[5] Males reach puberty earlier than females (6–8 weeks of age in males, 8–12 weeks in females).

Gestation in Chinese hamsters is approximately 20.5 days. Chinese hamster neonates are also born with incisors present.[5] Hair begins to become visible at day 3 to 4, and the haircoat is complete by day 7. The eyes and ears open at around day 10 to

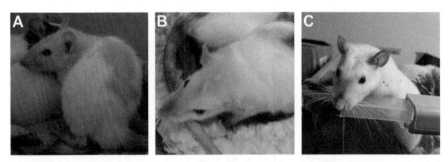

Fig. 2. Photographs showing the normal development of coat pattern in an approximately 6-8-week-old Siamese rat (A and B; photos taken a few days apart) and the final coat pattern in an adult Siamese rat (*C*). These rats initially have tan coloration, which is gradually replaced by a light color over the body with dark points. The coloration development is temperature-dependent with dark points developing at cooler area of the body.

14. Weaning occurs at day 21 to 25. In males, the testicles descend at day 30.[5] Chinese hamsters are sexually mature at 8 to 12 weeks. Aggression between females tends to develop around this time, and therefore, individuals may need to be separated.

The gestation period for Campbell's hamsters and winter white hamsters is approximately 18 days. The pups are born with closed eyes; the eyelids separate at day 10 to 14.[14] Pups are weaned at 3 weeks of age.[5] Sexual maturity occurs at 6 to 8 weeks.[15] In contrast to Syrian and Chinese hamsters, *Phodopus* hamsters are social and can be kept in pairs.[5]

Gerbils

Gestation in Mongolian gerbils is 24 to 27 days.[2,16,17] Similar to other Myomorpha rodents, the young are born hairless with the eyes and ears closed.[17] The eyes open at day 16 to 18.[17] Nursing occurs for approximately 3 to 4 weeks.[16,17] Sexual maturity occurs at 70 to 84 days in males and 70 to 90 days in females.[16]

Guinea Pigs

The gestation period in guinea pigs is 59 to 72 days with an average of 68 days.[18] Guinea pigs have a hemomonochorial labyrinthine placenta which allows for maternal antibody transfer.[19,20] They are born precocial (fully furred, with all teeth erupted, eyes open, and able to walk within an hour).[20] The birth weight of a guinea pig pup varies between 60 to 100 g depending on the litter size.[21,22] Guinea pig pups will nurse for 3 to 4 weeks but will start eating solid food within days (**Fig. 3**).[20,21] Once weaned, the pups grow 25 to 50 g/week until 2 months of age.[23]

Guinea pigs are sexed based on the appearance of their anogenital region, with females having a "Y" shape and males having a dotted "i" shape (with the dot being the penile urethra) (**Fig. 4**).[20] Sexual maturity occurs at 60 days in females and 90 days in males.[24]

Chinchillas

The gestation period for a chinchilla is 105 to 118 days.[25] Like guinea pigs, chinchillas have a hemomonochorial labyrinthine type placenta allowing for passive immunity and are born precocial (**Fig. 5A**).[25,26] The birth weight is between 30 to 50 g and their

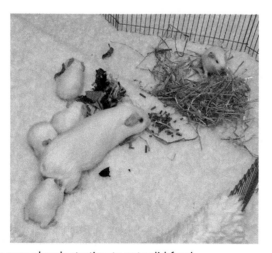

Fig. 3. Guinea pig pups already starting to eat solid food.

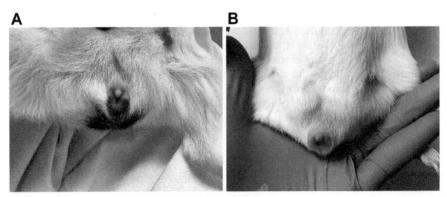

Fig. 4. Sexing juvenile guinea pigs based on the appearance of the anogenital region. (*A*) An approximately 3-month-old strain 2 guinea pig. The female has a "Y" shape. (*B*) An approximately 3-month-old Dunkin-Hartley guinea pig. The male has a dotted "i" shape (with the dot being the penile urethra). Photographs courtesy of Andrea Varela-Stokes, DVM, PhD.

growth rate is 3.6 g per day in the first month, 1.56 g per day from the second to sixth month, and 0.65 g per day from the sixth to twelfth month.[25,27] Kits may not nurse immediately, but will nurse for 6 to 8 weeks, and begin to eat solid foods at 1 week (**Fig. 5**B).[25,28] Once weaned, the kits are independent from their mother.[29] Hairs of a chinchilla kit are single and transition to adult hair (multiple hairs out of a single follicle) before 2 months of age (**Fig. 5**C).[30]

Sexing chinchillas is based on the anogenital distance, which is smaller in females. Although this distance is smaller in neonates, the relative differences are still visible.[29] Female chinchillas have a large urinary papilla that should not be confused with a penis. Testicles descend within 2 weeks of age.[31] Like other hystrichomorph rodents, chinchillas are not considered to have a true scrotum and the testicles are located in a parascrotal sac.[25,32] Sexual maturity occurs at 240 to 270 days in males and 120 to 180 days in females.[25]

Degus

Gestation in degus is 87 to 93 days.[33] Degus have a hemochorial chorioallantoic placenta allowing for passive immunity.[34,35] Like guinea pigs and chinchillas, degus

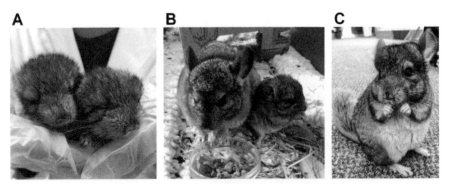

Fig. 5. Juvenile chinchillas at various ages. (*A*) Neonatal chinchillas. (*B*) Chinchillas will start to eat solid food at 1 week of age. (*C*) A 2-month-old chinchilla demonstrating an adult hair-coat (multiple hairs out of a single follicle).

are born precocial.[36] The birth weight varies between 13.5 to 14.6 g and the pup gains 1 to 1.5 g per day in the first 2 weeks of life.[35] Pups remain in their nesting site until 2 weeks of age, at which time they begin to eat solid foods and move around the cage.[37] Degu pups may begin to eat solid foods as early as 6 days and are weaned between 4 to 6 weeks of age.[35]

Sexual maturity can vary between 4 to 6 months, with 3 months being average when provided optimal diets.[34,38] Sexing of degus is similar to chinchillas; male degus are also 10% larger than females and have penile spines when sexually mature.[36,37]

HUSBANDRY
Hand-Rearing

Hand-rearing of orphaned rats and mice is difficult due to the fact that young are born altricial.[4] Paintbrushes or intravenous catheters can be used for syringe-feeding neonatal rats and mice.[11] The milk composition of rodents differs from cows' milk and tends to be more energy-dense.[11] Both altricial and precocial orphan neonates require provision of additional heat and should be weighed daily to ensure appropriate weight gain.[11,29,39]

Guinea pigs are passive nursers; sows will allow access to teats but will not encourage nursing.[24] However, they are gentle mothers and generally accept foster pups.[20] If a pup is weak, losing weight, or orphaned, fostering or hand-feeding is recommended.[20] Pups that have not received the sow's milk in the first 3 to 4 days of life have poorer survival.[24] Guinea pigs nurse multiple times a day and so hand-raised guinea pigs require 1 to 2 mL of milk replacer every 2 hours until 5 days of age and then feedings every 4 hours until weaning.[23,24] Guinea pig milk is high in carbohydrates and has higher protein than fat levels.[40] This milk composition is closest to that of cat milk.[20] In addition to milk, guinea pig pups will require vitamin C supplementation (30 mg/kg/day), access to young guinea pig pellets, and access to adult fecal pellets for coprophagy for intestinal inoculation.[20,24] Hand-raised pups will require anogenital stimulation in the first week of life to urinate and defecate.[20,24]

Orphaned chinchillas can be fostered onto a female with a small litter of kits of similar age or to a female with recently weaned kits.[41,42] Successful cross-species transfer to lactating guinea pigs has also been reported.[42] Should a lactating female not be available, hand-rearing can be successful. Neonates should be hand-fed every 4 hours at minimum during the day and once to twice overnight until 4 days of age.[29] Like guinea pigs, anogenital stimulation is required until the kits are urinating and defecting on their own.[43] Diarrhea and bloat can occur with large quantities of milk.[44] As chinchillas get older, nightly feeding can be discontinued, and daytime feeding intervals increased.[45] Although equal parts of evaporated milk to water have successfully been used to hand-rear chinchillas,[25] canine milk replacer with added lactase has a profile more like chinchilla milk and reduces the risk for gastrointestinal upset.[29,46] The reported minimal suckling period for survival of a chinchilla kit is 25 days,[30] but they can be weaned at 2 to 3 weeks when hand-rearing.[47]

Orphan degu pups can be fostered to nursing mothers as they are known to nurse co-nesting young.[48] However, monitoring is required as they do use olfactory cues to discriminate their pups from co-nesting and unfamiliar pups.[49] If nursing degu mothers are not available, hand-rearing can be pursued. Neonate degus are unable to regulate their temperature until 3 weeks of age and require heat support.[34] Like other precocial rodent species, they can be raised without colostrum.[35] Degu milk is more concentrated than chinchilla and guinea pig milk, with milk fat being the main energy source.[35,50]

Canine milk replacer with added vegetable oil and *Lactobacillus* can be used to feed orphans for 10 to 14 days.[35]

Feeding

Young rodents in general should start to eat solid food by 2 weeks of age.[4,16,17] Some species may start to eat solid food slightly earlier, such as mice at approximately 9 days of age, chinchillas at 7 days of age, and guinea pigs within a few days of birth.[11,25]

As stated earlier, rats and mice begin to wean at around 3 weeks of age. They can be offered free access to solid food at this age and can transition to milk being offered via a bowl at this point.[11] Weaning in mice and rats is complete around 28 days of age. Weaned rats require a higher protein diet compared to adult rats; in adults a lower protein is recommended due to the high prevalence of chronic progressive nephrosis in aged rats.[10]

Young guinea pig pups should have free access to juvenile guinea pig pellets (alfalfa-based) and alfalfa hay until 6 months of age, when they are transitioned to an adult diet consisting primarily of grass hay and limited adult guinea pig pellets.[21,23,51] Dietary vitamin C is required post-weaning (30 mg/kg/day) and throughout adulthood (10–25 mg/kg/day).[24] Although some pelleted diets are formulated with vitamin C (L-ascorbyl-2-polyphosphate) that has proven to be stable for more than 6 months, large quantities of pellets would have to be consumed to meet the daily requirements.[20,24,52] Therefore, additional supplementation through vitamin C tablets or vitamin C-rich produce such a bell peppers is recommended.

During weaning and juvenile stages, chinchillas can be free fed pelleted diets (alfalfa-based) formulated for their species, as well as equal parts alfalfa hay and grass hay.[29] As they mature, pellets should be offered in limited quantities with free choice grass hay.[29]

Once weaned, juvenile degus can be offered a rodent breeder pelleted diet (such as Prolab RMH 2000, LabDiet, Purina Mills Inc., Richmond, IN 47374, USA) and alfalfa hay until 10 weeks of age, at which time they are transitioned to a low-energy high-fiber diet consisting primarily of grass hay.[38] High carbohydrate food items such as root vegetables and fruits should not be offered as degus easily enter a hyperinsulinemic state, leading to diabetes mellitus, cataracts, and renal damage.[53]

Chinchilla and guinea pig pelleted diets resulted in high mortality when fed to young degus, while a rodent breeder diet (eg, Prolab RMH 2000) resulted in healthy pups with high survival and growth rates.[38] From 10 weeks of age into adulthood, degus should be provided a rodent diet (such as Laboratory Rodent Diet 5001, LabDiet, Purina Mills Inc.) in addition to hay, as this diet allowed for good body maintenance, while feeding chinchilla pellets resulted in weight gain.[38] These recommendations are based on evaluation of a laboratory colony. Evaluation of commercially marketed pelleted degu diets could not be found.

Housing and Social Behavior

Cages for housing neonate or juvenile animals may have different requirements from those used for housing adults. For example, bar spacing may need to be narrower in cages for young rodents to avoid escape or injury. Large adult male rats can be kept in cages with 1-inch (2.54-cm) bar spacing, such as ferret cages. However, young and small rats require 0.5-inch (1.27-cm) bar spacing. The use of appropriate bedding material is also critical; any type of fabric that can fray or has loops such as terry cloth or towels should be avoided due to the risk of limb entrapment.[39]

Rats are very social animals and should be kept in groups of 2 or more following weaning.[54] Female mice can generally be kept in groups, but male mice tend to be aggressive toward each other and usually must be housed singly.[55]

The sociability of hamsters varies with species.[3] Syrian hamsters are solitary and should be housed individually to avoid aggression.[2,3] Pregnant females should be kept separately from other hamsters and be disturbed as little as possible for at least 1 to 2 weeks before and after parturition to prevent them from cannibalizing or neglecting the pups.[5] Winter white hamster are more social and can be housed in pairs or groups if introduced when young.[3] Roborovski hamsters are social and can be housed in groups.[3] Chinese hamsters can be aggressive and should be housed alone.[2,3]

Gerbils are social and in the wild live as family groups including a breeding pair and offspring from previous litters who help care for the younger pups.[17] Males also assist in caring for the young, which is unusual among rodents.[17] Due to their social nature, gerbils housed singly may develop aggression and anxiety.[17] Cannibalism of the young is less common in gerbils compared to hamsters, but the dam should similarly be undisturbed before and after parturition.[17]

Guinea pigs do not use nest boxes; instead, pups stay close to the sow for warmth and protection.[20] Deep, plastic-bottomed, wire-topped cages with recycled paper bedding and loose hay are recommended for housing.[20,24] Narrow bar spacing is important as pups can squeeze between wire bars.[20] Guinea pigs prefer to drink from bottles, so these should be provided as behavioral enrichment.[56] Guinea pigs are social and should be housed in pairs or groups,[24] although some young males may fight when reaching sexual maturity.[20]

Neonatal chinchilla kits reside in a nest box and their mothers sit on top of them to keep them warm.[41,57] To reduce stress on the dam, minimal handling of the kits in the first 7 to 10 days is recommended.[29] Sires are friendly and protective of the kits.[25] The kits are social with each other, but maturing males may fight.[29] Chinchillas are social animals and should be housed as same-sex pairs or in small groups.[57] Solid-bottom cages with narrow cage bar spacing are required to avoid tibial fractures.[25] Chinchillas have low water intake and prefer to drink from dishes, but care should be taken to prevent neonatal drowning.[58,59] While chinchillas normally require dust baths for proper coat maintenance, the dust could potentially promote mastitis; therefore, dust baths should be avoided during late pregnancy and lactation.[57,60]

Degus are social and live in groups. Males occasionally look after young and females do not display maternal aggression.[36,37] Young degus readily interact with each other independent of relatedness.[61] Social housing during the juvenile period is important to prevent irreversible behavioral deficits, including fear of conspecifics and difficulty handling.[37,38] In captivity, pups can be divided into groups of 2 or 3 individuals until at least 6 months of age, after which isolation is not noted to cause behavioral deficits.[37] However, due to their social nature, they should be housed in pairs at minimum. Solid bottom cages, with nonadherent bedding such as paper or corn cob for burrowing, are recommended. A running wheel is preferred by degus over polyvinyl chloride tubes and next boxes.[38] Degus have variable preferences to drinking water from a bottle or bowl.[58]

COMMON DISEASES OF JUVENILES
Gastrointestinal

Rats
Enterococcal enteropathy (also known as streptococcal enteropathy) can cause diarrhea and death in nursing rat pups.[9,62] Tyzzer's disease, caused by *C piliforme*, is most likely to be seen in recently weaned pups.[9] Clinical signs of *C piliforme* include anorexia, emaciation, diarrhea with mucus and blood, abdominal distension, and sudden death.[9] Hepatitis and myocardial lesions may be noted on necropsy.[62] *Campylobacter*

can cause mild diarrhea in young rats.[63] Rat rotavirus, the cause of infectious diarrhea of infant rats, may cause diarrhea and perianal irritation in rats less than 2 weeks of age, but little mortality.[9,62,63] This virus is rare and unlikely to be seen in pet rats. Pinworms in rats may be due to *Syphacia* spp. or *Aspicularis* spp.; infections are often subclinical but can lead to poor growth in young rats.[63] A study in rats and mice showed that topical selamectin was ineffective for pinworms (*Syphacia* spp.) infections, while fenbendazole-treated feed was effective.[64] Coccidiosis due to *Eimeria* spp. may also be asymptomatic in rats. Treatment with ponazuril was effective in a pair of one-month-old pet rats, 1 of which had diarrhea prior to treatment.[65]

Familial megacolon has been reported in juvenile rats, and presented as abdominal distension soon after weaning.[66] Other clinical signs include diarrhea, perineal staining, and death before 2 months of age.[66]

Mice

Salmonellosis may cause anorexia, weight loss, and lethargy, with or without signs of gastroenteritis. Clinical signs are more severe in young (suckling and weanling) mice compared to adults.[13] The disease can be contracted via contamination of food and water, wild rodents, and other animal species that can serve as carriers.[13] Salmonellosis is zoonotic. Clostridial disease can also be a cause of enteric disease in young mice. *Clostridium perfringens* type D can cause diarrhea or fecal impaction, paraplegia, and death in 2 to 3 week old mice.[13] *C. perfringens* can also cause necrotizing enteritis in weaned mice.[13] *Citrobacter rodentium* is the cause of transmissible murine colonic hyperplasia, and can cause diarrhea, rectal prolapse, and death in nursing or recently weaned mouse pups.[13]

A rotavirus can cause epizootic diarrhea of infant mice.[13] Clinical signs occur in mice less than 2 weeks of age and include diarrhea, fecal soiling of the coat, and weight loss.[13] Other viruses that can cause diarrhea in nursing mouse pups include intestinal coronavirus (mouse hepatitis) and reovirus 3.[13] Mice with rotavirus typically continue to nurse and recover from infection, while intestinal coronavirus often leads to death.[13]

Hamsters

Gastrointestinal disease is a common problem in pet hamsters.[2] The most concerning diarrheal syndrome in hamsters is proliferative ileitis caused by *Lawsonia intracellaris*.[2,5] This condition is known as "wet tail," but it should be noted that some laypeople and practitioners use the term "wet tail" more broadly to refer to any cause of diarrhea or even urogenital discharge or perineal soiling.[67] Hamsters from weaning age (3 weeks) to 10 weeks of age are most commonly affected.[2,5] Treatment involves hydration, nutrition, antacids, and antibiotics (such as tetracycline, enrofloxacin, or trimethoprim-sulfa,[2] or chloramphenicol, as is used to treat *L intracellularis* in ferrets[68]). The prognosis is guarded as the condition commonly leads to death in affected hamsters.[2,67]

Gerbils

Like other rodents, gerbils can develop Tyzzer's disease due to *C piliforme*. It is most common in weanlings but can also occur in adults.[63] Clinical signs may include lethargy, diarrhea, and death, with weight loss seen in more chronic infections.[63] Treatment involves antibiotic therapy (tetracycline or chloramphenicol) and supportive care.[63] Salmonellosis is more common in young (3- to 10-week-old) gerbils compared to adults.[63] Symptoms may include depression, poor hair coat, weight loss, diarrhea, and abdominal distension.[63] *Syphacia* pinworms have been reported in both adult and juvenile gerbils without clinical signs.[16]

Guinea pigs

Guinea pigs can also develop Tyzzer's disease from *C piliforme,* which tends to affect young and stressed animals in poor husbandry situations.[23,24] Transmission is via fecal-oral contamination of bedding and food.[23,24] Clinical signs vary from diarrhea to sudden death.[23,24] Guinea pig pups can be also be affected by *Escherichia coli* and salmonellosis.[23] Pups can be infected with *E. coli* via the umbilical cord and from nursing a sow with mastitis.[21,23]

Intestinal parasites, including *Eimeria caviae* and *Cryptosporidium wrairi,* occasionally cause weight loss and diarrhea in young guinea pigs.[23,24] These juvenile animals can clear their *C wrairi* infection spontaneously.[69]

Atresia ani, with and without a rectocutaneous fistula, has been reported in guinea pigs, and a surgical correction technique has been described for correction of the fistula.[70] Affected animals may present with tenesmus.

Chinchillas

Chinchillas less than 4 months of age have increased susceptibility to enteritis and dysbiosis[71] with *Clostridium perfringens, Salmonella enterica* serovar Enteritidis, and *S enterica* subspecies *arizonae* being commonly isolated.[72–74] In a retrospective evaluation of mortality in ranched chinchillas, enteritis was the leading cause of mortality in kits (154/375; 41%), with female kits having a higher incidence.[59] Hemolytic *E coli* was the most common cause of enteritis in that study.[59]

Giardia has a high prevalence in asymptomatic young farmed (100/170; 58.8%) and pet chinchillas (41/104; 39.4%) in Europe.[75,76] Similar studies have not been performed in North America. Treatment can be considered with fenbendazole, metronidazole, or tinidazole, but it should be noted that metronidazole and high-dose tinidazole have been associated with anorexia in chinchillas.[77–79]

A congenital diaphragmatic hernia and a cleft soft palate with absent nasal turbinates have been reported.[80,81] Congenital cleft palates have also been described in a neonate degu and guinea pig.[82]

Degus

Degu pups less than 3 months of age are prone to opportunistic *Pseudomonas* infections due to poor sanitation of water bottles.[34] Regular disinfection of bottles and acidification of the water (2.5 mL of 3.7% HCl per gallon of water) is recommended to prevent secondary diarrhea.[34,38]

Urogenital

Rats

Bladder threadworms due to *Trichomoides crassicauda* can be seen in rats 8 to 12 weeks of age.[83] The parasites can be asymptomatic or lead to urolithiasis and pyelitis.[83]

Respiratory

Rats

Rats in general are exquisitely prone to respiratory infections.[84] Rats housed in an inappropriate environment may present with respiratory signs at a younger age compared to those housed in an appropriate environment with adequate ventilation and regular cleaning.[85] Murine respiratory mycoplasmosis (caused by *Mycoplasma pulmonis*) is one of the most common respiratory infections in rats, but as it tends to develop chronically over long periods, early infections may not be appreciated. It can be transmitted horizontally or vertically to offspring via *in utero* transmission.[9] Young rats are typically asymptomatic and may be negative on serologic tests for several months after exposure.[9,10] In contrast to mycoplasmosis, which tends to increase in severity with age, *S pneumoniae* pneumonia is more severe in juvenile rats.[10] Young rats may die acutely; other possible clinical signs include dyspnea and purulent nasal discharge.[10] Bacteremia can develop.[9,10] Asymptomatic infection is also possible.[9] Treatment of streptococcal pneumonia involves beta-lactamase-resistant penicillins.[10] Thoracic neoplasia can present similarly to respiratory infections in rats, and has been reported even in relatively young rats.[84]

Mice
Sendai virus or murine respirovirus, a virus in the family Paramyxoviridae, is a cause of respiratory disease in rats and mice.[86] Adults may experience weight loss, dyspnea, and potentially death; mortality is more often seen in nursing pups.[10,13,86] Nursing pups may be protected by maternal antibodies until they are weaned.[13] Mycoplasmosis can occur in both young and adult mice, and rats serve as a reservoir for this infection in mice.[13]

Guinea pigs
Guinea pig pups are at risk for pneumonia in poor husbandry and diet conditions including stress, vitamin C deficiency, high ammonia, high humidity, and temperature extremes.[20,82] Common bacterial etiologies include *Bordetella bronchiseptica*, *M pulmonis*, and *S pneumoniae*.[24,82,87] Animals may clear their *Bordetella* and *Mycoplasma* infections, but some remain asymptomatic carriers.[82]

Chinchillas
Pneumonia is not common in pet chinchilla kits.[29] However, it was the second leading cause of mortality in chinchilla kits on fur ranches (98/375; 26%), with *Pasteurella multocida*, *Bordetella bronchiseptica*, *Staphylococcus aureus*, *Pseudomonas aeruginosa*, *Streptococcus* spp., *Klebsiella pneumoniae*, and *Listeria monocytogenes* most commonly isolated.[59] *K pneumoniae* was also isolated from an outbreak of respiratory disease and diarrhea in a fur farm.[88]

Cardiovascular

Gerbils
Congenital ventricular septal heart disease has been reported in neonatal gerbils.[16]

Chinchillas and degus
Heart murmurs of varying intensity are commonly found on routine examinations in chinchilla kits.[43,89] Chinchillas have a higher prevalence of physiologic heart murmurs when compared to other species.[90] However, echocardiography should be recommended if a grade 3 or higher murmur persists into adulthood.[90]

Congenital ventricular septal defects have been described in chinchillas and degus and resulted in death.[89,91]

Dermatologic

Rats
Ringtail, the formation of an annular constriction on the tail, has been described in young, unweaned rats and occasionally mice.[10] This condition may be related to humidity levels, temperature, genetics, and nutrition and is unlikely to be encountered in pet rats.[10,62] Dermatophytosis is occasionally seen in young rats (**Fig. 6**), although less frequently than in other pet rodent species such as guinea pigs and chinchillas (see later).

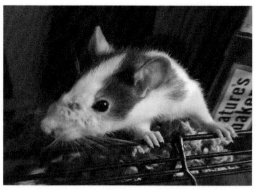

Fig. 6. Dermatophytosis in a 7-week-old male rat with facial alopecia, scaling, and erythema.

Mice

Corynebacteriosis due to *Corynebacterium kutscheri* can be asymptomatic or associated with anorexia, rough coat, oculonasal discharge, cutaneous ulceration, and arthritis. *Corynebacterium bovis* can also be associated with dermatitis.[13] Skin disease associated with corynebacteriosis can be fatal in nursing pups but tends to resolve in weanling mice.[13] Young mice can experience constriction of tail known as ringtail, similar to rats, as well as necrosis of the extremities due to constriction from bedding material.[13] Therefore, it is important that appropriate bedding material is used.

Hamsters

Lymphoma is a common neoplasm in hamsters. In older hamsters, non-viral-associated multicentric lymphoma may occur.[92] However, young hamsters can develop lymphoma secondary to hamster polyomavirus. If the infection is established in a colony, young hamsters are protected and older hamsters are occasionally affected. If the virus is introduced into a group that has not been previously exposed, it can have very high morbidity in young hamsters.[92] Lesions can affect the skin and lymph nodes, as well as abdominal organs.[92]

Gerbils

A dermatologic syndrome of unknown etiology has been reported in neonatal gerbils. The gerbils are born with patchy alopecia, lack of hair pigmentation, and poor growth.[93] *Staphylococcus aureus* dermatitis is typically seen in young gerbils and may have a high morbidity and mortality.[93]

Guinea pigs

The most common dermatologic condition seen in juvenile guinea pigs is dermatophytosis.[20,23] Both *Microsporum canis* and *Trichophyton mentagrophytes* have been isolated, with *T. mentagrophytes* being more common.[20,94] Lesions include circular areas of alopecia and scaling on the face, dorsum, and feet. Lesions can be pruritic.[95] Terbinafine is a more effective treatment than itraconazole and fluconazole in guinea pigs.[96] Heavy infestations of ectoparasites can cause weakness and secondary infections in guinea pig pups.[20] The most common ectoparasites include the fur mite *Chirodiscoides caviae,* the sarcoptic mite *Trixacarus caviae,* which causes severe pruritus, and fur lice (*Gliricola porcelli, Gyropus ovalis*), which can cause pruritus, alopecia, crusting, and unkempt fur.[21,23,97] Selamectin is effective in the treatment of *T. caviae* and imidacloprid 10%/moxidectin 1% is effective in treatment of *G. porcelli*.[98,99]

Chinchillas

Dermatophytosis is also seen in young chinchillas.[29] Although *T mentagrophytes* is more commonly reported, *Microsporum* has also been isolated.[100,101] The infection can range from subclinical to areas of patchy hair loss, erythema, and scaling, primarily around the base of the ears, around the nose, and on the forefeet.[25] Treatment is described elsewhere.[25]

Cases of *Streptococcus equi* subspecies *zooepidemicus* in young chinchillas have been described in literature.[102,103] These cases describe rapidly growing ventral cervical masses.[102,103] *S equi* subspecies *zooepidemicus* is considered an emerging pathogen of chinchillas.[104]

Degus

Degu and gerbil tails have thin overlying skin that is prone to degloving.[2,34] Degus also self-barber with stress, which can occur with social isolation as a juvenile.[105]

Musculoskeletal

Rats and hamsters

Avascular necrosis of the femoral head has been reported in young rats.[10] In all species, fractures can occur due to trauma. Depending on the severity of the fracture, fixation[106] or stabilization via external coaptation can be considered, but the patient should be monitored closely for chewing at the bandage.[107] Patient size can present difficulties when attempting fracture fixation, but surgical correction is possible even in rodent patients weighing less than 100 g.[106] In the case of severe fractures, amputation can be considered and is generally tolerated well by certain species, such as rats.[107]

Chinchillas and degus

Neonatal trauma has been reported in chinchilla kits from accidents and material aggression.[29] A retrospective review of chinchilla mortality in fur ranches found female kits were more likely to be attacked by adults (31/375; 8%).[59] Traumatic injuries in degu pups are also reported.[105,108]

Neurologic

Rats and mice

Pituitary tumors in rats may present with neurologic signs, including behavior changes, head tilt, ataxia, and proprioceptive deficits.[109,110] Although these tumors are much more common in older rats, with an average age of 23 months in affected rats, they have been reported in rats as young as 9 months of age.[111] A more likely cause of neurologic signs in a young rat or mouse would be bacterial otitis media.[10,112]

Gerbils

Seizures are very common in gerbils, occurring in 20% to 40% of animals and developing at around 8 to 12 weeks of age.[2,17] The seizures worsen up to 6 months of age but ultimately may resolve over time.[2,17] It is thought that the seizures are related to stress and may be prevented by handling young gerbils during the first 3 months of life, starting at 1 week of age.[17,107]

Chinchillas

Hydrocephalia has been reported in 3 newborn kits.[59]

Ophthalmic

Rats

Sialodacryoadenitis is caused by a coronavirus in rats. The classic clinical sign of cervical salivary gland swelling typically occurs in weaned or adult rats, while unweaned rats may experience conjunctivitis.[9,10]

Guinea pigs

Congenital conjunctivitis is reported in guinea pig pups, with C caviae being the primary pathologic agent.[113,114] The infection is passed from sow to pup during parturition.[114] Although the infection is self-limiting, treatment with ophthalmic tetracycline is recommended due to its zoonotic potential.[24] Corneal disease has been reported in Texel and Teddy guinea pig pups from their curly hair or eyelashes contacting the cornea.[20] This issue usually resolves as the pup grows.[20]

Degus

Congenital cataracts have been described in degus.[115]

PREVENTATIVE CARE
Vaccinations and Wellness Care

Typical pet rodent species do not require vaccinations,[4,10] but routine wellness care is recommended due to the shorter lifespans of some of these species and their propensity to hide signs of illness.[67] Pet rats, for example, are often presented once problems develop rather than for preventative care,[85] so there is a critical need to encourage clients to bring pet rodents in for wellness examinations soon after adoption.

Antiparasitics

Antiparasitics, such as selamectin, can be considered for ectoparasite infestations. As noted previously, topical selamectin was ineffective for treatment of pinworms in rats and mice.[64] Therefore, fecal flotation and treatment for endoparasites as needed is recommended.

Spay

Prophylactic spaying is not as commonly performed for pet rodents[85] as it is for dogs and cats. One study found that only 6.6% of female rats were spayed, and almost half of those spays were performed in rats with a previous history of mammary tumors, rather than prophylactically.[85] In a retrospective study of guinea pigs presented with urolithiasis, only 2 out of 84 female guinea pigs were spayed.[116] Another study reported that 4% of female guinea pigs were spayed.[117] Only 0.56% of female pet hamsters were reported to be spayed.[67] Despite low rates of prophylactic spaying in pet rodents, it is being increasingly recommended for some pet rodent species due to reported health benefits.

Rats

Ovariectomy is recommended in young female rats to reduce the risk of mammary and pituitary tumors. In rats ovariectomized at 90 days of age, the risk of subcutaneous tumors was approximately 6%, compared to 53% in intact females.[118] In addition, 66% of intact rats developed pituitary tumors, while only 4% of ovariectomized rats did.[118] Survival to 630 days was significantly greater for ovariectomized females compared to intact females.[118] Another study in which female rats were spayed at an older age (5–7 months) revealed similar findings, with the incidence of tumors declining from 73.8% to 5.3% in ovariectomized rats.[119] Flank ovariectomy is the method preferred by many veterinarians for altering female rats due to possible benefits, such smaller incisions, decreased risk of evisceration, and less pain. A study found decreased complication rates with flank ovariectomy compared to ventral midline ovariohysterectomy, although the result was not statistically significant.[120] As elective spaying has a low perioperative mortality rate in rats,[120,121] it should strongly be considered to prevent mammary tumors, pituitary tumors, and reproductive tract pathology. Flank ovariectomy should be recommended for female rats between 3 and 7 months of age. For older female rats, imaging of the reproductive tract could be considered prior to sterilization to determine whether an ovariohysterectomy or ovariectomy is indicated. Premedication protocols for spay and neuter of pet rats have been described.[122]

Mice
In contrast to rats, ovariectomy in mice does not appear to be protective against mammary neoplasia.[123] However, others report that ovariectomy may reduce the rates or delay in the onset of mammary tumors in certain strains of mice.[124] Therefore, it is unknown whether prophylactic spaying should be routinely recommended for mice.

Hamsters
Whether prophylactic spaying should be recommended in female hamsters is not straightforward. Reproductive problems can develop in females, and, in theory, spaying could prevent some of these issues. For instance, non-reproductive winter white hamsters can develop cystic ovaries.[5] Other reported reproductive disorders in hamsters include pyometra, endometrial hyperplasia, endometritis, uterine neoplasia, and granulosa cell tumors.[2] Male hamsters tend to have longer lifespans than female hamsters.[67] This may be due to the fact that atrial thrombosis, a common condition in hamsters, occurs at an earlier age in females compared to males.[125] Spayed females had even shorter lifespans, and it is thought that there may be a hormonal influence in the development of this disorder.[125]

Gerbils
Ovarian granulosa cell tumors are one of the most common neoplasms in gerbils.[126] They are often bilateral and have the potential to metastasize.[126] Gerbils can also develop ovarian cysts.[2,16] Therefore, prophylactic ovariectomy could be considered in female gerbils to prevent this condition.[2]

Guinea pigs
Prophylactic ovariectomy should be strongly considered in young female guinea pigs to reduce the risk of ovarian cysts (**Fig. 7**).[127] Ovarian cysts are very common in guinea pigs,[128–131] and the prevalence increases with age.[127,132] Laparoscopic ovariectomy in guinea pigs has been described,[133] but further studies are needed to determine if this approach is associated with a reduction in post-operative pain compared to a traditional flank ovariectomy. No benefit associated with laparoscopic over open ovariectomy was found in rabbits.[134] The decision whether to perform an ovariectomy or ovariohysterectomy in a guinea pig is based on the presence or absence of uterine disease. In a juvenile guinea pig with no known uterine disease, ovariectomy alone is likely reasonable. Guinea pig anatomy makes ovariohysterectomy more challenging compared to that of other species, as they have a very large cecum, a short mesovarium, deeply-positioned ovaries, and a friable ovarian ligament due to excessive adipose tissue.[123,135] Anecdotally, guinea pigs appear more prone to complications and death following ventral midline ovariohysterectomy compared to other species.[123,136–138] Alternatively, a flank ovariohysterectomy technique has been described and can be considered for both prophylactic spaying and for treatment for ovarian cysts.[139]

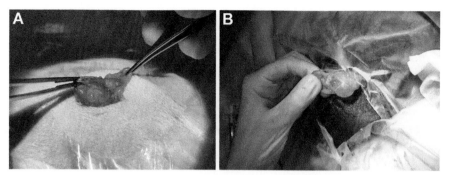

Fig. 7. Flank ovariectomy in guinea pigs. (*A*) Prophylactic flank ovariectomy in a young female guinea pig without ovarian cysts. (*B*) Therapeutic flank ovariectomy in a female guinea pig with a large ovarian cyst.

Chinchillas and degus

Though not commonly pursued, prophylactic ovariohysterectomy can be considered to prevent endometritis and pyometra in chinchillas and degus, as well as for population control.[25,105] Flank ovariectomies can be performed in a similar manner to other rodents.[31,140] Like guinea pigs, chinchillas store fat in their mesovarium, mesometrium, and broad ligaments.[31] Anecdotally, chinchillas seem to tolerate ovariohysterectomies better than guinea pigs do.

Neuter

Rats

Five percent of male pet rats were reported to be neutered.[85] Castration of male rats is less commonly recommended for health benefits compared to spaying female rats. One possible health benefit is preventing the development of urethral plugs.[123] Compared to male mice, which generally cannot be housed in groups due to aggression, intact male rats can often be housed together peacefully.[9] However, castration of male rats can be considered to reduce the risk of aggression between males, to help facilitate introduction between different groups of rats, or to allow males to be housed with intact females. Neutering dominant rats was shown to result in a significant decrease in aggression toward introduced, non-aggressive rats.[141] The decrease in aggression may be seen as early as 5 days after surgery, but it may take up to 5 to 6 weeks for aggression to fully decline in some rats.[141] Neutering to prevent aggression is generally more effective when performed at a younger age.[142] Male rats and other rodents should be separated from intact females for 8 weeks to reduce the risk of inadvertent pregnancy.[125]

Mice

Castration of male mice can be considered to allow them to cohabitate with intact females without the risk of breeding. Castration can also be considered to reduce aggression between group-housed male mice. Castration significantly eliminated bites and injuries and significantly reduced, but did not eliminate, aggressive behaviors in group-housed male mice.[143]

Hamsters

As Syrian hamsters are solitary animals, and other species of hamsters may be kept in single-sex groups, castration of males is typically not required for prevent reproduction.[67] A study showed a decreased lifespan in male hamsters following castration,

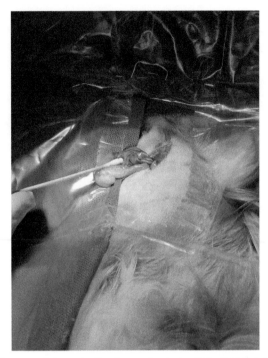

Fig. 8. Abdominal approach to castration in a guinea pig. Note that the guinea pig's head is at the bottom of the image.

which may be related to less protection against atrial thrombosis in castrated animals.[125] Reproductive disorders are uncommon in males so castration carries questionable health benefits.[2] Only 0.63% of male pet hamsters were reported to be neutered.[67]

Gerbils
Castration in gerbils can be considered to prevent pregnancy if housed with an intact female. Scent marking decreases in castrated males.[17] Testicular neoplasia has been reported in gerbils.[123]

Guinea pigs
Neutering of male guinea pigs can be considered to prevent breeding if housed in a mixed-sex group including intact females. Testicular tumors are rare in guinea pigs but have been described.[144] An abdominal approach to castration (**Fig. 8**) is preferred over a scrotal approach due to significantly lower infection rates compared to a scrotal approach.[145] Although only 10.9% of guinea pigs were reported to be neutered, it was significantly higher than the percent of female guinea pigs reported to be spayed.[117]

Chinchillas
Castration can be considered for mixed-sex groups or hormonal aggression. The procedure can also be considered to prevent disease such as infection or neoplasia, although no reports were found in literature. A single report of a semen-matrix calculus has been reported.[146] Therefore, routine castration is generally not considered. Chinchillas are prone to incisional picking and contamination.[31] Should castration be

pursued, an open paramedian or abdominal approach can be considered.[31] Closed castration is not recommended as the vaginal tunic is adhered to the surrounding tissues.[31] Studies are lacking on the best approach and true postoperative infection risks.

Degus

Degus hold their testicles intraabdominally or in the parascrotal sacs, as they do not have a true scrotum.[34] Castration to avoid conspecific aggression is recommended for males.[34] In a comparison of prescrotal and parascrotal methods, the prescrotal approach was found to reduce surgical time, although recovery times were not significantly different.[140]

SUMMARY

Rats, mice, hamsters, and gerbils are altricial and have relatively short gestation periods while guinea pigs, chinchillas, and degus are precocial and have longer gestation periods. Young rodents will typically start eating solid food by 1 to 2 weeks of age. The weaning age is 21 to 28 days in most rodents, but at an older age in chinchillas and degus. Most juvenile rodents can be sexed by the presence of larger anogenital distance in males. Tyzzer's disease (*C piliforme*) is an important disease of juvenile rodents. Proliferative ileitis (*L intracellularis*) is a common cause of diarrhea in young hamsters and has a guarded prognosis. Prophylactic ovariectomy should be considered in young rats, guinea pigs, and gerbils to prevent mammary tumors, ovarian cysts, and ovarian tumors, respectively.

CLINICS CARE POINTS

- Rats and mice are altricial, so hand-rearing of orphaned rats and mice is difficult. Orphaned guinea pigs and chinchillas can be fostered.
- *C piliforme*, *C perfringens*, salmonellosis, and *L intracellularis* are important gastrointestinal disorders in pediatric rodents.
- Dermatophytosis is a noted skin disorder of juvenile guinea pigs and chinchillas.
- Prophylactic ovariectomy should be discussed with the owners of female rats, guinea pigs, and gerbils.

DISCLOSURE

The authors declare that they have no known competing financial or commercial interests that could have appeared to influence the work reported in this paper. No funding was provided for this article.

REFERENCES

1. Yarto-Jaramillo E. Rodentia. In: Miller RE, Fowler ME, editors. Fowler's Zoo and Wild Animal Medicine. 8th edition. St. Louis, MO: Elsevier; 2015. p. 384–422.
2. Miwa Y, Mayer J. Hamsters and gerbils. In: Quesenberry KE, Orcutt CJ, Mans C, et al, editors. Ferrets, Rabbits, and Rodents: Clinical Medicine and Surgery. 4th edition. St. Louis, MO: Elsevier; 2020. p. 368–84.
3. Albright J, de Matos R. Hamsters. In: Tynes VV, editor. Behavior of Exotic Pets. West Sussex, UK: Blackwell Publishing; 2010. p. 127–37.

4. Keeble E. Rodents: biology and husbandry. In: Keeble E, Meredith A, editors. BSAVA manual of rodents and ferrets. Gloucester, UK: British Small Animal Veterinary Association; 2011. p. 1–17.

5. Hankenson FC, Van Hoosier GL. Biology and diseases of hamsters. In: Fox JG, Anderson LC, Loew FM, et al, editors. Laboratory animal medicine. 2nd edition. San Diego, CA: Elsevier; 2002. p. 167–2002.

6. Eshar D, Gardhouse SM. Prairie dogs. In: Quesenberry KE, Orcutt CJ, Mans C, et al, editors. Ferrets, rabbits, and rodents: clinical medicine and surgery. 4th edition. St. Louis, MO: Elsevier; 2020. p. 334–44.

7. Johnson-Delaney CA. Rodents: biology, husbandry and clinical techniques in more unusual pet species. In: Keeble E, Meredith A, editors. BSAVA manual of rodents and ferrets. Gloucester, UK: British Small Animal Veterinary Association; 2011. p. 96–106.

8. Faghihi H, Aftab G, Rajaei SM, et al. Evaluation of conjunctival microbiota in clinically normal Persian squirrels (*Sciurus anomalus*). J Zoo Wildl Med 2018;49(3):794–7.

9. Kohn DF, Clifford CB. Biology and diseases of rats. In: Fox JG, Anderson LC, Loew FM, et al, editors. Laboratory animal medicine. 2nd edition. San Diego, CA: Elsevier; 2002. p. 121–65.

10. Frohlich J. Rats and mice. In: Quesenberry KE, Orcutt CJ, Mans C, et al, editors. Ferrets, rabbits, and rodents: clinical medicine and surgery. 4th edition. St. Louis, MO: Elsevier; 2020. p. 345–67.

11. Fowler A. Hand-rearing small mammals: facts and fallacies. In: ExoticsCon 2019 Proceedings. St. Louis, MO: Association of Avian Veterinarians, Association of Exotic Mammal Veterinarians, and Association of Reptile and Amphibian Veterinarians; 2019. p. 459–68.

12. Hanson AF, Berdoy M. Rats. In: Tynes VV, editor. Behavior of exotic pets. West Sussex, UK: Blackwell Publishing; 2010. p. 105–16.

13. Jacoby RO, Fox JG, Davisson M. Biology and diseases of mice. In: Fox JG, Anderson LC, Loew FM, et al, editors. Laboratory animal medicine. 2nd edition. San Diego, CA: Elsevier; 2002. p. 35–120.

14. Keller DL. Small mammals: hamsters - ocular disorders. In: Mayer J, Donnelly TM, editors. Clinical veterinary advisor: birds and exotic pets. St. Louis, MO: Saunders; 2013. p. 293–5.

15. Keller DL. Small mammals: hamsters - abdominal distension. In: Mayer J, Donnelly TM, editors. Clinical veterinary advisor: birds and exotic pets. St. Louis, MO: Saunders; 2013. p. 285–7.

16. Donnelly TM, Quimby FW. Biology and diseases of other rodents. In: Fox JG, Anderson LC, Loew FM, et al, editors. Laboratory animal medicine. 2nd edition. San Diego, CA: Elsevier; 2002. p. 247–307.

17. Parker ADF, Tynes VV. Gerbils. In: Tynes VV, editor. Behavior of exotic pets. West Sussex, UK: Blackwell Publishing; 2010. p. 117–26.

18. Gresham V, Haines V. Management, husbandry, and colony health. In: Suchow M, Stevens K, Wilson R, editors. The laboratory rabbit, Guinea pig, hamster, and other rodents. London, UK: Academic Press; 2012. p. 603–19.

19. Enders AC, Blankenship TN. Comparative placental structure. Adv Drug Deliv Rev 1999;38(1):3–15.

20. Bishop CR, Burgess ME. Reproductive physiology, normal neonatology, and neonatal disorders of cavies (guinea pigs). In: Lopate C, editor. Management of pregnant and neonatal dogs, cats, and exotic pets. Ames, IA: John Wiley & Sons, Inc; 2012. p. 239–58.

21. Martinic G, Harkness J, Wagner J. The biology and medicine of rabbits and rodents. 4th edition. Philadelphia, PA: Williams & Wilkins; 1995.

22. Weir B. Notes on the origin of the domestic guinea-pig. Symp Zool S 1974;34: 437–46.

23. Huerkamp M, Murray K, Orosz S. Guinea pigs. In: Laber-Laird K, Flecknell P, Swindle M, editors. Handbook of rodent and rabbit medicine. Oxford, UK: Butterworth-Heinemann; 1996. p. 91.

24. Pignon C, Mayer J. Guinea pigs. In: Quesenberry KE, Orcutt CJ, Mans C, et al, editors. Ferrets, rabbits, and rodents: clinical medicine and surgery. 4th edition. St. Louis, MO: Elsevier; 2020. p. 270–97.

25. Mans C, Donnelly TM. Chinchillas. In: Quesenberry KE, Orcutt CJ, Mans C, et al, editors. Ferrets, rabbits, and rodents: clinical medicine and surgery. 4th edition. St. Louis, MO: Elsevier; 2020. p. 298–322.

26. Mikkelsen E, Lauridsen H, Nielsen PM, et al. The chinchilla as a novel animal model of pregnancy. R Soc Open Sci 2017;4(4). https://doi.org/10.1098/rsos. 161098.

27. Neira R, Garcia X, Scheu R. Descriptive analysis of reproductive and growing performance of chinchillas (*Chinchilla lanigera grey*) in confinement. Av Prod Anim 1989;14:109–19.

28. Brower M. Practitioner's guide to pocket pet and rabbit theriogenology. Theriogenology 2006;66(3):618–23.

29. Burgess ME, Bishop CR. Reproductive physiology, normal neonatology, and neonatal disorders of chinchillas. In: Lopate C, editor. Management of pregnant and neonatal dogs, cats, and exotic pets. Ames, IA: John Wiley & Sons, Inc; 2012. p. 295–307.

30. Spotorno AE, Zuleta CA, Valladares JP, et al. *Chinchilla laniger* [sic]. Mamm Species 2004;758(758):1–9.

31. Saunders R. Soft tissue surgery of the chinchilla. In Pract 2013;35(8):446–59.

32. Kondert L, Mayer J. Reproductive medicine in guinea pigs, chinchillas and degus. Vet Clin North Am Exot Anim Pract 2017;20(2):609–28.

33. Weir BJ. The management and breeding of some more hystricomorph rodents. Lab Anim 1970;4(1):83–97.

34. Jekl V. Degus. In: Quesenberry KE, Orcutt CJ, Mans C, et al, editors. Ferrets, rabbits, and rodents: clinical medicine and surgery. 4th edition. St. Louis, MO: Elsevier; 2020. p. 323–33.

35. Hankel J, Fehr M, Kamphues J. The degu, a desert inhabitant, as a "new" pet - Part 2: reproduction, rearing of degu orphans, sex determination and castration. Kleintierpraxis 2019;64(1):27–36.

36. Donnelly T, Bergin I, Ihrig M. Biology and diseases of other rodents. In: Fox J, Otto G, Pritchett-Corning K, et al, editors. Laboratory animal medicine. 3rd edition. Elsevier; 2015. p. 285–349.

37. Palacios AG, Lee TM. Husbandry and breeding in the *Octodon degus* (Molina 1782). Cold Spring Harb Protoc 2013;2013(4):350–3.

38. Colby L, Rush H, Mahoney M. Degu. In: Suckow M, Stevens K, Wilson R, editors. The Laboratory Rabbit, Guinea Pig, Hamster, and Other Rodents. Academic Press; 2012. p. 1031–53.

39. Miller EA. Natural history and medical management of squirrels and other rodents. In: Hernandez SM, Barron HW, Miller EA, et al, editors. Medical management of wildlife species: a guide for practitioners. Hoboken, NJ: John Wiley & Sons; 2020. p. 169–84.

40. Oftedal O. Milk composition, milk yield and energy output at peak lactation: a comparative review. Symp Zool S 1984;51:33–85.

41. Richardson V.C.G., Chinchillas. In: Diseases of small domestic rodents, 2nd edition, 2003, Blackwell Publishing; Oxford, UK, 1–53.

42. Webb R. Chinchillas. In: Benyon P, Cooper J, editors. Manual of exotic pets. Ames, IA: Iowa State University Press; 1991. p. 15–22.

43. Saunders R. Veterinary care of chinchillas. In Pract 2009;31(6):282–91.

44. Houston J. Chinchilla care. High Point: Owens Press; 2010.

45. Weir B. Chinchilla. In: Hafex E, editor. Reproduction and breeding techniques for laboratory animals. Philadelphia, PA: Lea & Febiger; 1970. p. 209–23.

46. Volcani R, Zisling R, Sklan D, et al. The composition of chinchilla milk. Br J Nutr 1973;29(1):121–5.

47. Johnson-Delaney C, Harrison L. Special rodents: chinchillas. In: Johnson-Delaney CA, editor. *Exotic companion medicine handbook for veterinarians.* Lake Worth, FL: Wingers Publishing; 1996. p. 1–17.

48. Jesseau SA, Holmes WG, Lee TM. Communal nesting and discriminative nursing by captive degus, *Octodon degus.* Anim Behav 2009;78(5):1183–8.

49. Jesseau SA, Holmes WG, Lee TM. Mother-offspring recognition in communally nesting degus, Octodon degus. Anim Behav 2008;75(2):573–82.

50. Veloso C, Kenagy GJ. Temporal dynamics of milk composition of the precocial caviomorph *Octodon degus* (Rodentia: Octodontidae). Rev Chil Hist Nat 2005; 78(2):247–52.

51. Oxbow Animal Health. Guinea pig lifepsan and life stages. Published 2019. Available at: https://oxbowanimalhealth.com/blog/guinea-pig-life-stages. Accessed June 19, 2023.

52. De Rodas BZ, Maxwell CV, Davis ME, et al. L-ascorbyl-2-polyphosphate as a vitamin C source for segregated and conventionally weaned pigs. J Anim Sci 1998;76(6):1636–43.

53. Ardiles AO, Ewer J, Acosta ML, et al. *Octodon degus* (Molina 1782): A model in comparative biology and biomedicine. Cold Spring Harb Protoc 2013;2013(4): 312–8.

54. Neville V, Mounty J, Benato L, et al. Pet rat welfare in the United Kingdom: The good, the bad and the ugly. Vet Rec 2021;189(6).

55. Latham N. The mouse. In: Tynes VV, editor. Behavior of exotic pets. West Sussex, UK: Blackwell Publishing; 2010. p. 91–103.

56. Balsiger A, Clauss M, Liesegang A, et al. Guinea pig (*Cavia porcellus*) drinking preferences: do nipple drinkers compensate for behaviourally deficient diets? J Anim Physiol Anim Nutr 2017;101(5):1046–56.

57. Hsu C, Chan M, Wheler C. Biology and diseases of chinchillas. In: Fox J, Otto G, Pritchett-Corning K, et al, editors. Laboratory animal medicine. 3rd edition. San Diego, CA: Elsevier; 2015. p. 387–409.

58. Hagen K, Clauss M, Hatt JM. Drinking preferences in chinchillas (*Chinchilla laniger*), degus (*Octodon degu*) and guinea pigs (*Cavia porcellus*). J Anim Physiol Anim Nutr 2014;98(5):942–7.

59. Martino PE, Bautista EL, Gimeno EJ, et al. Fourteen-year status report of fatal illnesses in captive chinchilla (*Chinchilla lanigera*). J Appl Anim Res 2017; 45(1):310–4.

60. Harkness JE, Turner PV, VandeWoude S, et al. Harkness and Wagner's biology and medicine of rabbits and rodents. 5th edition. Ames, IA: Blackwell; 2010.

61. Villavicencio CP, Márquez IN, Quispe R, et al. Familiarity and phenotypic similarity influence kin discrimination in the social rodent *Octodon degus*. Anim Behav 2009;78(2):377–84.
62. Rat. In: Barthold SW, Griffey SM, Percy DH, editors. Pathology of laboratory rodents and rabbits. 4th edition. Ames, IA: John Wiley & Sons; 2016. p. 119–71.
63. Ward ML. Rodents: digestive system disorders. In: Keeble E, Meredith A, editors. BSAVA manual of rodents and ferrets. Gloucester, UK: British Small Animal Veterinary Association; 2011. p. 123–41.
64. Hill WA, Randolph MM, Lokey SJ, et al. Efficacy and safety of topical selamectin to eradicate pinworm (*Syphacia* spp.) infections in rats (*Rattus norvegicus*) and mice (*Mus musculus*). J Am Assoc Lab Anim 2006;45(3):23–6.
65. Marroquin SC, Eshar D, Browning GR, et al. Diagnosis and successful treatment of *Eimeria* infection in a pair of pet domestic rats (*Rattus norvegicus*) with ponazuril. J Exot Pet Med 2020;33:31–3.
66. Lipman NS, Wardrip CL, Yuan CS, et al. Familial megacecum and colon in the rat: a new model of gastrointestinal neuromuscular dysfunction. Lab Anim Sci 1998;48(3):243–52.
67. O'Neill DG, Kim K, Brodbelt DC, et al. Demography, disorders and mortality of pet hamsters under primary veterinary care in the United Kingdom in 2016. J Small Anim Pr 2022;63(10):747–55.
68. Hoefer HL. Gastrointestinal diseases of ferrets. In: Quesenberry KE, Orcutt CJ, Mans C, et al, editors. Ferrets, rabbits, and rodents: clinical medicine and surgery. 4th edition. St. Louis, MO: Elsevier; 2020. p. 27–38.
69. Chrisp CE, Reid WC, Rush HG, et al. Cryptosporidiosis in guinea pigs: an animal model. Infect Immun 1990;58(3):674–9.
70. Jiménez RR, Badia XV, Clivillé AM, et al. Surgical treatment of rectocutaneous fistula in a juvenile guinea pig (*Cavia porcellus*) using a rectal pull-through technique. J Exot Pet Med 2020;35:44–7.
71. Harkness J. A practitioner's guide to domestic rodents. Lakewood, CO: American Animal Hospital Association; 1993.
72. Moore RW, Greenlee HH. Enterotoxemia in chinchillas. Lab Anim 1975;9(2):153–4.
73. Mountain A. *Salmonella arizona* in a chinchilla. Vet Rec 1989;125(1):25.
74. Yamagishi S, Watanabe Y, Tomura H. Septic infection of a companion chinchilla with *Salmonella enteritidis*. J Jpn Vet Med Assoc 1997;50:345–8.
75. Gherman CM, Kalmár Z, Györke A, et al. Occurrence of *Giardia duodenalis* assemblages in farmed long-tailed chinchillas *Chinchilla lanigera* (Rodentia) from Romania. Parasit Vectors 2018;11(1).
76. Veronesi F, Piergili Fioretti D, Morganti G, et al. Occurrence of *Giardia duodenalis* infection in chinchillas (*Chincilla lanigera*) from Italian breeding facilities. Res Vet Sci 2012;93(2):807–10.
77. Thomas L, Doss G, Mans C. Presumptive metronidazole benzoate induced anorexia in two healthy chinchillas (*Chinchilla lanigera*). J Exot Pet Med 2021;36:52.
78. Mans C, Fink DM, Giammarco HE, et al. Effects of compounded metronidazole and metronidazole benzoate oral suspensions on food intake in healthy chinchillas (*Chinchilla lanigera*). J Exot Pet Med 2021;36:75–9.
79. Tournade CM, Fink DM, Williams SR, et al. Effects of tinidazole on food intake in chinchillas (*Chinchilla lanigera*). J Am Assoc Lab Anim Sci 2021;60(5):587–91.
80. Vetere A, Bertocchi M, Moggia E, et al. Concomitant congenital diaphagmatic hernia (CDH) and bilateral bacterial glomerulonephritis in a pet chinchilla

(*Chinchilla lanigera*). BMC Vet Res 2021;17(1). https://doi.org/10.1186/s12917-021-03085-4.

81. Ozawa S, Mans C, Miller JL, et al. Cleft palate in a chinchilla (*Chinchilla lanigera*). J Exot Pet Med 2019;28:93–7.

82. Ardiaca García M, Montesinos Barceló A, Bonvehí Nadeu C, et al. Respiratory diseases in guinea pigs, chinchillas and degus. Vet Clin North Am Exot Anim Pract 2021;24(2):419–57.

83. Hoefer H, Latney L. Rodents: urogenital and reproductive system disorders. In: Keeble E, Meredith A, editors. BSAVA manual of rodents and ferrets. Gloucester, UK: British Small Animal Veterinary Association; 2011. p. 150–60.

84. Fouriez-Lablée V, Vergneau-Grosset C, Kass PH, et al. Comparison between thoracic radiographic findings and postmortem diagnosis of thoracic diseases in dyspneic companion rats (*Rattus norvegicus*). Vet Radiol Ultrasound 2017; 58(2):133–43.

85. Rey F, Bulliot C, Bertin N, et al. Morbidity and disease management in pet rats: a study of 375 cases. Vet Rec 2015;176(15):385.

86. Mohd-Qawiem F, Nawal-Amani AR, Faranieyza-Afiqah F, et al. Paramyxoviruses in rodents: a review. Open Vet J 2022;12(6):877–87.

87. Brunner H, James WD, Horswood RL, et al. Experimental *Mycoplasma pneumoniae* infection of young guinea pigs. J Infect Dis 1973;127(3):315–8.

88. Bartoszcze M, Matras J, Palec S, et al. *Klebsiella pneumoniae* infection in chinchillas. Vet Rec 1990;127(5):119.

89. Hoefer HL. Clinical management of the chinchilla and hedgehog. In: Proceedings of 11th Annu Avian Exot Anim Med Symp; 1996:87-91.

90. Pignon C, Sanchez-Migallon Guzman D, Sinclair K, et al. Evaluation of heart murmurs in chinchillas (*Chinchilla lanigera*): 59 cases (1996-2009). J Am Vet Med Assoc 2012;241(10):1344–7.

91. Sanchez JN, Summa NME, Visser LC, et al. Ventricular septal defect and congestive heart failure in a common degu (*Octodon degus*). J Exot Pet Med 2019;31:32–5.

92. Orr H. Rodents: neoplastic and endocrine disease. In: Keeble E, Meredith A, editors. BSAVA manual of rodents and ferrets. Gloucester, UK: British Small Animal Veterinary Association; 2011. p. 181–92.

93. Longley L. Rodents: dermatoses. In: Keeble E, Meredith A, editors. BSAVA manual of rodents and ferrets. Gloucester, UK: British Small Animal Veterinary Association; 2011. p. 107–22.

94. Kraemer A, Mueller RS, Werckenthin C, et al. Dermatophytes in pet Guinea pigs and rabbits. Vet Microbiol 2012;157(1–2):208–13.

95. Meredith A, Johnson-Delaney C. BSAVA manual of exotic pets: a foundation manual. Gloucester, UK: British Small Animal Veterinary Assoication; 2010.

96. Mieth H, Leitner I, Meingassner J. The efficacy of orally applied terbinafine, itraconazole and fluconazole in models of experimental trichophytoses. J Med Vet Mycol 1994;32(3):181–8.

97. White SD, Sanchez-Migallon Guzman D, Paul-Murphy J, et al. Skin diseases in companion guinea pigs (*Cavia porcellus*): A retrospective study of 293 cases seen at the veterinary medical teaching hospital, University of California at Davis (1990-2015). Vet Derm 2016;27(5). 395-e100.

98. Eshar D, Bdolah-Abram T. Comparison of efficacy, safety, and convenience of selamectin versus ivermectin for treatment of *Trixacarus caviae* mange in pet guinea pigs (*Cavia porcellus*). J Am Vet Med Assoc 2012;241(8):1056–8.

99. Kim SH, Jun HK, Yoo MJ, et al. Use of a formulation containing imidacloprid and moxidectin in the treatment of lice infestation in guinea pigs. Vet Dermatol 2008; 19(3):187–8.

100. Donnelly TM, Rush EM, Lackner PA. Ringworm in small exotic pets. Semin Avian Exot Pet 2000;9(2):82–93.

101. Gonçalves GAM. Ringworm by *Microsporum canis* in a long-tailed chinchilla (*Chinchilla lanigera*). Acta Vet Bras 2015;9(3):274–8.

102. Mitchell CM, Johnson LK, Crim MJ, et al. Diagnosis, surveillance and management of *Streptococcus equi* subspecies *zooepidemicus* infections in chinchillas (*Chinchilla lanigera*). Comp Med 2020;70(4):370–5.

103. Berg CC, Doss GA, Mans C. Streptococcus equi subspecies zooepidemicus infection in a pet chinchilla (*Chinchilla lanigera*). J Exot Pet Med 2019;31:36–8.

104. Martel A, Donnelly T, Mans C. Update on diseases in chinchillas: 2013–2019. Vet Clin North Am Exot Anim Pract 2020;23(2):321–35.

105. Jekl V, Hauptman K, Knotek Z. Diseases in pet degus: A retrospective study in 300 animals. J Small Anim Pract 2011;52(2):107–12.

106. Yarto-Jaramillo E, Sánchez C, Çitaku I. Surgical correction of a closed comminuted diaphyseal fracture of the humerus in a pet golden hamster (*Mesocricetus auratus*). J Exot Pet Med 2023;45:22–5.

107. Hollamby S. Rodents: neurological and musculoskeletal disorders. In: Keeble E, Meredith A, editors. BSAVA manual of rodents and ferrets. Gloucester, UK: British Small Animal Veterinary Association; 2011. p. 161–8.

108. Beregi A, Felkai F, Seregi J, et al. Medullary fixation of a tibial fracture in a three month old degu (*Octogon* [sic] *degus*). Vet Rec 1994;134(25):652–3.

109. Vannevel JY. Clinical presentation of pituitary adenomas in rats. Vet Clin North Am Exot Anim Pract 2006;9(3):673–6.

110. Mayer J, Sato A, Kiupel M, et al. Extralabel use of cabergoline in the treatment of pituitary adenoma in a rat. J Am Vet Med Assoc 2011;239(5):656–60.

111. Dębiak P, Wilczyńska A, Ziętek J, et al. Computed tomography in diagnosing pituitary tumours in rats - the authors' own observations. Med Weter 2019;75(10): 622–6.

112. Santagostino SF, Omodho LA, Francis A, et al. Pathology in practice. J Am Vet Med Assoc 2019;254(2):221–4.

113. Lutz-Wohlgroth L, Becker A, Brugnera E, et al. Chlamydiales in guinea-pigs and their zoonotic potential. J Vet Med A Physiol Pathol Clin Med 2006;53(4):185–93.

114. Mount DT, Bigazzi PE, Barron AL. Infection of genital tract and transmission of ocular infection to newborns by the agent of guinea pig inclusion conjunctivitis. Infect Immun 1972;5(6):921–6.

115. Worgul B, Rothstein H. Congenital cataracts associated with disorganized meridional rows in a new laboratory animal: the degu (*Octodon degus*). Biomedicine 1975;23(1):1–4.

116. Edell AS, Vella DG, Sheen JC, et al. Retrospective analysis of risk factors, clinical features, and prognostic indicators for urolithiasis in guinea pigs: 158 cases (2009-2019). J Am Vet Med Assoc 2022;260(S2):S95–100.

117. Harrup AJ, Rooney N. Current welfare state of pet guinea pigs in the UK. Vet Rec 2020;186(9):282.

118. Hotchkiss CE. Effect of surgical removal of subcutaneous tumors on survival of rats. J Am Vet Med Assoc 1995;206(10):1575–9.

119. Planas-Silva MD, Rutherford TM, Stone MC. Prevention of age-related spontaneous mammary tumors in outbred rats by late ovariectomy. Cancer Detect Prev 2008;32(1):65–71.

120. Frerichs K, Lennox AM, Bocchine A. Comparison of post-surgical complication rates and potential confounding factors in two common approaches for elective altering in female rats (*Rattus norvegicus*). J Exot Pet Med 2022;43:11–5.
121. Khelik I, Studer K, Brandão J, et al. Prevalence and outcome of routine and emergency reproductive surgery in female pet rats presented to a veterinary teaching hospital. J Exot Pet Med 2022;41:9–13.
122. Rondeau A, Langlois I, Pang DS, et al. Development of a sedation assessment scale for comparing the sedative effects of alfaxalone-hydromorphone and ketamine-midazolam-hydromorphone for intravenous catheterization in the domestic rat (*Rattus norvegicus*). J Exot Pet Med 2020;35:117–22.
123. Szabo Z. Soft tissue surgery: rodents. In: Quesenberry KE, Orcutt CJ, Mans C, et al, editors. Ferrets, rabbits, and rodents: clinical medicine and surgery. 4th edition. St. Louis, MO: Elsevier; 2020. p. 467–82.
124. Dutton M. Selected veterinary concerns of geriatric rats, mice, hamsters, and gerbils. Vet Clin North Am Exot Anim Pract 2020;23(3):525–48.
125. Bennett RA. Rodents: soft tissue surgery. In: Keeble E, Meredith A, editors. BSAVA manual of rodents and ferrets. Gloucester, UK: British Small Animal Veterinary Association; 2011. p. 73–85.
126. Malbrue RA, Arsuaga CB, Jay AN, et al. Pathology in practice. J Am Vet Med Assoc 2017;250(9):989–92.
127. Minarikova A, Hauptman K, Jeklova E, et al. Diseases in pet guinea pigs: a retrospective study in 1000 animals. Vet Rec 2015;177(8):200.
128. Bertram CA, Müller K, Klopfleisch R. Genital tract pathology in female pet guinea pigs (*Cavia porcellus*): a retrospective study of 655 post-mortem and 64 biopsy cases. J Comp Pathol 2018;165:13–22.
129. Quattropani SL. Serous cysts of the aging guinea pig ovary. I. Light microscopy and origin. Anat Rec 1977;188(3):351–60.
130. Shi F, Petroff BK, Herath CB, et al. Serous cysts are a benign component of the cyclic ovary in the guinea pig with an incidence dependent upon inhibin bioactivity. J Vet Med Sci 2002;64(2):129–35.
131. Keller LSF, Griffith JW, Lang CM. Reproductive failure associated with cystic rete ovarii in guinea pigs. Vet Pathol 1987;24(4):335–9.
132. Nielsen TD, Holt S, Ruelokee MLMF. Ovarian cysts in guinea pigs: Influence of age and reproductive status on prevalence and size. J Small Anim Pract 2003;44(6):257–60.
133. McCready J, Beaufrère H, Singh A, et al. Laparoscopic ovariectomy in guinea pigs: a pilot study. Vet Surg 2020;49(Suppl 1):O131–7.
134. Kabakchiev C, Singh A, Dobson S, et al. Comparison of intra-and postoperative variables between laparoscopic and open ovariectomy in rabbits (*Oryctolagus cuniculus*). Am J Vet Res 2021;82(3):237–48.
135. O'Malley B. Guinea pigs. In: O'Malley B, editor. Clinical anatomy and physiology of exotic species: structure and function of mammals, birds, reptiles and amphibians. 1st edition. London, UK: Saunders; 2005. p. 197–208.
136. Bean AD. Ovarian cysts in the guinea pig (*Cavia porcellus*). Vet Clin North Am Exot Anim Pract 2013;16(3):757–76.
137. Deresienski D. Ovarian cyst in a guinea pig. Exot DVM 1999;1(1):33.
138. Redrobe S. Soft tissue surgery of rabbits and rodents. Semin Avian Exot Pet 2002;11(4):231–45.
139. Rozanska D, Rozanski P, Orzelski M, et al. Unilateral flank ovariohysterectomy in guinea pigs (*Cavia porcellus*). New Zeal Vet J 2016;64(6):360–3.

140. Malbrue RA, Arsuaga-Zorrilla CB, Bidot W, et al. Evaluation of orchiectomy and ovariectomy surgical techniques in degus (*Octodon degus*). J Exot Pet Med 2019;30:22–8.
141. Albert D, Walsh M, Gorzalka B, et al. Testosterone removal in rats results in a decrease in social aggression and a loss of social dominance. Physiol Behav 1986;36(3):401–7.
142. Flannelly K, Thor D. Territorial aggression of the rat to males castrated at various ages. Physiol Behav 1978;20(6):785–9.
143. Vaughan LM, Dawson JS, Porter PR, et al. Castration promotes welfare in group-housed male swiss outbred mice maintained in educational institutions. J Am Assoc Lab Anim Sci 2014;53(1):38–43.
144. Kharbush RJ, Steinberg H, Sladky KK. Surgical resection of a testicular seminoma in a guinea pig (*Cavia porcellus*). J Exot Pet Med 2017;26(1):53–6.
145. Guilmette J, Langlois I, Hélie P, et al. Comparative study of 2 surgical techniques for castration of guinea pigs (*Cavia porcellus*). Can J Vet Res 2015;79(4):323–8.
146. Higbie CT, DiGeronimo PM, Bennett RA, et al. Semen-matrix calculi in a juvenile chinchilla (*Chinchilla lanigera*). J Exot Pet Med 2019;28:69–75.

African Pygmy Hedgehog Pediatrics

Daria Hinkle, DVM[a],*,
David Eshar, DVM, MBA, DABVP (ECM), DECZM (SM & ZHM)[b]

KEYWORDS

- African pygmy hedgehog • Pediatrics • Breeding • Hand-rearing • Neonates

KEY POINTS

- Hedgehogs are prone to cannibalism and abandonment of newborns, requiring proper husbandry and assessment of their comfort with handling.
- Knowledge of developmental milestones and expected weight gain are important for identifying neonates needing intervention.
- Hand-rearing of hedgehog neonates is difficult and cross-fostering to another dam is recommended when available.
- Similar to other small mammals, orphaned neonatal hedgehogs require heat support, frequent feedings with appropriate milk replacer, and physical stimulation for elimination.

 Video content accompanies this article at http://www.vetexotic.theclinics.com.

INTRODUCTION

Hedgehogs belong to the family *Erinaceidae* and are well known for their dorsal cutaneous spines and ability to roll into a ball for protection.[1] Although multiple species of hedgehog exist, the African pygmy hedgehog (*Atelerix albiventris*) is the most frequently owned in North America and will be the only species discussed in this review. The African pygmy hedgehog is native to Africa and was originally only available in zoos and through importation into North America but is now commonly available from both breeders and pet stores.[2] Hedgehogs are considered an insectivorous species that feed mostly on invertebrates with occasional plants, eggs, or small vertebrates.[1] Adults in the wild are generally solitary, and males are not involved in raising the young. Most captive hedgehogs are kept solitary unless housed together for breeding or a dam with nursing pups, also known as hoglets.[2,3] The risk of

[a] Department of Surgical Sciences, School of Veterinary Medicine, University of Wisconsin-Madison, 2015 Linden Drive, Madison, WI 53706, USA; [b] Wildlife Hospital of Israel, Zoological Center Ramat Gan, 1 Sderat Hatsvi, Ramat Gan 5225300, Israel
* Corresponding author.
E-mail address: dghinkle@wisc.edu

Vet Clin Exot Anim 27 (2024) 221–227
https://doi.org/10.1016/j.cvex.2023.11.005
1094-9194/24/© 2023 Elsevier Inc. All rights reserved.

cannibalism by the dam and difficulty in hand-rearing pups make neonatal care challenging in this species.[2]

BREEDING

Hedgehogs are easily sexed by external genitalia with the prepuce located midway up the abdomen on males and the vulva located close to the anus in females. Mature males may show obvious subcutaneous testicular bulges.[2,4,5] Although female African pygmy hedgehogs may be sexually mature at 2 to 3 months, it is recommended to wait until at least 6 to 8 months of age before breeding.[2,5] Males reach sexual maturity at 6 to 8 months of age.[2,4] A male and female pair, or multiple females with one male, may be housed together to encourage breeding.[2,3] In the wild, females are seasonally polyestrus,[6] and young are born in November but breeding occurs year-round in captivity.[3] The estrous cycle ranges from 3 to 17 days followed by 1 to 5 days of diestrus. African pygmy hedgehogs show evidence of being induced ovulators.[1,6,7]

Neonatal health begins with the health and husbandry of the breeding pair. In North America, African pygmy hedgehogs are affected by wobbly hedgehog syndrome, a fatal progressive paralysis disease with a prevalence ranging from 3.32% to 10%.[8,9] The disease is suspected to have a genetic component but clinical signs may not be evident for years and carriers may be subclinical.[9] Breeding of affected hedgehogs or those of close relation should be avoided.[8]

PREGNANCY

Breeding females should be weighed weekly, and a weight gain of 50 g within 3 weeks generally indicates pregnancy.[2,5] Swelling of the abdomen and mammary development may also be noted in the week leading up to parturition.[1] The gestation period is 34 to 37 days in African pygmy hedgehogs. Energy requirements during pregnancy and lactation are up to 3 times that of normal requiring access to greater quantities of food and to more calorically-dense food, such as canned high protein cat food.[2] Calcium supplementation may also be considered.[4] Pregnant females must be isolated before parturition to decrease the risk of cannibalism of the young by either the male or dam.[2,3,5] In the authors' experience, fully mature fetuses may not obviously show on survey radiographs and an abdominal ultrasound should always be performed when ruling out pregnancy.

PARTURITION

The birthing enclosure should be easily cleaned and not include wire because it may lead to traumatic injuries. Soft absorbent bedding such as wood shavings, newspaper, or recycled shredded paper is recommended, and cloth or any fiber threads are avoided because of the potential for limb entanglement or strangulation.[2] There must be a hidebox available for comfort and security of the dam to create a nest.[2,3] The ambient temperature should be 24°C to 29°C (75°F–85°F).[5]

Parturition generally occurs late at night or early in the morning and occurs over minutes to hours.[3,4] Dystocias are considered rare but can be addressed similar to other small mammals. Premature births are also rare but carry an extremely poor prognosis even with intensive care.[2] Risk for infanticide or abandonment of newborns is high in stressed individuals, and the nest should not be disturbed. Dams should remain undisturbed for a few days before and 5 to 10 days after the birth unless the dam is well conditioned to handling.[2-4]

FIRST 24 HOURS

African pygmy hedgehogs have an average birth weight of 8 to 13 g with an average of 3 to 5 pups but litter size can range from 1 to 7 pups.[6] Some recommend the umbilicus be treated with iodine or chlorhexidine if accessible[2]; however, the risk of cannibalism from handling newborns is high.[1] Strict sanitation of bedding without disturbing the nest adequately decreases the risk of umbilical infection with limited risk of infanticide.[2] At birth, the pup's skin is swollen and edematous to cover their spines. Within the first few hours, the fluid is absorbed and short nonpigmented spines emerge.[1] Dams will lay in the supine position with pups nursing in the prone position, likely to avoid harming the dam with their spines.[2,5] Colostrum is available in the first 24 to 72 hours following birth, and all efforts should be made to keep pups with the dam during this time to ensure intake. Although less is known about colostrum in hedgehogs specifically, it is shown to decrease the risk of early infection. Healthy young will be huddled beneath the dam and nursing regularly, with good dams licking and nuzzling them. Intervention is necessary for babies that lay separate from the others, seem weak or restless, or are overly vocal.[2]

NEONATAL DEVELOPMENT

Pups are born hairless with closed eyelids and sealed pinnae (**Fig. 1**).[4] At 2 to 3 days of age, a second set of darker spines emerge,[2,3] and ears open about day 10.[4] At 10 to 14 days, pups begin to gain the ability to roll up, and at 14 to 18 days, their eyes open and fur begins to grow.[2] Pups will exhibit innate behaviors of hissing and self-anointing even before their eyes open (see Video 1).[3] At 3 weeks, they begin exploring outside of the nest, and the first set of teeth emerge. By this age, handling is less risky because pups can be introduced to solid food and would require less-intensive hand-rearing. At 4 to 5 weeks, the pups are able to roll up completely and generally leave their dam between 4 to 6 weeks.[2] Their adult teeth erupt between 7 and 9 weeks,[3] and by 3 months old, they will have reached adult size.[2] Young must be separated from the dam before sexual maturity, or there is risk of inbreeding.[3]

  Weight gain is an important marker of appropriate development. Ideally weight is obtained with the same gram scale and recorded daily on all pups and is generally possible with well-socialized dams. Consideration may be given to forego obtaining early weights for pups of highly stressed dams that are at higher risk for infanticide or abandonment. African pygmy hedgehogs grow by 1 to 2 g per day for the first 10 days, then 4 to 5 g per day for the next few weeks, and finally 7 to 9 g per day until they reach their mature weight.[2,3] Decreased weight gain indicates the need for intervention in an individual or litter. Failure of lactation may be an underrecognized problem affecting the entire litter with possible causes including lack of oxytocin, underdevelopment of young dams, toxemia, mastitis, and stress. Pups will require cross-fostering or hand-rearing until the underlying cause can be treated or they are weaned.[2]

HAND-REARING

Hand-rearing hedgehogs can be difficult, and whenever a dam with similarly aged litter is available, attempts to cross-foster are recommended. Cross-fostering is generally successful but the risk for infanticide of either set of pups remains present.[2,4] Weak or neglected pups without a cross-foster available will require supportive care and milk replacer. Potential risks of hand-rearing include aspiration pneumonia from syringe or tube-feeding, bloat, and a weakened immune system from lack of colostrum intake.

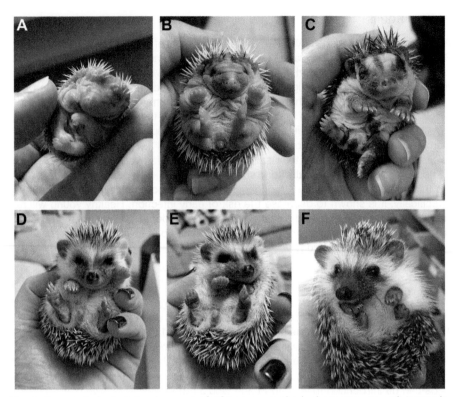

Fig. 1. Expected physical development of African pygmy hedgehog pups at week intervals. (*A*) At 2 hours of age, white spines are visible and the pup is hairless with closed eyes. (*B*) At 1 week of age, darker spines are visible. (*C*) At 2 weeks of age, eyes are generally still closed, (*D*) but by 3 weeks of age, eyes have opened and fur is growing in. (*E*) Continued growth and elongation of the face can be seen at 4 weeks of age, and (*F*) 5 weeks of age. (*Courtesy of* Jenna R. Perlick, Batavia, Illinois.)

Pups must be kept warm with an ambient temperature of 32°C to 35°C (90°F–95°F) until 3 weeks of age. Reports of normal body temperature for neonatal hedgehogs varies from 32.9°C to 36°C (91.2°F–96.8°F) but is noted to be lower than other domestic species. Neglected pups that are presented hypothermic must be warmed to normal temperature during the course of 1 to 3 hours before feedings can be provided.[5]

Feedings should occur every 2 to 4 hours.[4,5] Hand-raised individuals can be nursed in the prone position as they would nurse naturally. Those with an adequate suckle reflex can be fed with a syringe (**Fig. 2**) or dropper and should be fed until they refuse more. Any pups with a weak or absent suckle will require gastric tube feeding, with 5% of bodyweight per feeding recommended.[5] If additional hydration is needed, subcutaneous fluids can be provided in the space below the mantle. Physical stimulation to urinate and defecate by massaging the anus with a moistened cotton ball is necessary after each feeding. A daily record should be kept of weight, feedings and amounts, and urination and defecation quality to monitor trends.[2]

African pygmy hedgehog milk content has not been researched. Analysis of European hedgehog (*Erinaceus europaeus*) milk shows a lower carbohydrate content

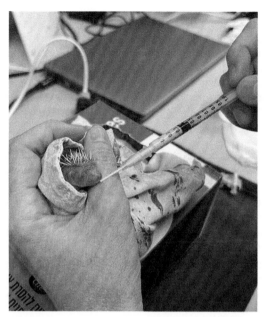

Fig. 2. Syringe feeding of a neonatal European hedgehog (*E europaeus*) being hand-reared. A 1-mL syringe attached to an intravenous catheter with the stylet removed is used to provide milk replacer. (*Courtesy of* Jenna R. Perlick, Batavia, Illinois.)

than that of canine milk[5] and only trace amounts of lactose. No commercially available product is targeted for hedgehogs, and the homemade recipe developed based on milk analysis has not reportedly been used in neonates.[10] Commercial canine milk replacer with a small amount of lactose-digesting product is easy to prepare and has been used successfully for hand-rearing neonatal hedgehogs.[2]

WEANING

Weaning is performed between 4 and 6 weeks of age. Solid foods can be introduced after the first set of teeth have emerged around 3 weeks of age, such as puppy or kitten kibble with or without milk formula mixed in.[2,4,6] The pups can then be slowly transitioned to a commercial insectivore diet supplemented with gut-loaded insects and occasional small amounts of fruit or vegetables.[4] Young hedgehogs might develop certain food preferences, and it is therefore advised to have them introduced to a large variety of appropriate food items (eg, insects, commercial cat kibble, fruit, and vegetables). Water must be available at all times, and although some hedgehogs will learn to use sipper bottles, others require a shallow bowl of water.[2,3]

NEONATAL DISEASES

Bacterial, fungal, and parasitic infections can be addressed as they would be in an adult hedgehog, with consideration to preferably refrain from using antimicrobials that are known to affect cartilage development in other species (eg, enrofloxacin).[5] No vaccinations are currently recommended for young or adult hedgehogs.[2] Ensuring good husbandry and educating about prevention of obesity and dental disease will help set up young hedgehogs for a healthy life.

SUMMARY

Breeding African pygmy hedgehogs can be challenging due to the high risk of infanticide and difficulty hand-rearing pups. Proper husbandry for the dam and pups including enclosure type, temperature, nutrition, and stress reduction will increase the chance of success. When hand-rearing is required, close attention to weight gain, feedings, and eliminations will allow for adjustments and proper intervention.

CLINICS CARE POINTS

- Dams must be isolated from male hedgehogs and should be undisturbed for 5 to 10 days after parturition unless they are well conditioned to handling.
- Orphaned pups may be cross-fostered to a dam with a similar-aged litter and is generally successful.
- Weight gain is an important marker for appropriate growth, and hand-raised individuals should be weighed daily.
- Hypothermic pups must be warmed before feeding with normal neonatal temperatures ranging from 91.2°F to 96.8 F.
- Hedgehog milk contains only trace amounts of lactose and a lactase-digesting product should be added to their milk replacer.

DISCLOSURE

The authors do not have any commercial or financial conflicts of interest, or any funding sources to disclose.

SUPPLEMENTARY DATA

Supplementary data to this article can be found online at https://doi.org/10.1016/j.cvex.2023.11.005.

REFERENCES

1. Doss GA, Carpenter JW. African pygmy hedgehogs. In: Quesenberry K, Orcutt C, Mans C, et al, editors. Ferrets, rabbits, and rodents: clinical medicine and surgery. 4th edition. St. Louis, MO: Elsevier Saunders; 2021. p. 401–15.
2. Smith AJ. Neonatology of the hedgehog, (Atelerix albiventris). J Small Exot Anim Med 1995;3:15–8.
3. Wissink-Argilaga N. Veterinary care of African pygmy hedgehogs. In Pract 2020; 42:151–8.
4. Burgess ME, Bishop CR. Reproductive physiology, normal neonatology, and neonatal disorders of hedgehogs. In: Lopate C, editor. Management of pregnant and neonatal dogs, cats, and exotic pets. 1st edition. Hoboken, NJ: Wiley-Blackwell; 2012. p. 273–81.
5. Santana EM, Jantz HE, Best TL. Atelerix albiventris (Erinaceomorpha: Erinaceidae). Mamm Species 2010;42:99–110.
6. Johnson D. African pygmy hedgehogs. In: Meredith A, Delaney CJ, editors. BSAVA manual of exotic pets. 5th edition. Hoboken, NJ: Wiley; 2010. p. 139–47.
7. Bedford JM, Mock OB, Nagdas SK, et al. Reproductive characteristics of the African pygmy hedgehog, Atelerix albiventris. J Reprod Fertil 2000;120:143–50.

8. Graesser D, Spraker TR, Dressen P, et al. Wobbly hedgehog syndrome in African pygmy hedgehogs (*Atelerix spp.*). J Exotic Pet Med 2006;15:59–65.

9. Gonzalez GA, Balko JA, Sadar MJ, et al. Retrospective evaluation of wobbly hedgehog syndrome in 49 African pygmy hedgehogs (*Atelerix albiventris*): 2000–2020. J Am Vet Med Assoc 2023;261:1–6.

10. Landes E, Zentek J, Wolf P, et al. Investigation of milk composition in hedgehogs. J Anim Physiol Anim Nutr 1998;80:179–84.

Sugar Glider Pediatrics

Colin T. McDermott, VMD, DABVP (Reptile and Amphibian Practice), CertAqV

KEYWORDS

- Sugar gliders • *Petaurus breviceps* • Thermoregulation • Neonatal development
- Marsupial reproduction • Hand rearing

KEY POINTS

- Pediatric diseases of sugar gliders are sparsely documented and appear to be uncommon. A thorough understanding of the normal reproductive anatomy and physiology will aid the clinician in diagnosing and treating any abnormal conditions related to breeding and raising young.
- Due to the small size of joeys at birth, close monitoring is challenging and primarily relies on monitoring the health and activity of the dam.
- The best way to ensure the health of the joey is to ensure proper health and nutrition in the parents, specifically the dam, prior to parturition and during lactation.
- Early eviction from the pouch may occur due to a number of factors. In these cases, human intervention and support feeding are indicated.

INTRODUCTION

Sugar gliders (*Petaurus breviceps*) are small, nocturnal marsupials native to northern, southern, and eastern Australia, New Guinea, and the surrounding islands.[1–4] There are currently 7 recognized subspecies, separated primarily based on their geographic location and physical characteristics (**Box 1**).[1,3,5] Recent molecular evidence from Australian sugar gliders suggests 2 additional, distinct species under what is currently considered *P breviceps*.[6] Further molecular studies may change our understanding of these species and subspecies.[7,8]

Natural History

Sugar gliders are primarily found in open areas within woodlands or forests throughout their natural range.[3] As arboreal species, they will utilize branches and plant material to climb between trees while feeding at night, inhabiting tree hollows that may be up to 14 m above ground.[9] Sugar gliders are social animals, living in groups of up to 12 individuals in the wild (5–7 on average). Wild groupings generally consist of a dominant

Department of Veterinary Clinical Sciences, Jockey Club College of Veterinary Medicine and Life Sciences, City University of Hong Kong, 1B-403 To Yuen Building, 31 To Yuen Street, Kowloon Tong, Hong Kong 999077, China
E-mail address: c.mcdermott@cityu.edu.hk

Vet Clin Exot Anim 27 (2024) 229–244
https://doi.org/10.1016/j.cvex.2023.11.006
1094-9194/24/© 2023 Elsevier Inc. All rights reserved.

Box 1
Recognized subspecies of the sugar glider, *Petaurus breviceps*.

Petaurus breviceps breviceps[a]

P breviceps longicaudatus[a]

P breviceps ariel[b]

P breviceps flavidus

P breviceps tafa

P breviceps papuanus

P breviceps biacensis

[a] Individuals in Australia currently described as *P breviceps breviceps* and *P breviceps longicaudus* have been suggested to be redesignated to *P breviceps* or *P notatus* based on their geographic distribution.[1]

[b] Individuals currently described as *P breviceps ariel* have been suggested to be redesignated to *P ariel*.[1]

Summarized from sources: Cremona T, Baker AM, Cooper SJB, et al. Integrative Taxonomic Investigation of *Petaurus breviceps* (Marsupialia: Petauridae) Reveals Three Distinct Species. Zool J Linn Soc. 2020;191(2):503-527. Kubiak M. Chapter 9 Sugar Gliders. In: Kubiak M, ed. *Handbook of Exotic Pet Medicine*. John Wiley & Sons, Incorporated; 2021:125-140.

---

male, 1 to 2 nondominant males, and multiple females. Sugar gliders engage in vocal communication as well as scent marking to identify their territory and individuals within their social grouping. Dominant males will mark the territory and group members with secretions from the frontal, gular, and paracloacal scent glands. Females may scent mark with their pouch secretions during estrus.[4] Urine marking also occurs and has been noted in male and female sugar gliders.[4] Group members nest communally in insulated leaf-lined cavities, either in trees or in artificial nest boxes, if provided.[3] Reported territory size ranges from 0.5 to 4 ha, depending on the size of the group and level of forest fragmentation in the area.[2–4] After weaning, males disperse from the colonies to establish their own territory.[3]

Sugar gliders are omnivorous, with a seasonally varied diet in the wild. The natural diet of sugar gliders has been the focus of several publications and has been summarized in several reviews and textbooks.[10–13] In short, sugar gliders feed on several plant exudates, including acacia gum, eucalyptus sap, and other various nectars, saps, manna, and honeydew, in addition to insects and arachnids. They have also been reported to prey on nesting birds.[14] Previous studies have shown seasonal variation in diets, where plant exudate material was a higher percentage of the diet in winter and a preferential change to eating more insects in summer, even when exudates were more available during that time.[10] In the wild, sugar gliders have been observed foraging for their food approximately 55% to 60% of their waking hours in the evening.[2]

The metabolic rate of sugar gliders is approximately two-thirds the rate of comparably sized eutherian mammals.[15,16] In addition to lower metabolic rates, sugar gliders can utilize torpor as a means of conserving energy during decreased temperatures, decreased food availability, or adverse weather.[9,17] During torpor, the body temperature may drop to 15°C (59°F) or below (normal rectal temperature (36.2 ± 0.4°C [97.2 ± 0.7°F]), with a concurrent drop in heart rate and respiratory rate. The use of torpor during adverse weather events in the wild resulted in a reduction of metabolic energy expenditure of 67% during deep torpor, similar to laboratory studies.[9] Shallow torpor of a shorter duration in response to mild changes resulted in a decreased energy expenditure of closer to 9%.[9] Arousal from torpor is slower than comparably sized eutherian mammals (eg, rodents like mice and chipmunks), and appears to rely on aerobic and anaerobic metabolism.[17] Additional mechanisms may provide wild sugar gliders the ability to adjust their metabolism to maximize thermoregulatory heat production in the winter, resulting in a conservation of overall metabolic energy expenditure.[18] A full discussion of metabolism in sugar gliders is beyond the scope of this article, and the reader is directed to a previous review article.[12]

Sugar Gliders in Captivity

The exportation of sugar gliders from Australia was banned in 1959 and currently enforced under the Wildlife Protection (Regulation of Exports and imports) Act 1982.[4,19] The captive population of sugar gliders in the United States appears to have originated from West Papua and New Guinea, based on recent molecular data.[19] Although the majority of sugar gliders are produced for the US pet trade through captive breeding, there is still an active trade in wild-caught sugar gliders throughout parts of their range, including Indonesia.[20] The extent of the illegal trade in sugar gliders is not well documented.

Sugar gliders can be maintained in colonies similar to in the wild or as pairs. Due to their social nature, sugar gliders should not be housed singly.[3,4] Of particular interest in the captive management of sugar gliders, there have been a number of recent studies outlining specific diet recommendations. The reader is directed to previous articles on captive diets for sugar gliders.[12,21–23]

In a controlled environment in captivity, torpor is generally unlikely and, when observed, is seen at a lower frequency than in wild populations.[24] In instances where the temperature drops below the normal range, owners may observe decreased activity and feeding in their pet sugar gliders. If this is observed, temperatures should be checked and brought back into the normal range prior to any other interventions.

REPRODUCTIVE ANATOMY AND PHYSIOLOGY
Male Reproductive Anatomy

The reproductive anatomy of male sugar gliders is typical of most marsupials. Intact males have a pendulous scrotum cranial to the cloaca. The scrotum is generally tucked close to the body but may be significantly extended out from the body, especially during anesthesia for castration.[25] The scrotal width may increase during the breeding season, although this change may not be clinically evident or significant.[26] The penis is bifid, with the tip of the urethra at the base of the bifurcation. Males have an elongated prostate and 2 paired bulbourethral glands.[3]

The male has 2 dermal scent glands, used in marking territories and conspecifics. The frontal gland is located over the frontal bone between the eyes, and the gular scent gland is found along the ventral neck/chest (**Fig. 1**). The size and activity of these scent glands is associated with testosterone levels.[26] When concentrations of testosterone are elevated during the breeding season, the size and activity of the sebaceous and apocrine cells in the glands increase. The dermal glands can be categorized into 3 stages of activity based on their appearance (**Table 1**).[1]

In addition to the dermal glands, sugar gliders have 3 sets of paired paracloacal glands, which produce a white to yellow milky discharge.[3,27] Although both sexes have these paracloacal glands, they are more developed in males.[3] The dorsal

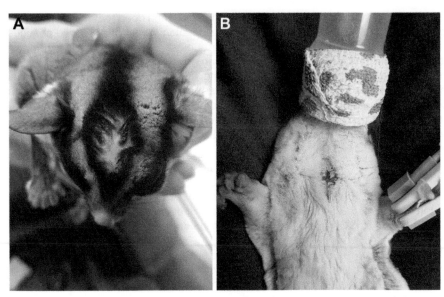

Fig. 1. The frontal (A) and gular (B) scent glands in a mature intact male sugar glider. Note the region of alopecia and oily discharge from each of the glands.

paracloacal gland enlarges under the influence of testosterone during the breeding season.[26]

Female Reproductive Anatomy

The female reproductive anatomy is typical of marsupials. A recent anatomic study has been published with detailed dissection and schematics of the female reproductive anatomy.[28] The reproductive tract of female sugar gliders consists of paired ovaries, oviducts, uteri, and cervices. The paired uteri are elongated and fusiform. Cervices terminate into the vaginal sinus or vaginal cul-de-sac, the connecting point between the single short median vagina and 2 elongated, U-shaped lateral vaginae (collectively termed the vaginal apparatus). The cranial portion of each lateral vagina is separated from one another at the vaginal sinus by a longitudinal septum. The

Table 1
Levels of dermal gland activity and associated life stages in male sugar gliders

Dermal Glands	Description	Life Stage
Little to no activity	Little or no staining of the hair, no hair loss over the gland.	Inactive glands in immature males or castrated males.
Medium activity	Some staining around the hair, some hair loss, waxy product visible.	Mature, sexually active males, out of breeding season or subordinate males in a colony.
High activity	Significant staining to the hair, alopecia present, waxy discharge in the surrounding hair	Mature, sexually active dominant males

Adapted from Jackson S. Possums and Gliders. In: Jackson S, ed. *Australian Mammals: Biology and Captive Management.* CSIRO PUBLISHING; 2003:204-244:chap 8.

caudal opening to the lateral vaginae connects to the urogenital sinus. The urogenital sinus opens caudally into the urogenital opening, along with the colon.[28]

The median vagina connects the caudal portion of the vaginal sinus and the cranial portion of the urogenital sinus. In nulliparous sugar gliders, the median vagina is reduced or closed off. The median vagina is more prominent and open during pregnancy to provide a birth canal for the joey.[28]

Externally, mature females have a well-developed pouch (marsupium) with 4 teats. The pouch is classified as a type 5 configuration pouch based on Russell (1982)[29], where the mammae are completely covered by a fold of skin and the pouch is formed so it opens anteriorly. The pouch can vary in appearance based on the stage of maturity and reproduction. In nulliparous females, the pouch is shallow and almost closed. The teats are reduced at less than 1 mm in length. Prior to the breeding season, there may be patches of black waxy secretions in the pouch.[30] By the start of the breeding season, the lips of the pouch become more turgid and thickened and the pouch deepens. At the same time, the internal lining becomes pink with small white glands.[30] If the female does not successfully breed by the end of the season, the pouch returns to the nulliparous state.[30] When pregnant, the skin folds become more prominent and the internal lining of the pouch becomes more pink and glandular. For females that have been previously bred but are not currently pregnant or nursing, the pouch is considered small but distinct, with slightly elongated teats (>1 mm).[1] The epipubic bones that are found in other marsupials are absent in sugar gliders.[3]

Reproductive Physiology

In the wild, sugar gliders are seasonally polyestrous and polygynous. **Table 2** summarizes the main life history and reproductive data for sugar gliders. Females reach sexual maturity at 8 to 12 months and the estrus cycle is 29 days. Males reach sexual maturity later, at 12 to 15 months. One dominant male will mate with multiple females in the group, with minimal opportunities for breeding for the subordinate males. The normal breeding season in the wild in Australia is from June to November,[4] although this may vary by location. For example, Jackson[31] reported births in a population in North Queensland year-round. If resources are abundant or if the female loses the first litter, females may produce up to 2 litters per breeding season in the wild.[31,32] In captivity, where resources may be plentiful, breeding may occur throughout the year without a defined breeding season.[4] While embryonic diapause has been documented in other marsupials, there is no definitive evidence of embryonic diapause or postpartum estrus in sugar gliders.[4,32]

A previous study in captive sugar gliders described a colony with a dominant male and a supportive relationship with 1 of his male offspring.[33] Field studies provide evidence that this cooperation of adult males and sons is likely an artifact of captivity.[1,34]

As with other marsupials, there is a smaller metabolic investment in pregnancy and a higher energy requirement and metabolic drain during lactation.[35] In the first few weeks of lactation, the field metabolic rate for lactating females with 1 or 2 young was similar to males and nonlactating females.[36] In the early stages of lactation, the rate of milk consumption in the young is low. As the young develop during the later stages of nursing (days 70–110 after birth), the increased metabolic rate and accelerated growth of the young increase the metabolic expenditure of the dam for lactation.[37]

Despite being considered easy to breed in captivity, there are minimal reports of reproductive behaviors in sugar gliders. Females in estrus may show subtle signs of receptivity to breeding, including a change in vocalizations and increased scent marking from the pouch.[4,13] Receptive males may show more interest in the female

Life History Data for Sugar Gliders	
Table 2	
Life history data for sugar gliders	
Average lifespan (wild) (years)	
Male	4–5
Female	5–7
Max lifespan years (captive)	
Male	15
Female	7
Adult weight (grams)	
Male	100–160
Female	80–135
Thermoneutral zone	27–31°C (81–88°F)
Cloacal temperature	32°C (89.6°F)
Rectal temperature	36.2 ± 0.4°C (97.2 ± 0.7°F)
Basal metabolic rate	2.54 (weight in kg)$^{0.75}$
Birth season (wild)	April–November
Litter size	1–2 most common, up to 4 reported
Litters per year	1–2, up to 4 possible
Sexual maturity (months)	
Males	12–15
Female	8–12
Estrus cycle (days)	29
Gestation (days)	15–17
Postpartum estrus	No
Embryonic diapause	No

Jackson, Stephen M. (2007). Australian Mammals: Biology and Captive Management. CSIRO Publishing.

glider, chasing her and licking the area around her cloaca.[13] Both sexes may also become irritable and fight in the initial stages of breeding.[3,16] Pregnancy may go unnoticed, or owners may notice that the female is restless with a change in attitude to be less interactive.

Preparing for Parturition

Anyone considering breeding sugar gliders should review the genetics of the male and female to ensure they are not directly related, and that there are no known genetic disorders in the lines they are breeding. There has been an increase in the number of color morphs available in recent years.[3] As seen with other species, certain lines and morphs may carry undesirable genetic traits along with the desired color patterns. For example, certain lines of mosaic color variations may produce sterile males.[3] The US Department of Agriculture does not currently regulate small-scale breeding of sugar gliders, but a permit is needed for breeders that have 4 or more breeding females (https://www.aphis.usda.gov/animal_welfare/downloads/graybook.pdf). National and state regulations may vary, so any potential breeders are recommended to review national and state laws prior to any breeding attempts.

Before potential breeding, husbandry should be optimized to reduce stress in both the male and female sugar gliders. Cage size should be adequate for the number of gliders.

Minimum cage size for an adult pair is 36 × 24 × 36 inches (91.4 × 60.9 × 91.4 cm) and with more space needed for each additional glider in the colony.[3] Adequate branches for climbing and cover should be provided to provide visual security. A nest box must be provided and should be appropriately sized for the number of sugar gliders in the colony, at a minimum of 6 × 6 inches (15.2 × 15.2 cm). In the wild, nesting areas in tree hollows are lined with leaves for insulation. In captivity, hard wood shavings or paper products may be used, making sure to avoid cloth or fabrics with frayed strings that could cause toe or limb constrictions.[3,13] Nest boxes should be cleaned every 1 to 2 weeks. This cleaning should occur before parturition if possible, to avoid disturbing the dam in the early stages of rearing the joeys. Environmental temperature should remain stable in the thermoneutral zone (27–31°C or 81–88°F) to prevent any potential signs of torpor.[38] A well-balanced diet should be offered to ensure the nutritional status of the dam.[12,21–23]

All introductions should be done well in advance of potential breeding. Ideally, the male and any breeding females should be accustomed to one another and cohabitating in a suitable enclosure prior to any breeding attempts. For new introductions, signs of acceptance to the group would be scent marking by the dominant male on the female and the environment.[4] New males should not be introduced into established colonies with a dominant male to prevent fighting between the males. The introduction of a single sugar glider to an established colony should be supervised closely, as the established group may become aggressive in defending their territory.[3,4]

Normal Joey Development

A general timeline for gestation, birth, and development of the joey has been well described for sugar gliders.[30–32,37] There are multiple ways that this timeline has been presented in the literature, in days or weeks of development, and split into major times frames: gestation, in-pouch, and out-of-pouch, for example. For simplicity, the timeline in the following section is described in the number of days after birth. **Table 3** summarizes the main milestones and time points for the maturation of the joey.

Following successful breeding, there is a short gestation period of 15 to 17 days. When joeys are born, they are approximately 0.2 g and extremely altricial. The dam can give birth to 1 to 3 joeys at a time, but 2 joeys are most common. Joeys have developed forelimbs and a relatively well-developed olfactory system that allow them to migrate from the cloaca up to the pouch.[35] The dam may assist the joeys by licking the region from the cloaca to the pouch and wetting the fur with its saliva. The migration may only take a matter of minutes and is not commonly observed. Once in the pouch, each joey will attach to 1 of the 4 teats. The sides of the mouth are fused, and the tongue is formed to accommodate the teat in the oral cavity. Once the joey is attached, the teat swells, sealing the mouth around the teat. Joeys should stay continually attached to the dam for a minimum of 40 days, although the average time frame is reported as 50 to 60 days.[30,38] By this time, the mouth has fully developed and the joey may spend time in the pouch detached from the teat. Joeys may emerge from the pouch for short periods of time from days 50 to 60.

Growth of the joey follows a sigmoidal growth curve. Initial growth is slow, until approximately 60 days of age. From days 60 to 110, sugar glider joeys grow an average of 1 g per day.[37] In this time frame, the eyes will open, fur covers the body, and animals will generally resemble adults by 110 days, at which point they are able to leave the nest on their own. The rate of growth is generally consistent whether there are 1 or 2 joeys in the pouch.[37]

From birth to at least 95 to 100 days of age, sugar glider joeys are poikilothermic, unable to regulate their own body temperature. This is likely associated with an

Table 3
Timeline of the development of sugar glider joeys from birth to the subadult stage

Age (days)	Weight (grams)	Head Length (mm)[a]	Leg Length (mm)[b]	Notes
1	0.2	5.7	-	Birth, migration to the pouch
12–14	-	-	-	The pouch or scrotum can start to be distinguished
16	-	-	-	Ears free at tips
20	0.8	11	6	Ears free from the head and pointed forward; papillae of mystacial vibrissae (whiskers) visible
25	-	-	-	Ears directed backwards
30	1.6	14	9	Fine fur over the head and muzzle, ears lightly pigmented
35	-	-	-	Mystacial vibrissae erupt, ears pigmented
40	3.2, 4.5–5	17	12	Start to pigment on shoulders; eye slits present; ear pigmented
50	6.2	20	16	Typical detachment from the teat and emergence from the pouch from days 50–60
60	8–18	-	-	Intermittently detached from the teat, dorsal stripe, fur, and gliding membrane developing
70	12–22	-	-	Fully furred, more of the body out of the pouch. Can be left in the nest box while the dam forages
74–80	17–29	-	-	Eyes begin to open
80	18–35, 35–44	-	-	Fur lengthens
90	-	-	-	Complete fur coverage, light fur on the abdominal area, the tail continues to fill out
100	54, 20–45	-	-	Emerging from nest, start to eat solids. Able to thermoregulate.
120	78	-	-	Weaning, feed up to 20% body weight in solids
130	-	-	-	
200	100	-	-	Subadult

[a] Head length is the straight distance from the tip of the rostrum to the back of the skull.
[b] Leg length is the straight distance from above the stifle to the hock.
Data summarized from other resources.[3,30,32,38,45]

underdeveloped thyroid gland, small body mass, and lack of hair coat until later development.[37] By day 56, they can maintain their own body temperature at ambient temperatures above 25°C (77°F). By 100 days, joeys are able to maintain a constant body temperature at ambient temperatures between 15 to 30°C (59–86°F). In the time that gliders are in pouch, the body heat from the dam allows them to maintain a relatively steady temperature. From when they can first leave the pouch (days 50–60) until approximately day 110, they are reliant on the body heat of fellow colony members and insulation from the nest box to maintain their body temperature. When the dam leaves the nest to forage, other colony members may remain with the young in the nest box. If the young leaves the nest box and emit a call, other colony members have been observed returning the young to the nest.[37] Paternal care of out-of-pouch young has been documented in the wild and can occur in captive colonies.[39]

Sugar gliders will wean completely at approximately 120 to 130 days. Joeys may start to show mild interest in solid food items after emergence from the nest to explore but rely on milk from the dam until weaning.[35] In the wild, young remain with colonies until they are dispersed at 7 to 10 months of age, prior to sexual maturity in males.

VETERINARY EXAMINATION OF JOEYS

Veterinary examination and intervention are not commonly needed in the development of the joeys. Dystocia has not been reported in sugar gliders and is highly unlikely given the size of the joeys at birth. Pregnancy detection methods have not been described and are unlikely to be productive in most clinical cases due to the short gestation period and the altricial state of the young at parturition.

From birth to days 50 to 60, the joey is completely within the pouch, making examination difficult. Roberts (1991)[40] described a technique of using an otoscope cone and light source to examine the joeys in the pouch; however, this required restraining the dam in a plastic tube restraint device. The female sugar glider was habituated to the restraint device and period of restraint prior to breeding in order to reduce the stress of handling during the observation period. If needed, endoscopic equipment could be used in place of the otoscope cone for improved visualization, provided that there was no additional heat produced from the tip of the endoscope.

In some cases, anesthesia may be needed to immobilize the dam either to examine the young in the pouch or to examine the dam. The use of anesthesia has been associated with detachment of joeys from the teats and is a risk that should be considered before recommending an anesthetized examination for females with joeys in pouch.[3,13]

DISEASES AFFECTING YOUNG SUGAR GLIDERS

There is a paucity of peer-reviewed information on pediatric diseases in sugar gliders. This is likely due to a combination of the relatively low pet population of sugar gliders compared to other exotic companion mammals and the inability to monitor the joey closely during early stages of development. It can be presumed that "failure to thrive" joeys may have congenital or acquired diseases that may go undetected, leading to failure of attachment and early infant death. At early stages of development in the pouch, the joey is dependent on passive immunity from maternal immunoglobulins, which are absorbed unchanged across the gut epithelium. In contrast to eutherian mammals, this passive immunity persists for a longer period of time postbirth, until the joey detaches from the nipple in many marsupials. No lymphoid tissue is present in marsupials at birth, and it develops within the first week of life. This reliance on maternal immunoglobulins may lead to the rapid development of acquired infections in neonatal sugar gliders, especially if they need to be raised on milk replacer.[35] Therefore, it is essential to ensure that the dam remains healthy and is not immune compromised in any way prior to parturition. Infections in the pouch or urogenital tract of the dam may lead to a higher risk of infection in the joey.

Infectious Diseases

Mastitis/pouch infection
Mastitis and pouch infections have been described in sugar gliders[3,13,41] Females may be presented for exudate at the pouch opening with a possible pungent or foul odor. If joeys are present, they may stop feeding or detach from the teat. A full examination of the pouch and milk production is warranted, often requiring general anesthesia. The infected teats may be red, inflamed, or swollen with no milk production. Various species of bacteria as well as *Candida* yeast have been identified in cases of mastitis and pouch infection. Samples from the skin of the pouch and the milk should be collected for cytology and culture. The affected dam should be treated with topical or systemic antimicrobials based on the results, and the joey may also require treatment, depending on their condition. Topical cleaning of the pouch can be performed with 2% chlorhexidine.[3] If the joeys are unable to remain in the pouch, they should be removed and hand reared.

Reproductive tract infection
Ascending infections of the reproductive tract have been reported in female sugar gliders. Signs of reproductive tract infection may be nonspecific, with anorexia, depression, and abdominal swelling. Cloacal discharge may or may not be present.[3] If discharge is present, cytology may reveal signs of infection. Medical management may be preferable over surgical excision due to the unique anatomy of the female reproductive tract. Reported bacterial isolates from reproductive infections include *Staphylococcccus aureus*, *Streptococcus* sp, *Escherichia coli*, and *Proteus* sp, among others.[42] Recently, a case of reproductive tract infection with *Kocuria kristinae* was diagnosed and medically managed in an adult female sugar glider.[43] Depending on the type and severity of infection, systemic spread may cause disease in nursing joeys. If reproductive tract disease is diagnosed, the joey may need to be removed and hand reared.

Sugar glider "ick"
The protozoa *Simplicimonas* sp (Tritrichomonadae) has been implicated in an emerging disease of sugar gliders. Affected furred, in-pouch joeys are found covered in a sticky exudate and show signs of diarrhea. Joeys may be lethargic, dehydrated, and anorexic. Death can occur rapidly depending on the severity of the signs. Fecal wet mounts of the joey or the dam may show the organism, and fecal PCR may provide identification of the organism. Treatment with metronidazole benzoate at 25 mg/kg by mouth for 14 days may effectively clear the infection, but there is concern for possible carrier states in adult sugar gliders. More research is needed on this disease to make specific recommendations for the management of the colony, but it is currently recommended to treat all adults in the colony with metronidazole when detected in joeys.[3]

Noninfectious Conditions

Nutritional diseases
Malnutrition in the dam can result in poor milk production or quality, resulting in poor growth rates of the joeys, or possible detachment or infection. In dams fed protein-restricted diets (8%) during the prenatal period under experimental conditions, neonatal

sugar gliders were found to have a decreased weight compared to those on normal protein (32%) diets. The offspring of the protein-restricted females also showed decreased ability to perform visual pattern discrimination in laboratory testing compared to controls.[44] For dams fed excessive fat during pregnancy and lactation, lipid deposits may form within the eyes of the juveniles, affecting their vision. Proper nutrition for the dam is essential to avoid these issues.[3]

Once the joey has been weaned and has moved on to solid food, a balanced diet with an adequate calcium to phosphorous ratio and vitamin D3 should be provided to prevent nutritional secondary hyperparathyroidism.[3,21–23]

Trauma
The joey may be traumatized by overgrooming, maternal aggression from the dam due to external stressors, or eviction from the pouch by a yearling joey.[3,13] When joeys are out of the pouch and exploring, they are at risk for potential band constrictions around the limbs with loose string, hair, or fabric. Treatment for traumatic wounds is similar to treatment in adult animals. The cause of the underlying trauma should be identified and addressed. Supportive treatment should be initiated to correct any fluid losses and maintain proper body temperature. Depending on the severity of the trauma, appropriate analgesia and systemic or topical antibiotics may be warranted.[3]

Hypothermia and hyperthermia
As the joeys cannot thermoregulate until they are about 110 days old, joeys are at high risk for hypothermia. Any joey that has been evicted from the pouch is at high risk and should be treated promptly. Unfurred joeys should be maintained in an ambient temperature of 32°C (89°F). Furred joeys should be maintained at 28°C (82°F).[3]

Sugar gliders are also prone to hyperthermia due to their metabolism.[15] Hyperthermia may occur following the failure of a heating element or if the joey is expelled from the pouch in direct sunlight or under a heat source. Any animal suspected of hyperthermia should be immediately moved into an enclosure with the appropriate ambient temperature for the development stage and monitored closely. Avoid rapid cooling in unfurred joeys, as hypothermia may result.

HAND REARING JOEYS

Hand rearing may be necessary in cases where the joeys cannot stay on the dam. In the wild, this commonly occurs due to maternal death from traumatic injury or if the joeys are found ejected from the pouch due to a stressful event, for example, when a dam is chased by a predator and the joey is left behind or ejected from the pouch. In captivity, these events are less likely. However, there still may be a need to hand rear young following the death of the dam, ejection from the pouch due to stressful events, mastitis or pouch infection, or evidence of poor maternal care from the dam.

For any joeys that are found out of the pouch, they should be immediately triaged and assessed for signs of trauma, breathing difficulties, hypothermia, shock, or wounds. Prior to any treatment or feeding, joeys should be warmed to an appropriate temperature to combat hypothermia. Unfurred joeys should be maintained in an ambient temperature of 32°C (89°F). Furred joeys should be maintained at 28°C (82°F).[13,45]

For unfurred joeys, the skin should be moistened with topical barrier creams like Sorbolene cream, Keri lotion,[13] or lanolin[46] to hydrate the skin and mimic the moist conditions of the pouch. When joeys are expelled from the pouch, rapid dehydration may occur. Hydration of the joey can be achieved with oral fluids, or in severe cases, with subcutaneous fluids.[45]

If the young are ejected early from the pouch due to a stressful event or sudden change, it may be possible to replace the joey either back on the teat or back within the pouch. The dam should be restrained and the joey should be placed back on the teat within the pouch. If needed, a piece of tape can be placed across the body at the level of the pouch opening to keep the pouch closed for a period to time. The dam will then groom off the tape when placed back in her enclosure. In cases of repeated eviction, the pouch can be loosely sutured closed to prevent eviction, or the joey should be removed from the dam and hand reared.[3,13]

If the joey cannot be replaced on the teat or in the pouch, then they will need to be hand reared. If the age of the joey is not already known, age can be estimated based on the weight and physical characteristics listed in **Table 3**. As a general rule, the prognosis is poor to grave for hand rearing unfurred joeys.[45] If the joey is furred, then there is a good prognosis with proper care.

Young joeys can be maintained in a cotton sock or fleece bag to mimic the pouch. The ambient temperatures should be maintained at the appropriate temperature for the stage of development (see the earlier paragraphs) to ensure proper digestion and metabolism. Stress must be reduced with any attempts at hand rearing. Extended periods of stress may lead to treatment failure, secondary infections, and death of the joey.[45]

Joeys can be fed from the end of a syringe, from a bottle and appropriately sized teat, or lapping from a spoon depending on their condition and stage of development. Prior to the introduction of milk replacers, high-energy fluids can be administered in the first 24 to 48 hours to joeys that may be more dehydrated. These fluids include oral electrolyte solutions such as Pedialyte (Abbott Laboratories) or other electrolyte or glucose replacers.[1,45] Once the joey is adequately hydrated, then a milk replacement formula can be introduced.

Milk Formulations and Feeding

Major constituents of milk vary by the species of marsupial. The milk constituents of sugar gliders are 31% to 38% total solids, 11% carbohydrates, 22% lipids, 8% protein, 2,300 mg/L calcium, and 1.6 mg/L iron.[1] The composition of the milk will change over time, generally increasing in lipids and solids later in lactation as the energy needs of the joeys increase.[1] Marsupial milk is low in lactose and providing lactose-rich milk will result in diarrhea and rapid dehydration of the joey.[35]

Various milk replacers have been described for use in juvenile sugar gliders. Common low-lactose formulas include Wombaroo (Wombaroo Food Products, Glen Osmond, South Australia, Australia), Biolac (Biolac Milk Products, Ulladulla, New South Wales, Australia), and Di-Vetelact Low Lactose Milk Replacer (Sharpe Laboratories, Vaucluse, New South Wales, Australia). These companies produce various formulas for different species and stages of development, and feeding instructions are provided for each formula.[35] A summary of previously reported feeding regimens is given in **Table 4**. Additional information on milk replacers and rearing orphaned joeys has been discussed in various textbooks in more detail.[1,35,45]

Unfurred young should be fed every 2 to 3 hours. Recently furred young may be fed less often, every 4 hours. This can gradually be reduced to once or twice daily before weaning, depending on the growth of the young. Formula can be warmed to 35°C (95°F) prior to feeding.[12]

Joeys should be weighed daily to monitor growth. Feeding frequency and amount may need to be adjusted to ensure proper growth compared to known growth rates in sugar glider young. Other data to record include general activity level, defecation and urine frequency and character, and amount of food offered and consumed.[1]

Table 4
Summary of milk replacement formulas and reported feeding schedules for sugar gliders

	Puppy Esbilac formulation for sugar gliders	
Age (days)	**Weight (grams)**	**Total Daily Intake (mL)**
1	0.2	-
20	0.8	0.2
35	2.0	1.0
40	3.2	0.6–1.5
60	12	2.5–3
70	20	4
80	35	6–8
90	44	7
100	54	8–10
120–130	78	Feed up to 20% body weight in solids
200	100	Feed up to 20% body weight in solids

Age (days)	**Feed (mL/day)**	**Wombaroo Possum Milk Replacer**
20	0.7	Formula<0.8
30	1.1	Formula<0.8
40	1.8	Formula<0.8
50	3	Formula<0.8
51–53	4 (3 mL<0.8 + 1 mL>0.8)	Transition from formula<0.8 to formula>0.8
54–56	4 (2 mL<0.8 + 2 mL>0.8)	Transition from formula<0.8 to formula>0.8
57–59	4 (1 mL<0.8 + 3 mL>0.8)	Transition from formula<0.8 to formula>0.8
60	3	Formula>0.8
70	4	Formula>0.8
80	6	Formula>0.8
90	7	Formula>0.8
100	8	Formula>0.8

1 scoop puppy Esbilac powder (Pet Ag, Inc, Hampshire, IL, USA).
3 scoops Pedialyte (Abbott Laboratories, Columbus, OH, USA) (initially, if dehydrated) or plain water[12].
Adapted from Johnson-Delaney CA. Sugar Gliders. In: Quesenberry KE, Orcutt CJ, Mans C, Carpenter JW, eds. *Ferrets, Rabbits, and Rodents* (Fourth Edition). 4th ed. W.B. Saunders; 2021:385-400:chap 27; Barnes M. Sugar Gliders. In: Gage L, ed. *Hand-Rearing Wild and Domestic Mammals.* Blackwell Publishing; 2002:55-62:chap 9.*Adapted from* Brust DM, Mans C. Chapter 7 - Sugar Gliders. In: Carpenter JW, Marion CJ, eds. *Exotic Animal Formulary (Fifth Edition).* W.B. Saunders; 2018:432-442.

Initially, there may be no weight gain or a possible minor weight loss in the first 2 days of feeding. The weight should slowly start to increase after the second day of formula.[45]

Proper hygiene should be observed to reduce the risk of nosocomial or secondary infection. Wash hands with an appropriate antiseptic prior to and after handling the joey and before prepping any food items for the joey. Food should be prepared with boiled water cooled to the appropriate temperature before feeding. Clean all feeding syringes, bottles, and nipples after each use, and sanitize prior to each use.

Joeys can be stimulated to urinate and defecate before or after feedings by applying warm water to the cloaca on a small piece of cotton. This can aid in reducing urination and defecation in the pouch, maintaining a cleaner environment. Cloacal prolapse and urethral swelling have been noted following excessive stimulation in some marsupials, and should be avoided.[1] If these complications occur, examination and replacement of tissues should be performed as soon as possible to reduce the long-term effects of the tissue prolapse.

SUMMARY

Sugar glider reproductive anatomy and physiology are unique compared to the common exotic companion mammals in the pet trade. As with most species, proper husbandry and management of the adults are essential for healthy offspring. When problems occur during nursing and the development of the joey, quick identification of the issue and intervention can have a positive outcome.

CLINICS CARE POINTS

- Although veterinary evaluation of joeys is uncommon in clinical practice, a thorough understanding of the normal parturition and care of joeys is essential for the early identification of diseases.
- Providing a proper environment and diet for the dam is the best way to prevent pediatric diseases in joeys.
- Orphaned joeys can be challenging to care for due to their unique metabolism and inability to maintain body temperature. Owners that plan to breed sugar gliders should be informed about situations where intervention and hand feeding may be needed.

DISCLOSURE

The author has no conflicts of interest to disclose.

REFERENCES

1. Jackson S. Possums and gliders. In: Jackson S, editor. Australian mammals: biology and captive management. Clayton, Victoria, Australia: CSIRO Publishing; 2003. p. 204–44, chap 8.
2. Tyndale-Biscoe H. Pygmy possums and sugar gliders: pollen eaters and sap suckers. In: Tyndale-Biscoe H, editor. Life of marsupials. Clayton, Victoria, Australia: CSIRO Publishing; 2005. p. 185–218, chap 6.
3. Johnson-Delaney CA. Sugar Gliders. In: Quesenberry KE, Orcutt CJ, Mans C, et al, editors. Ferrets, rabbits, and rodents. 4th Edition. Clayton, Victoria, Australia: W.B. Saunders; 2021. p. 385–400, chap 27.
4. Johnson DH. Miscellaneous Small Mammal Behavior. In: Bradley Bays T, Lightfoot TL, Mayer J, editors. Exotic pet behavior: birds, reptiles, and small mammals. Philadelphia, PA: Saunders; 2006. p. 263–344.
5. Quin D, Smith A, Norton T. Eco-geographic variation in size and sexual dimorphism in sugar gliders and squirrel gliders (Marsupialia: Petauridae). Aust J Zool 1996; 44(1):19–45.

6. Cremona T, Baker AM, Cooper SJB, et al. Integrative taxonomic investigation of petaurus breviceps (marsupialia: petauridae) reveals three distinct species. Zool J Linn Soc 2020;191(2):503–27.

7. Malekian M, Cooper SJB, Norman JA, et al. Molecular systematics and evolutionary origins of the genus petaurus (marsupialia: petauridae) in Australia and New Guinea. Mol Phylogenet Evol 2010/01/01/2010;54(1):122–35.

8. Malekian M, Cooper SJB, Carthew SM. Phylogeography of the australian sugar glider (petaurus breviceps): evidence for a new divergent lineage in Eastern Australia. Austr J Zool 2010;58(3):165.

9. Nowack J, Rojas AD, Körtner G, et al. Snoozing through the storm: torpor use during a natural disaster. Sci Rep 2015;5(1):11243.

10. Smith AP. Diet and feeding strategies of the marsupial sugar glider in temperate Australia. J Anim Ecol 1982;51(1):149–66.

11. Howard JL. Diet of *Petaurus breviceps* (Marsupialia: Petauridae) in a mosaic of coastal woodland and heath. Aust Mammal 1989;12(1):15–21.

12. Johnson-Delaney CA. Captive Marsupial Nutrition. Vet Clin North Am: Exot Anim Pract 2014;17(3):415–47.

13. Burgess ME, Bishop CR. Reproductive physiology, normal neonatology, and neonatal disorders of sugar gliders. In: Lopate C, editor. Management of pregnant and neonatal dogs, cats, and exotic pets. 2012. p. 283–93, chap 17.

14. Heinsohn R, Webb M, Lacy R, et al. A severe predator-induced population decline predicted for endangered, migratory swift parrots (*Lathamus Discolor*). Biol Conserv 2015;186:75–82.

15. McLaughlin A, Strunk A. Common emergencies in small rodents, hedgehogs, and sugar gliders. Vet Clin North Am: Exot Anim Pract 2016;19(2):465–99.

16. Johnson-Delaney C. Marsupials. In: Meredith A, Johnson-Delaney C, editors. BSAVA manual of exotic pets : a foundation manual. Gloucester, UK: British Small Animal Veterinary Association; 2010. p. 103–26.

17. Fleming M. Thermoregulation and torpor in the sugar glider, *Petaurus breviceps* (Marsupialia:Petauridae). Aust J Zool 1980;28(4):521–34.

18. Holloway J, Geiser F. Seasonal changes in the thermoenergetics of the marsupial sugar glider, *Petaurus breviceps*. J Comp Physiol B Biochem Syst Environ Physiol 2001;171(8):643–50.

19. Campbell CD, Pecon-Slattery J, Pollak R, et al. The origin of exotic pet sugar gliders (*Petaurus breviceps*) kept in the United States of America. PeerJ 2019; 7:e6180.

20. Lyons J, Natusch D. Over-stepping the quota? the trade in sugar gliders in West Papua, Indonesia. Traffic Bull 2012;24:5–6.

21. Dierenfeld ES, Thomas D, Ives R. Comparison of Commonly Used Diets on Intake, Digestion, Growth, and Health in Captive Sugar Gliders (Petaurus Breviceps). J Exot Pet Med 2006;15(3):218–24.

22. Dierenfeld ES, Pernikoff D, Brewer P. Dietary Vitamin D3 Influence on Serum 25-Hydroxy Vitamin D Concentrations in Captive Sugar Gliders (Petaurus Breviceps). J Exot Pet Med 2018;27(4):48–52.

23. Dierenfeld ES. Feeding Behavior and Nutrition of the Sugar Glider (*Petaurus breviceps*). Vet Clin North Am: Exot Anim Pract 2009;12(2):209–15.

24. Geiser F, Holloway JC, Körtner G. Thermal biology, torpor and behaviour in sugar gliders: a laboratory-field comparison. J Comp Physiol B 2007;177(5):495–501.

25. Malbrue RA, Arsuaga CB, Collins TA, et al. Scrotal stalk ablation and orchiectomy using electrosurgery in the male sugar glider (*Petaurus breviceps*) and histologic

anatomy of the testes and associated scrotal structures. J Exot Pet Med 2018/04/01/2018;27(2):90–4.

26. Bradley AJ, Stoddart DM. The dorsal paracloacal gland and its relationship with seasonal changes in cutaneous scent gland morphology and plasma androgen in the marsupial sugar glider (*Petaurus breviceps* ; Marsupialia: Petauridae). J Zool 1993;229(2):331–46.

27. Johnson-Delaney CA. Reproductive medicine of companion marsupials. Vet Clin North Am: Exot Anim Pract 2002;5(3):537–53.

28. Yllera MDM, Alonso-Peñarando D, Lombardero M. Gross anatomy of the female reproductive system of sugar gliders (Petaurus Breviceps). Animals 2023;13(14): 2377.

29. Russell EM. Patterns of parental care and parental investment in marsupials. BIO Rev 1982;57(3):423–86.

30. Smith M. Observations on Growth of *Petaurus breviceps* and *P. norfolcensis* (Petauridae : Marsupialia) in Captivity. Wildl Res 1979;6(2):141–50.

31. Jackson SM. Population dynamics and life history of the mahogany glider, *petaurus gracilis*, and the sugar glider, *Petaurus breviceps*, in North Queensland. Wildl Res 2000;27(1):21–37.

32. Smith MJ. Breeding the sugar-glider in captivity; and growth of pouch-young. Int Zoo Yearb 1971;11(1):26–8.

33. Klettenheimer BS, Temple-Smith PD, Sofronidis G. Father and son sugar gliders: more than a genetic coalition? J Zool 1997;242(4):741–50.

34. Sadler LM, Ward SJ. Coalitions in male sugar gliders: are they natural? J Zool 1999;248(1):91–6.

35. McCracken H. Veterinary aspects of hand-rearing orphaned marsupials. In: Vogelnest L, Woods R, editors. Medicine of australian mammals. Clayton, Victoria, Australia: CSIRO Publishing; 2008. p. 13–38.

36. Nagy K, Suckling G. Field energetics and water balance of sugar gliders, *Petaurus breviceps* (Marsupialia:Petauridae). Austr J Zool 1985;33(5):683–91.

37. Holloway JC, Geiser F. Development of thermoregulation in the sugar glider *petaurus breviceps* (marsupialia: petauridae). J Zool 2000;252(3):389–97.

38. Brust DM, Mans C. Chapter 7 - sugar gliders. In: Carpenter JW, Marion CJ, editors. Exotic animal formulary. 5th Edition. St. Louis, MO: W.B. Saunders; 2018. p. 432–42.

39. Goldingay RL. Direct male parental care observed in wild sugar gliders. Austr Mammal 2010;32(2):177.

40. Roberts M, Kohn F. A technique for obtaining early life history data in pouched marsupials. Zoo Biol 1991;10(1):81–6.

41. Johnson-Delaney C. Presenting Problem: Pouch Infection and Mastitis in Sugar Gliders. LaFeberVet, https://lafeber.com/vet/presenting-problem-pouch-infection-mastitis-sugar-gliders/. Accessed 31 July 2023.

42. Johnson-Delaney CA, Lennox AM. Reproductive disorders of marsupials. Vet Clin North Am: Exot Anim Pract 2017;20(2):539–53.

43. Bassan T, Cobos A, Mallol C, et al. Reproductive tract infection caused by *Kocuria kristinae* in an entire female sugar glider (*Petaurus breviceps*). Vet Rec Case Rep 2022;10(4). https://doi.org/10.1002/vrc2.507.

44. Punzo F, Laird A, Pedrosa E. Prenatal protein malnutrition and visual discrimination learning in the sugar glider, *Petaurus breviceps*. J Mammal 2003;84(4):1437–42.

45. Barnes M. Sugar gliders. In: Gage L, editor. Hand-rearing wild and domestic mammals. Ames, IA: Blackwell Publishing; 2002. p. 55–62, chap 9.

46. Kubiak M. Chapter 9 sugar gliders. In: Kubiak M, editor. Handbook of exotic pet medicine. Incorporated: John Wiley & Sons; 2021. p. 125–40.

Macropod Pediatrics

Jon Romano, DVM

KEYWORDS

- Macropod • Marsupial • Pediatric • Neonate • Pouch young • Kangaroo • Wallaby
- Joey

KEY POINTS

- Neonatal macropods are born highly underdeveloped and require specialized care and environment for normal development.
- The composition of macropod milk changes throughout lactation and provides offspring with growth and immune factors.
- Hypothermia, hypoglycemia, and dehydration are common life-threatening medical conditions observed in pediatric macropods.

INTRODUCTION

Marsupials are an ancient and diverse mammal group that are distinguished from eutherian mammals by several unique distinguishing features mostly involving reproductive anatomy (females have paired uteri and vaginas) and strategy (short gestation period; young born at embryonic state; extended and sophisticated lactation period during which young remain in a pouch).[1] There are approximately 68 species of marsupials belonging to the Family Macropodidae, which includes kangaroos, wallabies, wallaroos, pademelons, and the quokka (*Setonix brachyurus*).[2]

Pediatric medicine is concerned with the health, growth, and development of young organisms. Given the unique biology of macropods, the following definitions will be used throughout this article.

Neonate: from birth to several weeks of age
Juvenile: passed the neonatal phase but not yet weaned
Pediatric or young: neonates, juveniles, and subadults
Pouch young (PY): marsupial young at the preemergent phase of development (includes all neonates and some juveniles)

The health issues of pediatric patients differ from those of adults of the same species. Furthermore, the pediatric patient's response to illness and stress varies with age, developmental stage, and method of rearing. Macropod young are highly altricial

Department of Veterinary Clinical Sciences, Exotics and Lab Animal Medicine, Long Island University College of Veterinary Medicine, 720 Northern Boulevard, Brookville, NY 11548, USA
E-mail address: Jon.Romano@liu.edu

Vet Clin Exot Anim 27 (2024) 245–261
https://doi.org/10.1016/j.cvex.2023.11.007
1094-9194/24/© 2023 Elsevier Inc. All rights reserved.

at birth and require specialized environmental conditions as they mature.[2] Additionally, the small patient size, unique physiology, and developing immunocompetency are important considerations when assessing the overall health and in the treatment of the macropod pediatric patient. In general, there is limited information concerning macropod pediatrics and further research is warranted.

POSTNATAL DEVELOPMENT

At birth, neonatal macropods resemble a eutherian embryo, weigh less than 1 g, and lack a functioning immune system.[2–4] Following parturition, the young crawls from the cloaca to the pouch where it attaches to a teat and continues to develop within the nonsterile environment of the pouch. Macropods are ectothermic at birth and rely on the stable pouch environment (temperature and humidity) for thermoregulation.[2,5] Once in the pouch, neonatal macropods suckle continuously. After approximately one-third of pouch life, suckling becomes progressively intermittent. Milk composition changes considerably throughout lactation, with a gradual increase in lipids, protein, and energy content and a decrease in carbohydrates observed as the young macropod matures.[2,6,7] **Table 1** provides a summary of reproductive parameters and postnatal milestones for various macropod species.

Respiratory System

The lung structure of neonatal macropods is less developed than that of eutherian mammals and is composed of short branching airways that terminate in large saccules with a small surface area.[2,8] Cutaneous respiration has been documented in neonatal macropods; however, their primitive lungs are capable of gas exchange.[2,9] Lung development varies between macropod species but is generally slow compared with eutherian mammals.[10] The first true alveoli, characterized as the presence of single-capillary septa, are observed 65 days postpartum in the tammar wallaby (*Notamacropus eugenii*), whereas a typical alveolized lung, characterized by the presence of respiratory bronchioles, alveolar ducts, and alveolar sacs, can be observed 142 days postpartum.[9]

Pediatric mammals tend to exhibit higher minute volumes during respiration, which is a compensatory mechanism in response to having less alveolar surface area compared with adults.[6] Pliable ribs and immature ventilatory muscles pose a greater risk for respiratory fatigue in pediatric patients.[6,11,12]

Cardiovascular System

Neonatal macropods have less ability to alter cardiac contractility and preload; therefore, cardiac output is preserved via increased heart rate and low systemic vascular resistance.[6] As with most pediatrics patients, pediatric macropods poorly tolerate changes in preload and afterload and are less able to tolerate blood loss when compared to adults.[6] Young animals have immature cardiovascular systems, which justify close monitoring of heart rate during clinical evaluations.[6,11,12] Persistent bradycardia in an ill pediatric patient that fails to resolve with stabilization is a poor prognostic indicator.[6] Neonatal marsupials possess a unique form of hemoglobin that allows them to thrive in the pouch environment, with lower oxygen and higher carbon dioxide.[6,13] Given these unique findings, care should be taken when evaluating neonatal macropod hematology.

Hepatic System

At birth, the macropod liver is the site of hematopoiesis.[2,14] Gradually, as the macropod matures within the pouch, hematopoietic activity declines in the liver and bone

Table 1
Reproductive parameters and postnatal milestones of various macropod species

Macropod Species	Estrus Cycle (Days)	Gestation (Days)	Permanent Pouch Exit (Days)	Weaning (Days)	Sexual Maturity (Months)	
					Female	Male
Woylie (*Bettongia penicillate*)	22–23	21	100	130	10–12	12
Yellow-footed rock wallaby (*Petrogale xanthopus*)	32–37	31–33	190–201	210–235	18	18
Parma wallaby (*Notamacropus parma*)	41–42.5	34 ± 35	210–212	270–320	9–16	13–22
Red-necked wallaby (*Notamacropus rufogriseus*)	32–33	29–30	270–300	360–517	360–517	11–24	13–19
Tammar wallaby (*N eugenii*)	28–32	25–30	250–270	270–330	8–9	12–24
Western gray kangaroo (*Macropus fuliginosus*)	30–39	28–33	300–310	540	14–36	29–31
Common wallaroo (*Osphranter robustus*)	32–45	32	255–260	281–400	18–24	18–24
Red kangaroo (*Osphranter rufus*)	34–35	33–38	235–250	330–365	14–20	20–36

Jackson, Stephen M. (2007). Australian Mammals: Biology and Captive Management. CSIRO Publishing.

marrow becomes the primary site of hematopoiesis.[2,14] During this process, the liver matures and is involved with gastrointestinal functions.

Variations in albumin levels have been demonstrated among different pediatric macropod species.[6,15] Due to the differences in albumin levels as well as immature hepatic function, care should be taken when prescribing drugs because protein-binding and hepatic metabolism may affect their pharmacokinetics.

Renal System

The renal function of macropods in the early pediatric stage is significantly limited and is compensated with continuous milk consumption within the pouch.[2,13,16] Furthermore, drugs affected by renal clearance should be used cautiously and only when the patient is properly hydrated.

Gastrointestinal System

Shortly after birth, neonatal macropods produce the gastric hormone ghrelin, which is important for regulating appetite.[2,16–18] Given the extreme altricial state of neonatal macropods and lack of a functional immune system, establishment of the gastrointestinal microbiome is thought to be important for normal gastrointestinal development as well as to protect the host from infection and colonization by pathogenic organisms. Recent studies have demonstrated a remarkably diverse microbiome in highly immature neonates still attached to the teat.[19,20] It is important to note that the composition of milk changes as the PY develops.[21–24] Late-stage milk and plant material consumed by the emerging PY is thought to influence forestomach maturation.[2,19,25] Juvenile macropods can benefit from exposure to fresh feces from healthy adults of the same species, and fecal transplant is a specific therapy that can be used if there are concerns for gastrointestinal dysbiosis.[2,26]

Integument

Neonatal macropods are furless with very thin skin, capable of cutaneous respiration.[2,9] In addition to having thin skin, the integument also has a large water component.[2] When hand-rearing PY, care must be taken to ensure the skin is protected. These animals must be maintained in a relatively humid environment and require regular application of moisturizer. If these husbandry measures are not met, neonatal/juvenile macropods are at risk of dehydration and skin damage. Furthermore, the high-water content of the skin can enhance the absorption of topical medications and toxins.[6]

Immune Function

Although marsupials are born without a functioning adaptive immune system into a nonsterile environment, there are several complementary protective mechanisms provided by the innate immune system and maternal protective strategies, including immune compounds in the milk, prenatal transfer of immunoglobulins, antimicrobial compounds secreted from the postreproductive pouch skin, and chemical/mechanical cleaning of the pouch and the PY.[2,6,7,27]

PEDIATRIC MACROPOD CONSULTATION
History

It is important to obtain a thorough history including detailed husbandry information, as with any case involving nontraditional species, especially those involving pediatric patients. Macropods have unique husbandry requirements and caretakers should attempt to replicate environmental factors, which play a major role in normal development.[6] Caretakers should also be knowledgeable of species-specific husbandry needs and milestones.[28] **Box 1** provides a summary of important information that should be gathered during a routine history of a pediatric macropod, as well as important aspects of the physical examination and common initial diagnostics. Caretakers hand-raising a young macropod should be encouraged to take detailed notes on growth, behavior, feeding, and urination/bowel movements.[2,29] Clinicians should inspect the feeding protocol/technique and equipment to minimize the risk of inappropriate food administration and common issues such as aspiration.[2,30] The condition of the artificial pouch and moisturizing protocol should be assessed for cases involving furless joeys. It is also clinically relevant to determine the length of time the young have been separated from the dam because young macropods will lose maternal immunoglobulins 4 to 6 weeks after being separated from the dam and rely on an underdeveloped innate immune system.[2,31]

Box 1
Key components of history, husbandry, physical examination, and initial diagnostics for pediatric macropod examination

History/Husbandry
- Verify species and stage of development
- Presenting complaint
  - Duration and clinical course (improving vs deteriorating vs stable)
- Previous medical problems and treatments
- If orphaned, reasoning (ie, maternal death, rejection, and illness)
- If orphaned/hand-reared, time since separated from mother
- Housing (incubator, indoors, and outdoors)
  - Description of artificial pouch
  - Temperature (artificial pouch and ambient)
- Hygiene schedule (bottles, pouch, and disinfectants used)
- Diet
  - Formula (type and dilution rate)
  - Feeding schedule (volume per feeding and frequency of feeding)
  - Feeding technique and equipment
- Skin care (type of moisturizer and frequency of application)
- Urination/Bowel movement history
- Contact with other animals (conspecifics, domestic, or wild animals)
- Proposed fate of animal (zoo collection, return to wild, or pet)

Physical examination
- Morphimetrics (body weight and body length)
- Behavior/Demeanor
- Body temperature
- Hydration status (mucous membranes, skin turgor, and peripheral circulation)*
- Vital parameters (heart and respiratory rate/pattern)
- Assessment of skin/hair coat
- Abdominal palpation/auscultation
- Inspect cloaca/anus and any feces/urine passed
- Eye/Ear examination
- Palpate cervical thymus (if present) and lymph nodes
- Assess gate if ambulatory and for limb injuries

Initial diagnostics
- Blood glucose and electrolytes (if history/examination reveals weakness, dehydration, or anorexia)
- Radiographs (if history/examination reveals trauma)

PHYSICAL EXAMINATION

Minimal physical restraint is typically required to perform a physical examination on pediatric patients. Sedation or anesthesia of the adult female may be required if the patient is still with the dam. The physical examination of a pediatric macropod should be performed in a warm, quiet environment, with prewarmed hands. If the patient is pouch dependent, most of the examination can be performed within the artificial pouch. An artificial pouch, is typically a sac created from soft, breathable fabrics, used to raise orphaned marsupials (**Fig. 1**). The artificial pouch should be of appropriate size for the species being hand raised.

Clinicians should verify the species, estimate the patients' age, and determine if behavior is appropriate for the stage of development. The age factor of marsupial patients is defined as a proportion of the total expected pouch life (ie, an age factor of 0.5 PY has completed 50% of the expected pouch life). Knowledge of species-specific growth trajectories and milestones are vital when determining an appropriate therapeutic plan.[28] As a general rule, a guarded to poor prognosis is associated with hand-rearing a PY macropod with an age factor less than 0.4 or if still in the fixed lactation phase.[6]

A thorough physical examination should investigate all body systems. Hypothermia, hypoglycemia, and dehydration are common findings in pediatric macropods and should be corrected as soon as possible.[2] Obtaining a blood sample to assess blood glucose and electrolytes is helpful when assessing critically ill patients. Generally, additional diagnostics including, diagnostic imaging, full blood work (hematology and biochemistry), fecal examination, cytology, may be performed once the patient is stabilized. Relevant clinical information can also be obtained by performing diagnostics on the pouch environment, such as culture of the pouch.

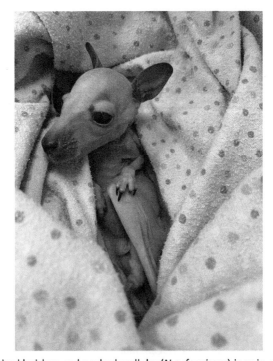

Fig. 1. A hand-raised hairless, red-necked wallaby (*N rufogriseus*) joey in an artificial pouch.

Whenever possible, pediatric macropods should be returned to a healthy dam capable of providing care rather than hand-rearing. To reduce the risk of PY being evicted from the pouch during the recovery phase, a partial temporary closure of the adult female's pouch can be accomplished using tape.

CLINICAL PATHOLOGY

At birth, the organ systems of neonates are incompletely developed and have reduced functional capacity.[6] As a result, enzyme levels and other metabolic products may vary, and clinicians should use caution when interpreting results if using reference ranges generated from adult animals.

In general, healthy juvenile macropods have lower red cell and globulin levels and elevated calcium, phosphorus, and alkaline phosphate levels compared to healthy adults. Unique fetal hematological characteristics have been observed, with some species demonstrating up to 100% nucleated erythrocytes at 1 day of age, which decreases over time.[6,13,32] Macropod young with evidence of dehydration should have renal function assessed via serum biochemistry and urinalysis.

PHARMACOLOGY/TOXICOLOGY

In general, there are limited studies investigating the effect of age on pharmacokinetics and toxicology.[33] Due to the immaturity of pediatric patient's organ systems, clinicians should exercise caution when prescribing drugs that undergo hepatic metabolism or renal elimination. Limited adipose tissue and increased water volume of pediatric patients may enhance the absorption of drugs and toxins compared to adults.[33] Clinicians should also be aware of species-specific variations that may affect the absorption/elimination of drugs or toxins. For example, juvenile brush-tailed rock-wallabies (Petrogale penicillata) have been documented to have higher albumin levels compared to adults, which may influence the bioavailability and half-life of certain drugs.[15] In general, the author prefers to use injectable drugs with macropods including pediatric patients. This limits the effect that dietary contents may have on administered drugs and minimizes the risk of dysbiosis.

NUTRITION

Milk is the primary source of nourishment for neonatal and juvenile macropods. The macronutrient composition of marsupial milk varies between species, and the concentration of the milk changes throughout lactation.[6,7,22,24] Marsupial milk also supplies growth and immune factors.[7,22] Studies have been conducted to determine the nutritional composition of milk from various macropod species and different phases of lactation. Macropods have been successfully hand-reared using various formulas, such as Wombaroo (Wombaroo Food Products, Glen Osmond, South Australia, Australia). The feeding protocol (volume and frequency), type of equipment and equipment hygiene, and appropriate environment (quiet, clean, secure, and stable temperature) are as important as the formula type used.[6,29,30]

Bovine colostrum supplements (ie, Impact bovine colostrum supplement, Wombaroo Food Products) are used by some caretakers as a nutraceutical to provide immunoglobulins to hand-reared young macropods throughout the nursing phase; however, there is little evidence to support cross-species protection.[6] After periods of anorexia/fasting, illness, or dehydration, species-appropriate formula should be diluted with water or electrolyte solutions. If well tolerated and the animal's condition continues to improve, the formula concentration can be gradually increased.

Species-appropriate solid food items (vegetation or forage) should be offered to young macropods at the time of emergence from the pouch. Many species are susceptible to gastrointestinal disorders, such as dysbiosis, at the time of weaning, and younger animals may benefit from exposure to healthy adult feces of the same species.[6,26] Alternatively, transfaunation can be achieved by mixing such feces in water or formula and fed as a slurry.

ANESTHESIA

Pediatric patients are at a higher risk of hypoxemia and hypercapnia, given the fact they have a greater tissue oxygen demand compared to adults.[34] Utilization of nonrebreathing anesthetic systems and a higher oxygen flow rate, minimizes these risks. Pediatric patients also have a higher minute volume, which can influence inhalant anesthetic absorption.[34] Factors that may influence the minute volume, including extreme temperatures, should be avoided.

Inhalant anesthetics, administered via mask induction, are most commonly used to anesthetize pediatric macropod patients. Anesthetized pediatric patients are predisposed to hypoventilation and airway collapse, especially with the use of respiratory depressant drugs such as opioids and inhalant anesthesia.[2] These findings warrant close monitoring and respiratory support during anesthetic procedures. Orotracheal intubation can be very challenging in pediatric macropods and the small diameter of the airways predisposes pediatric patients to obstruction.

Given the small size of the patient and limited glucose stores, prolonged fasting should be avoided before anesthesia. Merycism has been documented in macropods; therefore, measures should be taken to reduce aspiration pneumonia during procedures that use sedation or anesthesia, including elevating the head and tracheal intubation when appropriate.[35] It is recommended to check blood glucose every 30 minutes during and directly after anesthetic procedures, when feasible. Dextrose can be added to crystalloid fluids during prolonged anesthetic events to minimize the risk of hypoglycemia. Food should also be offered during recovery, as soon as it is safe to do so, to prevent hypoglycemia.

STABILIZING THE PEDIATRIC MACROPOD PATIENT
Hypothermia

Marsupials are ectothermic at birth and rely on the stable environment of the adult female's pouch for thermoregulation.[5] Marsupial young begin to transition to endothermy at least halfway through pouch life, and this is concurrent with the initiation of thyroid function.[2] Hypothermia is a common and life-threatening condition commonly observed in neonatal and juvenile animals, especially orphans. Rectal/cloacal or tympanic temperature can be used to determine body temperature. In general, the normal cloacal temperature of young macropods is 35.5°C to 37°C (95°F–98.6°F).[30] Hypothermia should be slowly corrected during 2 to 3 hours and the ideal ambient temperature for pediatric macropods is 32°C to 34°C (89.6°F–93.2°F).[2] Digestion may be impaired in the hypothermic patient, and therefore, these patients should not be fed until normothermy is achieved.[36] Given the lack of fur and the high surface area to body weight ratio, pediatric macropods can be rapidly warmed via external heat sources. Heating pads, forced heat blankets, and hot water bottles can be used to restore normothermy. In the author's experience, incubators and certain brooders provide the most stable environment for pediatric macropods, allowing for easier monitoring and control of monitoring of temperature and humidity. Care should be taken to avoid overheating when using these methods.

Hypoglycemia

Compared to adults, neonatal and juvenile animals have a higher demand for glucose, increased urinary loss of glucose, and decreased ability to synthesize glucose.[6,37,38] Therefore, younger animals have a higher risk of experiencing hypoglycemia, described as a blood glucose of less than 60 mg/dL (<3.3 mmol/L). If a hypoglycemic patient is alert and normothermic, glucose-containing fluids or formula may be offered orally. If the patient is unable to feed and immediate treatment is warranted, parenteral administration of 1 mL/kg of 12.5% dextrose followed by a constant rate infusion (CRI) of isotonic fluids supplemented with 1.25% to 5.0% dextrose.[2] The blood glucose of these patients should be monitored closely, if feasible.

Dehydration

Pediatric patients have higher fluid requirements compared to adults.[39] Decreased renal concentrating abilities, higher respiratory rate, and, depending on the species, higher metabolic rates result in increased fluid loss in these patients. Dehydration can quickly become life threatening, rapidly progressing to hypovolemia and shock if not addressed in a timely manner. Diarrhea and decreased feed intake are 2 common problems that can result in dehydration for the pediatric macropod patient. Alert, normothermic pediatric patients with evidence of mild dehydration can be treated with oral fluids or formula. If the animal is unable to nurse, warmed isotonic crystalloid fluids should be administered parenterally. Additionally, placement of a nasogastric or orogastric tube may be warranted in patients too weak to nurse. Intravenous fluid administration is warranted to treat severe dehydration. Large volumes of fluid administered during a short period are not tolerated well in pediatric patients. A bolus of 20 to 30 mL/kg of warm isotonic crystalloid fluid should be administered initially, followed by a CRI (60–80 mL/kg/d plus ongoing losses).[6]

Sepsis

Sepsis may develop secondary to traumatic wounds or infections of the respiratory or gastrointestinal tract. Clinical signs associated with sepsis are nonspecific and may include anorexia, decreased urine output, and cold extremities. The septic pediatric patient should be stabilized, providing heat and nutritional support. Ideally, antibiotic selection should be based on a culture and sensitivity; however, if empirical treatment is initiated, a broad-spectrum antibiotic should be selected.

Pain

Analgesia should be provided to any patient experiencing pain to facilitate normal feeding routine and physiologic functions. The judicious use of analgesics is warranted for painful conditions and procedures. Opioids should be reserved for conditions that cause moderate-to-severe pain, and patients should be monitored for respiratory depression and ileus.[40] Nonsteroidal anti-inflammatories are another commonly used analgesic; however, they should be avoided in a dehydrated patient.

COMMON PRESENTATIONS

Table 2 summarizes the most common conditions observed in pediatric macropod patients.

Infectious Diseases

Pediatric macropod patients may acquire infectious agents from the environment, from other animals (including via vertical transmission), or from human caretakers.

Table 2
Clinical signs, diagnostics, and treatment of common macropod pediatric conditions

Condition	Clinical Signs	Causes	Diagnostics	Treatment

Failure to thrive	• Poor weight gain
	• Poor skeletal growth
		• Malnutrition
		  ○ Inappropriate diet
		  ○ Inadequate food intake
		  ○ Incorrect temperature of formula
		  ○ Poor sucking reflex
		  ○ Inappropriate husbandry (ie, ambient temperature)
		  ○ Inappropriate feeding equipment
		  ○ Disease
		  ○ Stress
			• Detailed history
			• Investigate possible husbandry issues
			• Physical examination
			• Fecal examination
			• CBC/Chemistry
			• Work-up for systemic disease based on other clinical signs
				• Modification of diet
				• Modification of feeding technique and equipment
				• Nutritional support (ie, Nasogastric tube placement)
				• Supplement with bovine colostrum supplement
				• Improve husbandry conditions (ie, thermal support)
				• Treat underlying disease

Diarrhea (Noninfectious)	• Soft, loose, or watery fecal consistency incompatible with stage of development • Increased frequency of bowel movements • Cloacal/rectal prolapse	• Inappropriate diet • Poor feeding management (sudden diet changes, incorrect temperature of formula, excessive feed volumes, and irregular feeding routines) • Poor hygiene • Foreign body ingestion • Stress	• Detailed history including description and duration of diarrhea • Consider stage of development • Investigate possible husbandry issues • Abdominal imaging	• Correct hydration deficits • Consider electrolyte supplementation • Improve feeding management • Improve husbandry/hygiene • Transfaunation from a healthy adult from the same species • Application of barrier creams to cloaca to prevent dermatitis • Surgery for gastrointestinal (GI) obstruction

Condition	Clinical signs	Causes	Diagnostics	Treatment

Diarrhea (Infectious)	• Soft, loose, or watery fecal consistency incompatible with stage of development
	• Increased frequency of bowel movements
	• Cloacal/rectal prolapse
		• Bacteria
		  ○ *Escherichia coli*
		  ○ *Klebsiella*
		  ○ *Salmonella*
		  ○ *Clostridium*
		  ○ *Yersinia*
		  ○ *Campylobacter*
		• Fungal
		  ○ *Candida*
		  ○ *Torulopsis*
		• Protozoa
		  ○ *Eimeria*
		  ○ *Cryptosporidium*
		• Toxoplasmosis
			• Rule out noninfectious causes
			• Fecal examination
			  ○ Direct
			  ○ Gram stain
			  ○ Float
			• Fecal culture if not responsive to husbandry changes and supportive care
				• As above +
				• Treat specific pathogens if identified
				• If antibiotics are prescribed, consider prophylactic antiyeast therapy
				• Plasma transfusion from a healthy adult of same species
				• Transfaunation from a healthy adult from the same species

Acute abdomen	• Abdominal distension
	• Marked abdominal pain
		• Bloat
		• GI obstruction
		• Severe ileus
			• Review husbandry and nutrition
			• Physical examination
			• Abdominal imaging
			  ○ Radiographs ± contrast
			  ○ Ultrasound
				• Stabilize
				• Dietary modification
				• If fails to respond to medical therapy (fluids, analgesia, gastroprotectants, motility agents), consider surgical exploration

Skin disease	• Dry, rough, and cracking scaly skin • Localized inflammation • Alopecia/Poor hair coat • Cutaneous swelling	• Inadequate moisturization • Self-sucking of a body part • Inappropriate husbandry/pouch environment • Malnutrition • Ectoparasites • Bacterial, fungal, or viral lesion • Stress	• Signalment • History • Skin scrapes • Biopsy for histopathology and/or culture	• Correct husbandry/pouch environment • Routine application of moisturizer • Omega 3 supplementation • Provide a dummy (ie, teat) • Bandaging • Antimicrobials if appropriate

(continued on next page)

Table 2
(continued)

Condition	Clinical Signs	Causes	Diagnostics	Treatment
Traumatic fractures	• Lameness • Swelling • Inability to stand	• Trauma	• Assess environment for risk factors • Radiographs	• Reduce fractures according to small animal orthopedic principles • Euthanize if fracture type/location will result in significant dysfunction or result in welfare concerns

Pathologic fractures	• Lameness, swelling in the absence of a known traumatic event
	• Inability to stand
		• Metabolic bone disease
		  ○ Inadequate calcium intake (inappropriate formula)
		  ○ GI disease resulting in malabsorption
		  ○ Vitamin D deficiency
		  ○ Inadequate or improper exercise for stage of development
			• Obtain thorough history
			• Review husbandry practices (Mimicking the gradual emergence from the pouch is important for bone health)
			• Review nutrition
			• Nutritional analysis of feed
				• Fracture reduction
				• Pouch rest
				• Calcium/Vitamin D supplementation
				• Dietary correction
				• Euthanasia should be considered in severe cases

Respiratory disease	• May be subtle (ie, lethargy and inappetence) • Dyspnea • Nasal discharge • Respiratory stertor	• Rhinitis • Aspiration pneumonia • Infectious pneumonia	• Review history/husbandry • Physical examination • Radiographs of thorax • Culture and sensitivity • Endoscopy	• Oxygen therapy • Antimicrobials ideally on the bases of culture and sensitivity (oral, nebulized, and systemic)
Cataracts	• Clouding of the lens of one or both eyes	• Trauma • Nutritional issue • Metabolic disease • Infection • Congenital	• Review history/husbandry • Review nutrition • Thorough ophthalmic examination • Serum biochemistry • Urinalysis	• Rarely may resolve spontaneously • Surgery but prognosis is guarded due to high risk of postop complications in some cases depending on degree of pathology and surgical technique

| Oral disease | • Inappetence
• Facial swelling
• Oral plaques
• Loose or fractured teeth | • Candidiasis
• Malocclusion
• Dental or soft tissue bacterial infection | • Review history/husbandry
• Thorough oral examination (may require anesthesia) | • Fluid and nutritional support if unable or unwilling to feed
• Treat underlying problem |
| Sudden death | • Death without obvious clinical signs | • Various disease processes
  ○ Tetanus
  ○ Toxoplasmosis
  ○ GI accident
  ○ Trauma
  ○ Aspiration | • Review history/husbandry
• Necropsy examination | • Correct any predisposing factors to other animals in group on basis of necropsy examination results |

Adapted from Campbell-Ward M. Macropod Pediatric Medicine. In: Miller RE, Lamberski N, Calle P, eds. *Fowler's Zoo and Wild Animal Medicine: Current Therapy. Volume 9*. St. Louis (MO): Elsevier; 2019, pp. 500-505; with permission by Elsevier.

Young macropods have a reduced capacity to respond to infectious agents compared to adults due to their immature immune system. Hand-reared macropods do not receive the immunoglobulins from maternal milk and the pouch environment is difficult to replicate; therefore, these young animals have a higher risk of contracting infectious disease.

PREVENTATIVE MEDICINE

Various vaccines have been used in macropods. Emerging PY are typically vaccinated against clostridial organisms with a multivalent preparation marketed for livestock (ie, Vision CD-T; Merck Animal Health, De Soto, KS, USA), and then a booster is administered 4 to 14 weeks later.[6] Macropods can also be vaccinated for rabies using a killed vaccine in rabies-endemic countries (ie, Imrab 3, Merial Limited, Athens, Georgia, USA). Other vaccines that have been administered to macropods due to the presence of specific disease processes include a vaccine against *Dichelobacter nodosus* for oral necrobacillosis (lumpy jaw), a canine vaccine against *Bordetella bronchiseptica*, and an inactivated encephalomyocarditis virus vaccine.[2,41,42] Responses to vaccines are variable and sterile abscesses and swelling are commonly observed at the injection site.[1]

Although routine endoparasitic treatment or prophylaxis is considered unnecessary for most macropods, it is recommended to routinely screen for endoparasites, annually or biannually.[6,43] Treatment is reserved for individuals with high parasitic burdens or those that are clinically affected. Coccidia of the genus *Eimeria*, and less frequently *Isospora*, have been known to cause serious disease in macropods. Clinical disease is usually observed in juvenile macropods, less than a year in age, at the time of weaning when the young is exposed to contaminated pastures.[35] Coccidiosis commonly presents as a peracute form resulting in death with few clinical signs. Transmission is via ingestion. A definitive diagnosis of coccidiosis requires the identification of coccidial oocysts in a fecal float in conjunction with clinical signs. The recommended treatment of coccidiosis in macropods is toltrazuril 25 mg/kg, orally, once daily for 3 days.[35] Additionally, prophylactic antibiotics are typically administered to protect against secondary bacterial infection.[35] The prophylactic administration of plasma from immune adults to naïve juveniles as they become exposed to pastures has been successful at reducing morbidity and mortality.[35]

CROSS-FOSTERING

Cross-fostering is a complicated process and is usually reserved for cases involving threatened species. Cross-fostering is the process by which a young macropod is reared by a surrogate dam of a different taxon.[2,44] This technique provides an alternative to euthanasia for small unfurred orphans; however, it does necessitate the euthanasia of the surrogates PY. Ideally, a transferred PY remains within the pouch of the surrogate until the animal is weaned; however, cross-fostering is considered a success if the transferred PY can be raised to a stage at which hand-rearing could be confidently undertaken.

Several factors must be considered to achieve a successful cross-fostering including the relative size of the donor and surrogate females, size of PY at weaning, differences in length of pouch life between species, and size differences between the donor young and those of the surrogate species at transfer.[2,44] Additionally, adult females regulate milk composition and production irrespective of the age of the PY.[23] Therefore, transfer of a donor young to a female at a different stage of lactation can influence the growth and development of the PY.[25]

EUTHANASIA

Barbiturate overdose via intravenous injection is the preferred method of euthanasia.[45] Sedation or anesthesia may be warranted to minimize stress and facilitate intravenous access. Intraperitoneal or intrahepatic administration of barbiturates is an acceptable method of euthanasia in very small patients. Intraosseous injection is also acceptable if there is a preexisting catheter or if the animal is anesthetized before the injection. Manual methods of euthanasia performed by trained individuals including blunt force trauma and lethal shot for at-foot young are acceptable euthanasia methods if barbiturates are not available.[2]

SUMMARY

Pediatric macropod medicine is challenging given the unique anatomy, physiology, and reproductive strategy of macropods. To improve the care of pediatric macropods, clinicians should also be knowledgeable of species-specific husbandry requirements, understand normal postnatal development, and be aware of common medical conditions. Further research is warranted to improve the care and management of these animals in human care.

CLINICS CARE POINTS

- A thorough history including husbandry is warranted when examining a pediatric macropod patient.
- The macronutrient composition of marsupial milk varies between species and the concentration of milk changes throughout lactation.
- Hypothermia, hypoglycemia, and dehydration are common emergent findings in pediatric macropod patients and should be corrected as soon as possible.

DISCLOSURE

The author has nothing to disclose.

REFERENCES

1. Vogelnest L. Marsupilia (Marsupials). In: Miller RE, Fowler ME, editors. Fowler's zoo and wild animal medicine, 8. St. Louis: Elsevier/Saunders; 2015. p. 255–73.
2. Campbell-Ward M. Macropod pediatric medicine. In: Miller RE, Lamberski N, Calle P, editors. Fowler's zoo and wild animal medicine: current therapy, 9. St. Louis: Elsevier; 2019. p. 500–5.
3. Coulson G, Death C, Ritchie E, et al. Macropods. In: Smith B, Waudby H, Alberthsen C, et al, editors. Wildlife research in Australia: practical and applied methods. Clayton: CSIRO Publishing; 2022. p. 422–7.
4. Dawson T. Kangaroos. 2 edition. Collingwood: CSIRO Publishing; 2012.
5. Ferner K, Schultz J, Zeller U. Comparative anatomy of neonates of the three major mammalian groups (monotremes, marsupials, placentals) and implications for the ancestral mammalian neonate morphotype. J Anat 2017;231(6):798–822.
6. Campbell-Ward M. Pediatrics. In: Vogelnest L, Portas T, editors. Current therapy in medicine of australian mammals. Clayton: CSIRO Publishing; 2019. p. 249–65.
7. Stannard HJ, Miller RD, Old JM. Marsupial and monotreme milk—a review of its nutrient and immune properties. PeerJ 2020;8:1–31.

8. Makanya AN, Sparrow MP, Warui CN, et al. Morphological analysis of the postnatally developing marsupial lung: the quokka wallaby. Anat Rec 2001;262(3): 253–65.

9. MacFarlane PM, Frappell PB, Haase T. Respiratory characteristics of the tammar wallaby pouch young and functional limitations in a newborn with skin gas exchange. J Comp Physiol B 2021;191(6):995–1006.

10. Szdzuy K, Zeller U, Renfree M, et al. Postnatal lung and metabolic development in two marsupial and four eutherian species. J Anat 2008;212(2):164–79.

11. Farry T. Anesthesia for pediatric patients. In: Bryant S, editor. Anesthesia for veterinary technicians. Ames: Wiley-Blackwell; 2010. p. 267–74.

12. Sisak D. Anesthesia considerations: geriatric and pediatric patients. 2007. In: Proceedings of the international veterinary emergency and critical care symposium. 2007. Available at: https://www.vin.com/doc/?id=3861402&pid=0. Accessed June 12, 2023.

13. Sharman G. Adaptations of marsupial pouch young for extra-uterine existence. In: Austin C, editor. The mammalian fetus in vitro. Boston: Springer; 1972. p. 67–90.

14. Basden K, Cooper DW, Deane EM. Development of the blood-forming tissues of the tammar wallaby macropus eugenii. Reprod Fertil Dev 1996;8(6):989.

15. Barnes TS, Goldizen AW, Coleman GT. Hematology and serum biochemistry of the brush-tailed rock-wallaby (petrogale penicillata). J Wild Dis 2008;44(2): 295–303.

16. Wilkes GE, Janssens PA. The development of renal function. In: Tyndale-Biscoe CH, Janssens PA, editors. The developing marsupial: models for biomedical research. Berlin, Heidelberg: Springer; 1988. p. 176–89.

17. Pask AJ, Renfree MB. Molecular regulation of marsupial reproduction and development. In: Deakin JE, Waters PD, Graves JAM, editors. Marsupial genetics and genomics. Dordrecht: Springer; 2010. p. 285–316.

18. Menzies BR, Shaw G, Fletcher TP, et al. Early onset of ghrelin production in marsupial. Mol Cell Endocrinol 2009;299(2):266–73.

19. Chhour K, Hinds L, Jacques NA, et al. An observational study of the microbiome of the maternal pouch and saliva of the tammar wallaby, macropus eugenii, and of the gastrointestinal tract of the pouch young. Microbiology 2010;156(3): 798–808.

20. Chong R, Cheng Y, Hogg CJ, et al. Marsupial gut microbiome. Front Microbiol 2020;11:1–10.

21. Johnson-Delaney C. Captive marsupial nutrition. Vet Clin North Am Exot Pract 2014;7(3):415–57.

22. Green B, Merchant JC. The composition of marsupial milk. In: Tyndale-Biscoe CH, Janssens PA, editors. The developing marsupial: models for biomedical research. Berlin, Heidelberg: Springer; 1988. p. 41–54.

23. Trott JF, Simpson KJ, Moyle RLC, et al. Maternal regulation of milk composition, milk production, and pouch young development during lactation in the tammar wallaby (Macropus Eugenii). Biol Reprod 2003;68(3):929–36.

24. Nicholas K. Control of milk protein synthesis in the marsupial Macropus egenii: a model system to study prolactin-dependent development. In: Tyndale-Biscoe CH, Janssens PA, editors. The developing marsupial: models for biomedical research. Berlin, Heidelberg: Springer; 1988. p. 68–85.

25. Kwek JHL, De longh R, Digby MR, et al. Cross-fostering of the tammar wallaby (macropus eugenii) pouch young accelerates fore-stomach maturation. Mech Dev 2009;126(5–6):449–63.

26. Brust D. Gastrointestinal diseases of marsupials. J Exot Pet Med 2013;22(2): 132–40.
27. Edwards MJ, Hinds LA, Deane EM, et al. A review of complementary mechanisms which protect the developing marsupial pouch young. Dev Comp Immunol 2012;37(2):213–20.
28. Wombaroo: Growth and feed charts for macropods. Available at: https://www.wombaroo.com.au/product-category/native-wildlife/kangaroo/, 2023. Accessed June 8, 2023.
29. Booth R. Macropods. In: Gage L, editor. Hand-rearing wild and domestic mammals. Ames: Iowa State Press; 2002. p. 63–74.
30. McCracken H. Veterinary aspects of hand-rearing orphaned marsupials. In: Vogelnest RW, editor. Medicine of Australian mammals. Clayton: CSIRO; 2008. p. 13–38.
31. Deane EM, Cooper DW. Immunological development of pouch young marsupials. In: Tyndale-Biscoe CH, Janssens PA, editors. The developing marsupial: models for biomedical research. Berlin, Heidelberg: Springer; 1988. p. 190–9.
32. Clark P. Haematology of Australian mammals. Collingwood: CSIRO; 2004. p. 21–38.
33. Lu H, Rosenbaum S. Developmental pharmacokinetics in pediatric populations. J Pediatr Pharmacol Therapeut 2014;19(4):262–76.
34. Trachsel D, Erb TO, Hammer J, et al. Developmental respiratory physiology. Paediatr Anaesth 2022;32(2):108–17.
35. Vendl C, Munn A, Leggett K, et al. Merycism in western grey (Macropus fuliginosus) and red kangaroos (Macropus rufus). Mamm Biol 2017;86:21–6.
36. Jastrzebski P, Snarska J, Adamiak Z, et al. The effect of hypothermia on the human body. Pol Ann Med 2022;29(2):262–6.
37. Gattineni J, Baum M. Developmental changes in renal tubular transport - An orverview. Pediatr Nephrol 2015;30(12):2085–98.
38. Hume R, Burchell A, Williams FLR, et al. Glucose homeostasis in the newborn. Early Hum Dev 2005;81(1):95–101.
39. Macintire D. Pediatric Fluid Therapy. Vet Clin North Am Exot Pract 2008;38(3): 621–7.
40. Imam MZ, Kuo A, Ghassabian S, et al. Progress in understanding mechanisms of opioid-induced gastrointestinal adverse effects and respiratory depression. Neuropharmacology 2018;131:238–55.
41. Vogelnest L, Portas T. Macropods. In: Vogelnest L, Woods R, editors. Medicine of Australian mammals. Clayton: CSIRO; 2008. p. 133–226.
42. Smith J. Macropod Medicine. In: Proceedings of the American Association of Zoo Veterinarians. 2011. Available at: https://www.vin.com/doc/?id=5223076. Accessed Jun 8, 2023.
43. Cripps J, Beveridge I, Ploeg R, et al. Experimental manipulation reveals few subclinical impacts of a parasite community in juvenile kangaroos. Int J Parasitol Parasites Wildl 2014;3(2):88–94.
44. Taggart DA, Schultz D, Fletcher TP, et al. Cross-fostering and short-term pouch isolation in macropodoid marsupials: implications for conservation and species management. In: Eldridge C, editor. Macropods: the biology of kangaroos, wallabies and rat-kangaroos. Collingwood: CSIRO; 2010. p. 263–78.
45. American Veterinary Medical Association: AVMA Guidelinesfor the Euthanasia of Animals:2020 Edition. Schaumburg, Illinois, 2020. Available at: https://www.avma.org/sites/default/files/2020-02/Guidelines-on-Euthanasia-2020.pdf. Accessed June 9, 2023.

Psittacine Neonatology and Pediatrics

Mikel Sabater González, LV, MRCVS, CertZooMed, DipECZM (Avian)

KEYWORDS

- Neonatology • Pediatric • Psittaciformes • Avian • Preventive medicine

KEY POINTS

- Psittacine neonates are totally dependent on the constant care of a rearer for nutrition and thermoregulation. Additionally, they lack of a fully competent immune system, which makes them more predisposed to diseases than adult individuals.
- Neonatal rearing alternatives include parental and foster (including hand-rearing), each of which present advantages and disadvantages.
- Psittacine collections, including their nurseries, benefit from having well-designed facilities and following the principles of the closed aviary concept.
- Neonates and pediatric psittacine patients present anatomic and physiologic similarities but also differences when compared to adults of the same species. A good understanding of both is paramount for the correct prevention and management of medical disorders.
- Infecto-contagious diseases may affect neonates and adults differently and, therefore, may require different diagnostic and therapeutic approaches.

INTRODUCTION

Psittacine neonates are altricial (require nourishment and care), have high metabolic rates and low energetic reserves, and are born without feathers and with the eyelids and otic canals closed, which makes them totally dependent on the constant care of a rearer for nutrition and thermoregulation (**Fig. 1**). Additionally, they lack a fully competent immune system, which makes them more predisposed to develop some diseases than adult individuals.

Their health and development are influenced by multiple factors (eg, genetics, incubation, hatching, nutrition, environmental conditions, and diseases). Understanding these factors and controlling them as much as possible results in a healthier population.

This article aims to discuss the neonatological and pediatric care of psittacine chicks, the diagnosis and treatment of their most common disorders, and to provide minimal management guidelines to attempt to achieve a collection free of infecto-contagious disease.

Veterinary Specialist, Manor Vets Edgbaston, 371, 373 Hagley Road, Birmingham B17 8DL, UK
E-mail address: exoticsvet@gmail.com

Vet Clin Exot Anim 27 (2024) 263–293
https://doi.org/10.1016/j.cvex.2023.11.008
1094-9194/24/© 2023 Elsevier Inc. All rights reserved.

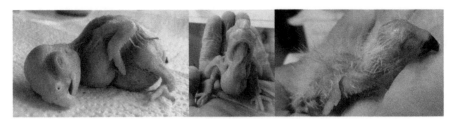

Fig. 1. Psittacine neonates are altricial, have high metabolic rates and low-energetic reserves, and are born without feathers and with the eyelids and otic canals closed.

PARENTAL REARING STRATEGIES

In ecology, the r/K selection theory classifies individuals based on the quantity and quality of their offspring. R-selected species reach sexual maturity relatively early, have short reproductive cycles, lay large clutches of eggs, and provide low parental care. This results in large offspring where individuals have to rely more on their instinctive survival abilities and have low probabilities of surviving to adulthood. Contrarily, K-selected species present longer life spans, reach sexual maturity later, and lay fewer eggs per clutch but parents invest more time rearing and teaching their chicks, which results in stronger social bonds and increases their chances of survival. Small psittacines such as budgerigars (Melopsittacus undulatus) are classified as predominantly r-selected species, whereas larger species such as macaws and cockatoos are considered predominantly K-selected species.[1]

Most psittacines are monogamous but polygynous, polyandrous, and polygynandrous species (eg, vasa parrots [Coracopsis spp], eclectus parrots [Eclectus spp], kakapos [Strigops habroptilus], or golden conures [Guaruba guarouba]) have been reported. Additionally, collaborative breeding, in which multiple females take care of the nestlings, has been reported in some species (eg, golden conures, monk parakeets [Myiopsitta monachus], or El Oro parakeets [Pyrrhura orcesi]). Behavioral studies in El Oro parakeet revealed that parents of this species show dominance over helpers but do not enforce them to provide alloparental care.[2]

NEONATE REARING ALTERNATIVES

Biological parent-rearing, foster-rearing (foster parents from the same or different species, including humans) or a combination of these 2 options are alternatives reported when rearing psittacine neonates and each of them presents advantages and disadvantages.

Parent-rearing requires less time and economic resources than most foster-rearing options. Moreover, parent-reared chicks show faster initial development when compared with foster-reared ones and have more chances to develop species-specific behaviors that may result in higher reproductive success.[3,4] A study in cockatiels (Nymphicus hollandicus) showed that (1) pairs containing hand-reared females were more likely to lay eggs and laid more eggs than pairs with parent-reared females but often laid them on the cage floor rather than in nest boxes, reducing hatching success; (2) pairs containing hand-reared males were less likely to produce fertile eggs, inspect nest-boxes or lay eggs in nest-boxes than pairs with parent-reared males; and (3) fledging occurred only in pairs containing parent-reared males. The authors suggested that early rearing experience was important for males to learn the characteristics of the opposite sex and for both males and females to learn the characteristics of nest sites.[4]

Disadvantages of parent-rearing include relying on breeding pairs that are not good parents and may traumatize the egg or the chick, a higher exposure of the chick to external hazards, and potential lower control over parental and environmental factors. Technological advances in nest monitoring and nest settings have significantly improved the control over the environment and reduced the stress of the chicks and parents associated with their monitoring.

Fostering has been reported in wild birds (eg, rainbow lorikeets [*Trichoglossus moluccanus*] raising scaly-breasted lorikeet [*Trichoglossus chlorolepidotus*] eggs after taking over the parent nest). The contribution of fostering to explain the presence of hybrid individuals (eg, scaly-breasted lorikeet × rainbow lorikeet, and gallarella [galah, *Eolophus roseicapilla*] × little corella [*Cacatua sanguinea*]) in some wild flocks has not been completely understood. Different fostering methods have been used to rear psittacine chicks. Eggs (preferably) or chicks may be moved from the parents' nest to a foster's nest, which may belong to the same or to a different species.

Fostering allows for an increased chick production. Depending on the species, the reproductive couple may produce more eggs. In determinate egg-layer species, the number of eggs laid in a clutch is determined at the onset of laying and cannot be changed by the external removal or addition of eggs. For example, cockatiels are determinate layers who lay between 3 and 8 eggs and stop laying when they reach their limit. Contrarily, indeterminate layers respond to either the removal or addition of eggs while laying by producing more or less eggs. However, this classification does not fully reflect the observations made in some species. For example, budgerigars, a species that lays an egg every 2 days and begins incubation with the first egg, are indeterminate if the first egg is removed shortly after it was laid but are determinate if the first egg remained in the nest, and unlike many altricial species, clutches of budgerigars hatch almost completely asynchronously.[5] Therefore, a reclassification of indeterminate layers was suggested: (1) removal indeterminacy, in which birds respond to egg removal by laying additional eggs; (2) addition indeterminacy, in which birds respond to egg addition by laying fewer eggs than normal; and (3) removal-and-addition indeterminacy, in which birds respond to egg removal by laying more eggs than normal and to egg addition by laying fewer eggs than normal.[5] Fostering also allows the use of infertile or suboptimal fertile couples as foster parents. Some highly domesticated species have shown excellent fostering skills. For example, there are anecdotal reports of double yellow-headed Amazon parrots (*Amazona oratrix*) rearing major Mitchell's cockatoos (*Cacatua leadbeateri*) to independence, rearing yellow-shouldered Amazon parrots (*Amazona barbadensis*) and one golden conure in the same nest, or an egg of a blue-fronted Amazon parrot (*Amazona aestiva*) fostered by gray parrots (*Psittacus erithacus*) and reared to independence.[6] Psittacines start incubation after a minimal number of eggs have been laid. In general, eggs are incubated by female psittacines but in some species (eg, cockatoos, blue lorikeet [*Vini peruviana*], and vernal hanging parrots [*Loriculus vernalis*]) both species feed the chicks. Most psittacine species will not incubate for more than 1 week past the expected hatch date. Although most eclectus parrot females only incubate eggs for one or 2 days past the incubation period of 28 days, some Amazon parrots continue to incubate eggs well past their incubation period. The case of a yellow-crowned Amazon parrot (*Amazona ochrocephala*; average incubation period of 27 days) incubating for 47 days a yellow-shouldered Amazon parrot egg has been also reported.[6]

The main disadvantage of fostering is that chicks may be carriers or may be exposed to trauma or infectious diseases during and after relocation. Placing an egg larger than the ones in the nest may reduce the chances of egg-breaking in parents prone to do this (eg, placing an infertile Amazon parrot egg in a blue-throated conure [*Pyrrhura cruentata*] nest).[6] When adding eggs to a nest, it is important to consider the number of eggs to add and the moment to do it. Gray parrots have an average clutch size of 3 eggs. Females tend to accept 1 or 2 additional eggs provided they are added while they are still laying. However, once the clutch is completed, adding more eggs is likely to be successful only if the same number of infertile or non-hatchable eggs are removed.[6] As expected, the best moment to add or remove eggs from a clutch is when the parents or foster parents leave the nest. The use of visual barriers preventing the psittacine parents from seeing humans when checking or making changes in the nests reduce their levels of stress.

Hand-rearing tends to produce, at least temporarily, more human-socialized chicks, a higher success rate (eg, saving weak or ill chicks and providing optimal environmental and nutritional conditions) and reduces the transmission of some contagious diseases. Studies in captive orange-winged Amazon parrots (*Amazona amazonica*) and cockatiels showed that early behavioral experiences, specifically being handled by humans during the nestling stage, can influence not only tameness but also immune status and, in cockatiels, adult reproductive performance.[4,7] Another study in orange-winged Amazon parrots incubated and hatched by wild-caught parents and handled by humans at various times (10–20 minutes a day from days 10–39 of age or 10–20 minutes a day from 40 days to fledging) revealed that they were tamer after fledging than the control group, which was only held for weight monitoring. In a second trial, handled chicks were handled for 30 minutes 4 times/week either from days 15 to 36 or 35 to 56, and results were similar to the first trial.[8] Another study in this species revealed that (1) until 6 months of age, parent-reared chicks human-held for 20 minutes 5 times a week between 2 and 8 weeks of age were groomed by their parents significantly more than parent-reared birds; (2) hand-reared birds were significantly less neophobic than parent-reared and parent-reared-human-held birds until 6 months of age; and (3) at 1 year of age, all the groups exhibited comparable levels of neophobia. The study concluded that development of neophobia in this species is not related to parental care but may be related to the level of novelty that the chicks experience during early life.[9] Finally, the influence of neonatal handling on behavior and immune function has been also assessed in this species. Chicks were gently handled for 10 minutes daily from 25 days of age until 38 days postfledging, whereas control chicks were not handled. Greater delayed-type hypersensitivity response to phytohemagglutinin-P injection and serum corticosterone levels were observed in nonhandled chicks.[10]

The main disadvantages of hand-rearing are the higher economical and time requirements. Additionally, a study performed in red-fronted macaws (*Ara rubrogenys*) and crimson-bellied conures (*Pyrhurra perlata*) revealed that hand-reared chicks showed growth-rate deficits when compared with parent-raised chicks.[3] However, this deficit was alleviated by allowing the parents to raise the chicks for the first week of life and beginning hand-rearing thereafter, suggesting that initial parental care seems to improve maintenance of normal growth rates in parrots.[3] Hand-reared gray parrots were more aggressive and more selective toward humans and begged for food more often than parent-raised ones. In addition, hand-reared chicks that were aged less than 5 weeks when removed from the nest developed stereotypies more often than chicks that stayed longer with their parents.[11]

Psittacines require exposure to individuals from the same species to develop species-specific identities (eg, social behaviors and communications and to establish their sexual preferences). However, learning differences have been reported between species. For example, vertical transmission of learned vocal signatures from both parents has been experimentally demonstrated in wild green-rumped parrotlets (*Forpus passerinus*), whereas Meyer's parrots (*Poicephalus meyeri*) use the male as their vocal tutor.[12,13]

Sexual imprinting refers to the process by which animals learn the characteristics of appropriate mates by learning the characteristics of their parents or siblings.[14] Galahs naturally cross-fostered to the sympatric major Mitchell's cockatoo imprint on their foster parents and only associate and mate with major Mitchell's cockatoos during adulthood.[15] In hand-reared cockatiels, serious deficits in reproductive behavior probably related to abnormal sexual and/or habitat imprinting have been reported.[4] Sexual imprinting also occurs in other parrot species (eg, budgerigars and Senegal parrots [*Poicephalus senegalus*]).[16]

Attempts to reintroduce a fostered chick to an established group of individuals should be performed under direct or remote monitoring and in facilities providing enough escape, protection, drinking, feeding, and resting alternatives to minimize stress and aggressions.

DESIGN AND MEDICAL MANAGEMENT OF A PSITTACINE NURSERY

Psittacine collections benefit from having well-designed facilities and following the principles of the closed aviary concept. However, the economical expenses related with this may be difficult to assume for small commercial and noncommercial collections.

In the wild, most parrots nest high over the ground in tree cavities already existing ranging from 0.5 to 1 m in depth and with entrance diameters proportional to their body size.[17] Some species (eg, *Brotogeris* spp and *Aratinga* spp) excavate holes in arboreal termite nests, whereas others (eg, golden-shouldered parrots [*Psephotellus chrysopterygius*] and red-faced lovebirds [*Agapornis pullarius*]) do it in terrestrial ones.[18] Cliff-nesting is observed in several species (eg, maroon-fronted parrot [*Rhynchopsitta terrisi*] and Lear's macaw [*Anodorhynchus leari*]). The rock parrot (*Neophema petrophila*) nests only in rock crevices just above the high-tide mark on the south Australian coast. Patagonian conures (*Cyanolyseous patagonicus*) and some of the *Bolborhynchus* spp dig burrows into banks or cliffs. Few species (eg, ring-necked parakeets [*Psittacula krameri*] and black-winged lovebirds [*Agapornis taranta*]) have adapted to nesting in gaps in masonry.[18] Very few species construct nests by carrying nesting material into cavities. The monk parakeet is able to build large communal stick nests (in which each pair has its own nest chamber), whereas lovebirds (*Agapornis* spp) carry materials, sometimes tucking them between their rump feathers, to line their nest-chambers. Some lovebirds (eg, Fischer's lovebirds [*Agapornis fischeri*] and yellow-collared lovebirds [*Agapornis personatus*]) and the hanging parrots (*Loriculus* spp) construct domed nests with grass.[18] Ground parrots (eg, *Pezoporus wallicus*, *Pezoporus flaviventris*, and *Pezoporus occidentalis*) and Antipodes green parakeets (*Cyanoramphus unicolor*) lay their eggs in a shallow depression on the ground beneath a bush or tussock.[18] Finally, keas (*Nestor notabilis*) and kakapos (*S habroptilus*) nest in rock crevasses, holes, and under logs.

To meet their resource requirements, parrots use resource selection strategies of hierarchical nest site selection to increase the likelihood of nest success, and plasticity in dietary and foraging strategies to track variable food resources.[17]

In order to successfully breed, captive psittacines require adequate nests and, in some occasions, additional materials to complete them. Artificial nest box shape preferences have been reported for different parrot species.[19]

Environmental control is not restricted to indoor facilities. Cooling and heating systems have been successfully used in outdoor nest boxes or facilities.[20] Thermostats, hygrometers, smoke detectors, and monitoring cameras are examples of widely affordable technological equipment that can be accessed, even remotely, and allow better monitoring and control of environmental conditions.

The nursery is one of the most important critical points of control in a successful production system, understanding production not only from the economical point of view but also from an ecological perspective. Therefore, an appropriate design and management of the nursery is paramount not only to optimize production but also to provide long-term sustainability to the breeding collection (eg, minimizing transmission of contagious diseases or suggesting the need of changes in the management of breeding stock). The application of new technological advances (eg, aforementioned monitoring systems or unidirectional negative pressure ventilation systems with biological filters) and large data recording and processing allows for a more efficient management of the nursery, which results in a more successful management of the collection.

The incubation and hatching areas should be physically separated from the nursery. Eggshell contamination with feces and/or dirt may allow access of microorganisms to the internal egg membranes and the developing embryo through the shell pores if the cuticle covering them is damaged. Therefore, eggs should be correctly disinfected (eg, with diluted F10 SC disinfectant [Health and Hygiene (Pty) Ltd., Randburg, South Africa] and alcohol) before accessing the incubation area.[21] Eggs and chicks coming from parents that have not been screened for contagious diseases should never be mixed with those coming from parents that have been screened until they have been tested negative. In addition, birds hatched in nests and birds hatched in incubators should not be mixed until tested negative for contagious diseases in which horizontal transmission has been proven.

To minimize transmission of contagious diseases, the nursery should be physically divided in separate areas: (1) chicks not tested for contagious diseases; (2) chicks tested but pending on results; and (3) birds tested negative. The flow of movement of chicks should always follow this order, whereas staff and the negative pressure airflow system filtered by bio-security filters should flow inversely unless each room has its own independent extraction system (**Fig. 2**). Each area of the nursery needs subdivisions separated by physical barriers (including biosecurity filters for air), individual ventilation, temperature, and humidity control, individual feeding areas with individual feeding tools, good water quality, nonporous and easy to disinfect walls, floors, and ceiling, back-up electrical system or electric alarm, adequate containers that can be readily disinfected and adequate substrate (**Figs. 3** and **4**). Additionally, a quarantine site and an area for ill chicks or chicks suspected to carry contagious diseases must be created separated from the nursery. Each of these areas must have an independent entry and an independent negative pressure ventilation system with biosecurity air filters and be fully equipped with all the requirements to take care (eg, food, water, food bowls, cleaning equipment, and so forth) and monitor the chicks (**Fig. 5**).

Nestlings from other collections should never be introduced in the nursery unless correctly quarantined and tested negative for contagious diseases before admission. Adequate pest and predator control protocols should be established. Humans should not be allowed to visit the nursery after having been in contact with birds that have not tested negative for contagious disorders. Barrier methods to prevent transmission of diseases should be used within the facilities and should be specific for each area. Rooms must be fogged routinely with an adequate disinfectant. Birds tested negative for contagious diseases should never be mixed with nontested birds. Potentially contagious birds should be immediately separated. Birds that leave the nursery and have

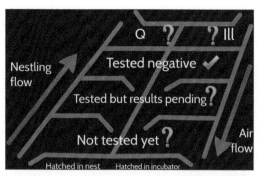

Fig. 2. Proposed ideal design of a psittacine nursery. Chicks hatched in the nest and those hatched in the incubator do not mix and advance to the following area once tested or confirmed (when possible) negative for infecto-contagious diseases. Staff must follow the inverse direction unless different members of the staff work at each section. Airflow should follow the inverse direction unless each room can have totally independent air extraction systems. The quarantine and the isolation areas have separated entrances.

not been individually isolated should not be reintroduced unless correctly quarantined and tested negative for contagious diseases.

Optimal chick growth requires correct environmental conditions for the species starting the moment the chick hatches. In general, neonates require environmental temperatures ranging from 34°C to 37°C (93°F–98°F) and humidity ranging from 24% to 76% for the first month and a half of life.[22] However, the precise conditions required may vary depending on the species and the age of the chick. Temperature and humidity supplementation must be reduced progressively until the bird is able to physiologically tolerate environmental conditions. The nest where the chick is kept must have the correct shape and be made of safe materials. Immediately after hatching, chicks can be placed in small containers lined with paper towels. This may allow for easy visual examination of droppings and provide a padded surface

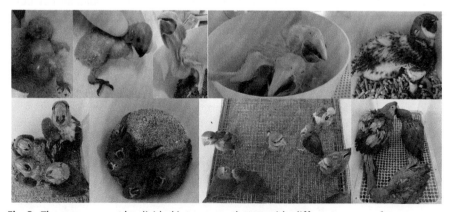

Fig. 3. The nursery must be divided into spaces that provide different ranges of temperature (note the temperature recorder in the right corner of the composite), humidity, and containment. The barriers must prevent air-borne transmission of diseases, and the air must be filtered by filtering face piece 2 (FFP2) or N95 filters. Once birds have tested negative for contagious diseases, chicks could be placed in a room in which they share the same air (bottom right).

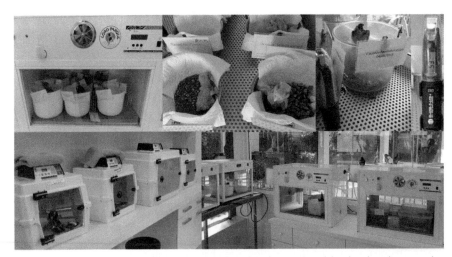

Fig. 4. Examples of containers (eg, feeding bowls, planters, and buckets), substrates (eg, kitchen paper, plastic mesh, paper pellets, wood chips, metal mesh, and combinations of these) and incubators useful when rearing psittacines.

in order to prevent trauma to their fragile bodies. After the first month and a half, chicks can be moved into larger containers lined with paper towels, mesh, or nontoxic substrate that is not easily ingested or aspirated (see **Fig. 4**).

A correct environmental design (eg, correct lighting, ultraviolet B light exposure, temperature, humidity, behavioral enrichment, and spaces that provide the sensation of protection) is also paramount for the healthy development of the individual.

A study in juvenile orange-winged parrots showed that behavioral enrichment reduced both the fear response to novel objects and the motivation to explore and interact with them and reduced fear responses to unfamiliar human handlers.[23] Another study in the same species showed that rotation of enrichment objects was more effective than providing enrichments alone in reducing neophobia but both enrichment object properties and individual differences should be carefully considered when providing behavioral enrichment.[24]

A study involving 80 captive bred nanday conure (*Aratinga nenday*) chicks of which 48 were assigned as test subjects concluded that enhancing their rearing environment

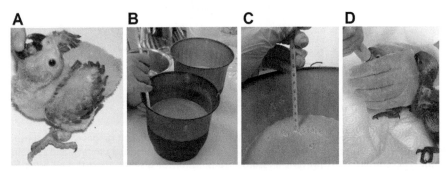

Fig. 5. (*A*) Feeding response assessment of a gray parrot; (*B, C*) Stirring a liquid diet and measuring its temperature before feeding it to chicks; (*D*) Syringe feeding of a juvenile gray parrot.

through enrichment and handling improved their psychological and physical well-being.[25]

Nutrition

Parents must be fed nutritionally complete species-specific diets including large amounts of fresh produce plus breeder pelleted diets. Additionally, controlled amounts of seeds, always proportional to the species size, can be offered. Vitamin and mineral supplements must be only supplemented when the minimal requirements of the species cannot be met. Caution must be taken not to overdose with vitamins and minerals. Reported embryonal abnormalities associated with nutritional deficiencies in the parents include fetal malformations associated with vitamin A deficiency; abnormal mineralization of bones and beak malformations associated with vitamin D, niacin, and biotin deficiencies; and incomplete abdominal closure associated with parental iodine deficiency.[26]

Scientific research in psittacine neonate nutrition remains relatively limited. The nutrition of 15 commercially available parrot hand-feeding formulas were compared with the average content of the crops of free-living scarlet macaw (Ara macao) chicks. The concentration of crude protein in the formulas was higher than that of the crop sample average, whereas the crude fat was lower than the average crop samples. More than 50% of the formulas had concentrations of potassium, magnesium, and manganese lower than the crop sample average.[27] Fatty acid profiles of crop contents of free-living nestlings of 5 psittacine species and of 15 commercial hand-feeding formulas have been studied.[28] The mean fatty acid concentration of the crop samples of each species ranged from 15% to 53% dry matter for crop samples and ranged from 6% to 22% for hand-feeding formulas. Long-chain fatty acids represented more than 92% of all fatty acids in the crop samples and more than 81% in the commercial formulas. Similar saturation profiles of crop samples were observed (ranging between 13% and 29% saturated fatty acids, 12% and 40% monounsaturated fatty acids, and 39% and 58% polyunsaturated fatty acids. All psittacines, except for the red-and-green macaw (Ara chloropterus), were within the range of values for hand-rearing formulas. Differences in the predominant saturated and monounsaturated fatty acids were observed between species, whereas linoleic acid was the most common polyunsaturated fatty acid in both avian species and commercial diets.

The type of diet must be selected based on its nutritional composition in order to provide the nutrients required and in the correct proportion to meet the nutritional requirements of the species. When the commercial diets available are not meeting the nutritional requirements, supplementation (eg, minerals, vitamins, fat, and so forth) must be considered.

Monitoring and comparing the growth rates for individuals of the same species maintained under similar environmental conditions is an invaluable tool to improve performance and to assess the response to dietary adjustments. Studies comparing growing rates with different hand rearing diets have been published.[29,30]

Adequate feeding practices should be established. The dry feeding formula must be stored in a dry, cool, and clean area. Opened dry food containers may need to be stored in the fridge or freezer based on manufacturer recommendations. The feeding formula must be carefully measured and mixed with clean warm water. The mixed formula must be warmed and contain 0% to 10% solids for chicks aged 1 day. The percentage of solids may be progressively increased to 23% to 27% by day 6 or 7 of life. Some breeders recommend to provide only isotonic hydroelectrolyte solutions supplemented or not with glucose (final solution of 5%) for the first day or first couple of days of life until the potential excess of fluid of the recently hatched chick has evaporated or reabsorbed. Supplementation with *Lactobacillus* spp is relatively common in some large breeding institutions. Feeding frequency must progressively decrease from 7 times a day for the first couple of days, to 4 or 5 times a day on day 3 of life, and to 3 times a day by the time pin feathers open, at which point solid food may be introduced. Chicks do not need to be fed during the night because they need to rest and empty their crops. In general, the amount of formula fed each time ranges approximately between 10% and 12% (eg, cockatoos may be fed 10% and macaws 12%–14%) of body weight. The use of microwaves to warm the formula is controversial because increased temperature is achieved at the core of the container and incorrect stirring after heating may result in uneven distributions of temperature within the formula that may result in incorrect temperature readings and digestive burns after administration. Alternatively, feeding formulas can be warmed using water baths or fluid warmers (eg, bottle warmers) The final temperature of the feeding formula may be checked and may vary between 38.9°C and 42.2°C (102°F and 108°F) depending on the species and age of the chick (see **Fig. 4**). Any unused formula should be disposed and not reused later. Chicks can be force-fed using individual syringes with or without syringe tips (useful in very small individuals), soft or hard feeding tubes, or spoons (the sides of the spoon may be bent dorsally in order to adjust better to the shape of the beak). A study in gray parrots' hand-fed using tubes showed that they were more aggressive and were in poorer health than chicks fed using syringes or spoons.[11] All the equipment directly contacting the chick must be disposable or suitable for sterilization or correct disinfection. If the feeding tool touches the chick, it must not be placed back into the feeding formula.

Solid food (eg, fruit, vegetables, or pellets) may be offered once chicks are fed twice a day. If food is placed at the bottom of the container or over a mirror to promote chick interest in it, care should be taken to prevent fecal contamination and ingestion. The size and hardness of the solid food provided must be in accordance with the size of the chick, in order to prevent impactions. Chicks must be inspected regularly to remove any remaining formula or soft food attached to the skin. Water bowls can be introduced when chicks are fed once a day and must be shallow enough to prevent drowning, securely fixed to prevent trauma and routinely disinfected and refilled to prevent microbial overgrowth. Chicks must be completely weaned only when able to eat enough by themselves.

MEDICAL CARE OF HAND-REARED PSITTACINE CHICKS
Systematic Analysis of Medical Records

Systematic and routine analysis of medical records allows an earlier detection of problems and a consequently an earlier response. Chicks should be individually identified (eg, microchipped, rings, nontoxic nail polisher, and so forth) and examined at least once a day. Complete medical histories for the individual, the parents, and siblings should be systematically recorded and reviewed. Important data to be recorded include but it is not restricted to daily accurate weight (before first feeding), environmental records (during incubation, hatching, and growing), dietary records (eg, composition), date of eye and ears opening, and date of first appearance of head, tail, and wing feathers. Traceability records (eg, locations, companions in the same enclosures, dates of movements, and so forth) are also important.

In general, weight loss may occur in the first 24 to 48 hours after hatching. Slow growth is expected until the fourth day of life. From day 5 to weaning, psittacine chicks tend to gain weight and fluctuations may be the consequence of feeding or environmental techniques. Usually, before weaning, the weight of the chick may exceed the adult average weight for the species. During weaning, loss of 10% body weight is considered acceptable provided the body weight before weaning was adequate (**Figs. 6 and 7, Table 1**). Weaning ages depend on the species but differences between parent-raised and hand-reared chicks from the same species have also been reported[31] (**Table 2**).

However, each species has different growth rates and behaviors, and when previous information is not available for a given species under a specific diet and environmental conditions, evaluating closer published resources may be useful to optimize their development (**Fig. 8**).[32]

Physical Examination and Medical Conditions Commonly Observed in Neonate Psittacines

Physical examination should be performed just before feeding. During physical examination, the chick may remain warm and bio-security measures (eg, gloves, coats, disinfectants, and so forth) should be applied. Chicks with food in the crop should be carefully handled to minimize risk of regurgitation and aspiration.

The levels of brightness, activity and response to stimuli, as well as gait should be assessed before and after handling the chick. Feeding response, vigorous swallowing movements on response to food administration, or applying gentle pressure on the commissures of the beak should also be evaluated (see **Fig. 4**). Weight should be systematically and accurately recorded at least once a day, ideally before the first feeding. Body condition should be evaluated by assessing the degree of muscle development (lower in nonflying chicks than in flying ones) and the amount of subcutaneous (SC) fat. Moreover, chicks must be routinely auscultated, palpated, and have their temperature checked. Small chicks can be transilluminated, if needed. Different species may show different gaits and behaviors. For example, cockatoos tend to sit on their hocks, whereas macaws prefer to lay down. Eyelids are first opened between 10 and 14 days of age in budgerigars and cockatiels; 10 and 21 days in cockatoos, conures, and lorikeets; 14 and 21 days in Amazon parrots; and 14 and 28 days in macaws. A small amount of clear discharge may be normal immediately after their opening.

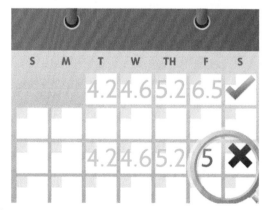

Fig. 6. Example of weight monitoring chart for 2 different chicks. The chick in the first row is apparently gaining weight normally, whereas the one in the third row is showing an abnormal weight gain. The following day, if the weight of the second chick has not increased, closer monitoring is indicated.

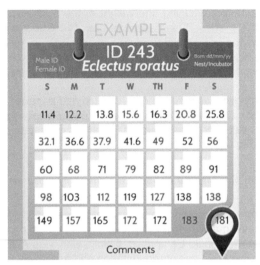

Fig. 7. Example of a normal weight record sheet for an eclectus chick.

Congenital (eg, bilateral anophthalmia in a budgerigar, cryptophthalmia, ankyloble-pharon, and entropion in cockatiels, and familial cataracts in scarlet macaws) and ac-quired ocular disorders have been reported.[33,34] Ears open at hatching in Old World psittacines. Eclectus parrots and macaws have their ear canals covered with a mem-brane that will open after a couple of days of life and after 23 days, respectively.[35] Occluded ear openings can be easily diagnosed visually but diagnostic imaging tech-niques may be useful to assess normality of the underlying structures before consid-ering its surgical opening.

Table 1 Example of normal weight gain in a macaw chick from birth to weaning						
Week 1	20.9	20.8	23.6	26.8	30.3	36	43.9
Week 2	54	64	75	81	90	103	115
Week 3	132	155	173	188	201	211	233
Week 4	264	289	333	357	383	396	433
Week 5	465	494	525	553	586	598	605
Week 6	643	673	684	733	736	749	812
Week 7	806	854	888	918	899	936	954
Week 8	980	995	1014	1026	1038	1070	1082
Week 9	1098	1099	1129	1118	1149	1146	1142
Week 10	1162	1160	1167	1152	1144	1136	1149
Week 11	1130	1125	—	—	—	—	—

Weight loss may be observed during the first couple of days of life. After this, the weight should increase, although external factors may contribute to 1 to 2 d of weight loss (eg, overfeeding or underfeeding 1 d, stress factors, and so forth). This should not be a problem if after 1 or 2 d the weight increases again. Weight loss may also be observed when the feathers are grown (transitory weight drop) or when the chick is weaned because they get more reluctant to accept forced feeding. Note that the normal weight for a weaned juvenile is species-specific and may be slightly lower than the maximum weight observed while force-fed.

Table 2
Weaning ages (in days) reported for parent-raised and hand-raised chicks of some psittacine species

	Parent-Raised	Hand-Raised
Budgerigar	30–40	30
Lovebird	45–55	40–45
Cockatiel	45–52	42–49
Conures	45–70	60
Lory/lorikeet	62–70	50–60
Galah	90–120	80–90
Small macaw	90–120	75–90
Ring-necked parakeet	55–65	
Gray parrot	100–120	75–90
Eclectus parrot	120–150	100–110
Amazon parrot	90–120	75–90
Medial size cockatoo	90–120	75–100
Large size cockatoo	120–150	95–120
Large macaw	120–150	95–120

Source: Sánchez-Migallón Guzmán D, Beaufrére H, Welle KR, et al. Birds. In: Carpenter JW, Harms CA. Carpenter's exotic animal formulary. Sixth edition. Elsevier 2022:223 to 444.

Integumentary system

The skin should be yellow to pink. Dehydration may be suspected in chicks with a dry, hyperemic, and sticky skin. SC edema, paleness, or dermatitis are abnormal and should be investigated. External parasites should be treated with fipronil, ivermectin, selamectin, and so forth. Integumentary disorders may be congenital (eg, polydactyly or syndactyly) or acquired. Toe constriction is normally a consequence of environmental humidity lower than 40% (**Fig. 9**).[36] If left untreated, the condition results in avascular necrosis of the digit tips due to the constriction. Treatment includes restoring hydration and surgical removal of the skin ring compromising the blood supply to the end of the toe, topical dimethyl sulfoxide, systemic anti-inflammatories, and sometimes external coaptation and/or topical or systemic antimicrobials.

The feathers of the head, wings, and tail are the first ones visible. The presence of stress bars is indicative of stress or metabolic disturbances on the day that portion of feather was growing.

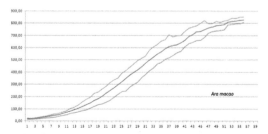

Fig. 8. Reference graph of weight gain over time (average [purple], maximum [blue], and minimum [orange]) for growing scarlet macaws (*Ara macao*) in a breeding collection. Please note these data should not be extrapolated to individuals of different species or of the same species fed a different diet or reared under different environmental conditions.

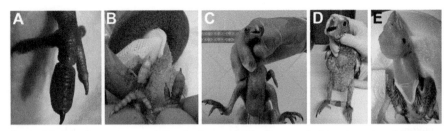

Fig. 9. (A) Skin ring toe constriction before and (B) after surgical treatment and bandage. (C) Splay leg before and (D) after external coaptation and (E) cervical external coaptation for the management of cervical lordosis.

Musculoskeletal system

The musculature of chicks is not completely developed, and their skeletons are not completely calcified making them more prone to fractures and luxations. The radiographic examination of the development of the skeleton and feathers of dusky parrots (*Pionus fuscus*) in relation to their behavior revealed that (1) chicks from 16 to 45 days of age (few days before cessation of bone growth) removed from the nest and placed alone on a flat surface would walk until restrained (whereas those in the nest they would just move very little); (2) at 50 days of age, they climbed to the nest entrance, retreating if scared; (3) from day 51 they flapped their wings vigorously inside the nest box; and (4) they emerged at 53 days of age when nearly all large feathers finished growing. The authors of this study suggested that premature exercise may be the cause of the high rate of juvenile osteodystrophy (eg, deformity of long bones such as the tibiotarsi) observed in hand-reared parrots (see **Fig. 9**).[37] Musculoskeletal disorders tend to manifest as abnormal posture at rest and/or when moving. Fractures may be the consequence of metabolic bone disease (nutritional secondary hyperparathyroidism) caused by nutritional imbalances (calcium, phosphorus, and vitamin D) and/or incorrect UVB light exposure. Fractures and dislocations in chicks tend to be managed in a conservatively (external coaptation) but the interval between bandage changes should be shorter than that of adults. Commonly observed disorders include splay leg due to lack of concavity of the nest, valgus of the long bones, stifle luxations and subluxations, and hip luxations. Further information about these disorders can be found in 2 recent publications.[38,39] This author had a case of keel partial agenesia in a gray parrot. Surgical treatment of this condition has been previously reported in this species (**Fig. 10**).[40]

Cardiovascular system

The heart rate ranges between 180 and 400 beats per minute. Congenital and acquired disorders have been reported (eg, ventricular septal defect and persistent

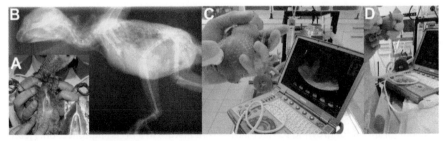

Fig. 10. (A, B) Keel partial agenesia in a gray parrot; (C, D) Cardiac disease and ultrasound-guided celomocentesis in a caique chick.

truncus arteriosus in an umbrella cockatoo [*Cacatua alba*] and a subvalvular septal defect and aortic hypoplasia in a Moluccan cockatoo [*Cacatua moluccensis*]).[41] Diagnostic imaging techniques and electrocardiography are useful to achieve antemortem diagnoses. The low level of calcification of the bones of very young birds may allow the assessment of the heart from echocardiographic windows not useful in adults such as intercostal or even through the keel (see **Fig. 10**).

Respiratory system

The respiratory rate in psittacine neonates is 20 to 40 respirations per minute. Congenital choanal atresia in the absence of concurrent congenital disorders choana has been reported in gray parrot chicks, one cockatoo, and one monk parakeet (unilaterally).[42,43] This author treated surgically a bilateral case in a hyacinth macaw (*Anodorhynchus hyacinthinus*) chick.

Upper respiratory infections are frequently consequence of food passing from the oral cavity although the choanal slit to the nasal cavity. Infections of the lower respiratory tract are also commonly observed. Aspiration pneumonia is more common in chicks near to weaning as they become more resistant to being hand-fed.[35] Affected chicks tend to show intermittent dyspnea and recurrent respiratory infections. Mild cases may manifest as rasp respiratory sounds after feeding, whereas in severe cases, sudden death may occur. Medical treatment (antimicrobials, anti-inflammatories, and supportive care) is normally required. Endoscopic removal of granulomas may be required in some cases.

Digestive system

Beak disorders are very common in hand-reared psittacines. Scissor beak is a lateral deviation of the rhinotheca leading to beak malocclusion. Although it may occur in any species of psittacine, it seems to be more common in macaws and cockatoos. Suggested causes include improper temperature during incubation, genetics, inadequate nutrition, or incorrect feeding techniques. Scissor beak correction is easier in young individuals because the bones and rhinotheca are actively remodeling. Diagnostic imaging techniques have been recommended as a prognostic aid before correction. Corrective procedures aim to change the forces that direct the anterior growth of the rhinotheca. Multiple corrective alternatives have been reported (ie, massage, corrective beak trimming, ramp prosthesis, and contralateral constant lateral tension [eg, transsinus pinning technique]). Transsinus pinning has been reported as a simple, effective, and rapid technique for correcting this malocclusion in macaw chicks aged younger than 16 weeks, and results can be expected in 2 to 4 weeks.[44] Scissor beak associated with prefrontal bone collapse is not yet amenable to treatment. These birds usually adapt to their disability and do well when regular beak trimmings are performed to maintain a functionally normal occlusion. Mandibular prognathism is the anteroposterior discrepancy between the upper and the lower beaks in which the lower beak is rostrally displaced in relation to the upper beak. This disorder is more commonly reported in cockatoos. The cause remains unknown and may include genetics, improper incubation, and feeding techniques. Correction techniques are based on forcing the tip of the upper beak upward and outward so that it rests over the edge of the lower beak in the most natural position. In very young chicks, gentle manual pressure applied outward to the maxillary tip placing it over the mandible for 10 minutes 6 to 8 times daily may be enough to correct the malformation. Once the beak hardens, surgical correction is preferred. Beak trauma is also commonly reported.[45] Additional information about the causes, diagnosis, and treatment of the previously mentioned conditions can be found elsewhere.[46]

The oral cavity should be examined paying special attention to the rule out blunted choanal papillae (which is suggestive of chronic upper respiratory discharge or hypovitaminosis A), foreign bodies, and abnormal growths (eg, choanal papilloma caused by herpesvirus infection).

The crop size is 2 to 3 times larger proportionally to body size in chicks when compared with adults. Motility should be observed and gently pinching the skin may promote it. Palpation is paramount for the detection of impacted content or foreign bodies. The crop should totally empty at least once a day (usually overnight). Crop stasis may be the consequence of improper management (eg, environmental inadequate conditions), aboral delayed transit time, or infectious disorders. Diagnostic techniques of utility include radiographs, contrast radiographs, ultrasonography, endoscopy, cytology, and microbiological cultures and sensitivity. The presence of few gram-negative bacteria in the absence of clinical signs does not require treatment unless clinical signs are observed. Medium-to-large amounts of gram-negative bacteria (more than 45%) or fungus (eg, budding yeasts) should be treated. Parasitic forms should never be observed. Local treatment may include the use of prokinetics, crop lavage, antibiotics, and/or antifungals. Systemic treatment may be required depending of the cause and severity of clinical signs. Other common conditions affecting the crop include ingluvitis, impactions, foreign bodies, pendulous crops, foreign body, crop wall trauma, and burns.[35] Depending on the size and nature of the impaction or the foreign bodies, these could be divided, lavaged, or extracted (eg, milked out through the oral cavity if the contents are not sharp or irritant, endoscopically or via ingluviotomy). Pendulous crops occur when crops are repeatedly overstretched to the point incorrect emptying occurs. When this happens, the use of a temporary "crop bra" made of tape, cohesive bandage or tissue may help to temporarily facilitate a correct emptying until the chick grows enough to consider the crop is proportional and correctly positioned to allow the normal passage of food. Regurgitation is common in hand-reared psittacines, and it can be caused by infectious diseases, inadequate food temperature, amount or consistency of food or feeding intervals, foreign bodies (eg, nesting material), stress, administration of some drugs (eg, trimethoprim-sulfa compounds or doxycycline), and/or incorrect handling of the chick or feeding technique, among others. Overfeeding has been suggested as the most common cause of regurgitation in hand-reared chicks.[47] Crop burns caused by excessive high temperature of hand-rearing formula can take up to 3 weeks to make a fistula. Immediately after burning, the chick becomes lethargic or agitated, hypo/anorexic, may present delayed transit times and/or regurgitate, and the skin covering the crop may evolve from showing erythema and swelling to becoming ulcerated with necrotic edges due to a fistula of the crop. Although medical treatment must be started immediately, surgery (excision of necrotic tissues and suture of the crop wall and skin in 2 separate layers) must be delayed, typically 3 to 5 days, until the extension of necrosis has completed. Supportive care must always be provided in case of crop disorders. Ingluviostomy tubes may be useful in the management of crop disorders. Aerophagy is commonly observed in chicks showing anxiety while fed or fed at a slower speed than required and should be differentiated from pathologic gas production by bacteria in the crop (**Fig. 11**).[35]

The digestive tract immediately after birth should be sterile until environmental bacterial progressively colonizes it. Normal bacterial flora in chicks include but are not restricted to Lactobacillus spp, Bacillus spp, Corynebacterium spp, nonhemolytic Streptococcus spp, Micrococcus spp, and Staphylococcus epidermidis. Microbial organisms in the food and water considered to have little effect on adult birds can cause life-threatening infections in neonates (eg, yeast, Escherichia coli, Klebsiella spp, Enterobacter spp, Pseudomonas spp, and Salmonella spp).[48] The study of gut microbiota by

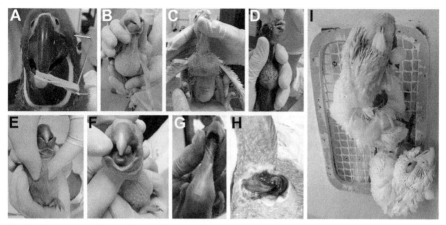

Fig. 11. Upper row (*A–D*) Surgical treatment of scissor beak, distended crop, crop bra, and crop swab for cytology. Lower row (*E–H*) Paper substrate foreign body in crop, foreign body manually milked out of crop to oral cavity, feeding tip in crop following accidental ingestion, and crop burn. (*I*) Ingluviostomy tubes placed in 2 cockatoo chicks.

amplicon pyrosequencing in hand-reared kakapos revealed a juvenile fecal microbiota enriched with particular lactic acid bacteria compared with the microbiota of adults, although the overall community structure did not differ significantly among different ages.[49]

Cloacal swabs are more representative than fecal swabs due to lower environmental contamination. No more than 5% to 8% of gram-negative bacteria, *Clostridium* spp, parasites, or yeasts should be observed in cloacal cytology. Parasitic forms should never be observed in fecal tests. Gastrointestinal obstruction, gastric or intestinal ulcers, intestinal torsion, intussusception, and cloacal prolapses have been reported and should be diagnosed and treated similar to in adults (**Fig. 12**).

Yolk-sac
The yolk-sac provides nutritional support to the developing embryo. The yolk sac is exterior to the body until 2 to 4 days before hatching, when it becomes internalized and the celomic cavity closes forming the navel. Most yolk should be absorbed within the first 5 to 7 days of life. The Meckel's diverticulum, a common congenital abnormality of the small intestine caused by the incomplete obliteration of the vitelline (omphalomesenteric) duct is commonly seen in asymptomatic individuals. Yolk-sac retention

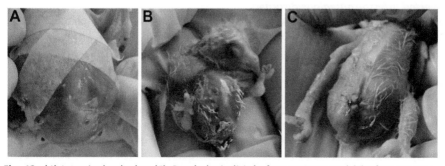

Fig. 12. (*A*) Intestinal volvulus; (*B*) Omphalovitelitis before surgery; and (*C*) after surgery.

may be consequence of noninfectious (eg, improper temperature, humidity, or feeding patterns) or infectious disorders. Infectious disorders may be primary or secondary (eg, infections of the navel not properly internalized before hatching [omphalo-vitellitis], bacterial contamination following fecal contamination of the shell). Chicks aged between 5 and 15 days may show decreased appetite, lethargy, celomic distension, impaired walking, dyspnea, and dehydration.[50] The presence of a yolk sac in a chick beyond 13 days of age supports a diagnosis of retained yolk sac.[50] Diagnosis can be confirmed by diagnostic imaging techniques. Microbiology of the yolk may be useful but sterile retentions are not uncommon. Yolk sac infections can originate from bacterial spreading from the oviduct of the female before the shell is formed, immediately after laying when air is sucked in through eggshell pores as the egg cools (which can facilitate bacterial penetration), or during the hatching process when the umbilicus may be exposed but incompletely sealed.[51] Treatment may be medical (eg, supportive care, disinfection with local antiseptics and use of topical or systemic antimicrobials, and so forth) and/or surgical (eg, unretracted yolk removal). Omphalitis refers to the infection (eg, E coli, Proteus sp, Streptococcus faecalis, or Clostridium sp) of the yolk sac, which may result in septicemia and death. Antiseptics (eg, povidone 10%) may be used to disinfect navels not internalized (see **Fig. 12**).

Hepatic system
Congenital extrahepatic biliary cysts have been reported in gray parrots. Idiopathic hepatomas or those secondary to blunt force trauma rupture of the liver causing hemorrhage have been reported in macaws. Affected birds may be paler (than normal due to anemia. Hepatomas are sometimes visible through the skin. Ultrasonographic examination may be useful to achieve a diagnosis. Blood transfusions may be required in severe cases of anemia. Hepatic lipidosis has been reported more commonly in cockatoos and Amazon parrots fed excessive amounts of formula or high-fat diets. Affected chicks may be dyspneic due to compression of the air sacs secondary to hepatomegaly. The liver is generally enlarged and paler than normal. A diagnosis may be suspected based on serum biochemistry and diagnostic imaging techniques. The definitive diagnosis is histopathological. Management requires diet correction, supportive care, correction of the any concurrent disorders, and hepatic protectants.[35]

Renal system
Droppings are usually polyuric due to the liquid diet fed. Renal disorders may be associated with cardiac disorders, severe dehydration, or hypervitaminosis D. Renal failure and gout are commonly reported. Diagnosis and management of renal disease in chicks is similar to that in adults.

Selected infecto-contagious disorders
Selected infecto-contagious disorders of epidemiologic impact for neonate and juvenile psittacines are reviewed and summarized in **Table 3**.

Diagnostics Techniques

Microbiology
Gram stain is a fast and cheap diagnostic method but its limitations must be considered when interpreting its results. Assuming a correct staining and experience of the reader performing this test and remembering the existence of Gram-variable bacteria, controversy may still occur when interpreting the results. For example, it is considered normal for a psittacine to have a mixed fecal bacterial population with a predominance (90%–100%) of gram-positive bacteria. In addition, the different strains of a bacterium

Table 3
Selected infecto-contagious diseases with epidemiologic impact for neonate and juvenile psittacines

Selected Infecto-Contagious Diseases with Epidemiologic Impact for Neonate and Juvenile Psittacines	
Avian gammapolyomavirus	E: Can infect different avian families. Incubation: ~2 wk. Deaths within 24–48 h (conures younger than 6 wk and macaws and eclectus younger of 14 wk). The transmission is horizontal through exposure to crop secretions, feces, urine, respiratory secretions, skin, or feathers or feather dust containing viral particles. Vertical transmission has been suggested in budgerigars. Adult birds typically are more resistant to infection and can seroconvert and shed the virus for up to 90 d, before clearing the infection CS: Weakness, pallor, hemorrhages, anorexia, dehydration, delayed crop emptying, regurgitation, vomiting, and depression. Survivors exhibit poor weight gain, polyuria, gut stasis, and abnormal feathers[22,26] AD: DNA probes of cloacal swab and blood samples and virus-neutralizing antibody tests of blood samples to identify birds previously exposed[51] PD: Macroscopic: Generalized pallor with SC and subserosal hemorrhage, splenomegaly, hepatomegaly, pericardial effusion, and/or ascites.[22,26] In nestlings, swelling and hemorrhage of the bursa may be observed.[52] Microscopic: Extensive hepatic and splenic necrosis. Virus inclusion bodies are mainly found in the spleen, mesangial cells of the kidney, and Kupffer cells of the liver but less-common locations (eg, feather follicles) may also occur. Occasionally, membranous glomerulonephritis.[26] Bursal necrosis and depletion of medullary lymphocytes (sometimes containing basophilic intranuclear inclusion bodies)[52] T: Specific treatment not available P: Quarantine, isolation, and testing. Vaccination (eg, an inactivated polyoma vaccine)[51]
Circovirus (Psittacine beak and feather disease)	E: All psittacines are susceptible. No one genotype is considered more virulent than another. Can affect birds of all ages but juveniles or young adult psittacine birds are more susceptible. Confirmed horizontal transmission after oral and/or intracloacal ingestion of the virus in feather dander or feces. Massively excreted in feather dander and feces. High concentrations can be detected in liver tissue, bile, crop secretions, feces, and feathers. Vertical transmission is suspected but not confirmed[53] CS: Acute form (more common in nestlings and fledgings): Depression (associated with leukopenia and anemia), green diarrhea, biliverdinuria, anorexia, regurgitation, and death due to hepatic necrosis. Pterylodynia with edematous and painful wing tips were also reported. Reports of African gray

(continued on next page)

Table 3 (continued)
Selected Infecto-Contagious Diseases with Epidemiologic Impact for Neonate and Juvenile Psittacines

	parrots dying within a week of showing clinical signs. Chronic form (long incubation period): Progressive feather loss with dystrophic feathers replacing normal ones, often without other clinical signs of illness. In Cacatuidae, the pulviplumes, are often the first feathers affected, and lack of feather dust can result in dull plumages and glossy or dark beaks and claws. The beak and nails may become hyperkeratotic and elongated, which may progress to osteomyelitis[53] AD: Low prealbumin and gammaglobulin concentrations. Viral excretion can be detected with PCR or hemagglutination assay as an antigen detection diagnostic test. Hemagglutination inhibition remains the gold standard for antibody detection. Positive birds must be isolated and retested in 90 d[53] PD: Macroscopic: Nonspecific. Often reflecting secondary infections. Major histologic changes are commonly limited to the primary and secondary lymphoid tissues. Immunohistochemistry and in situ hybridization can be used to demonstrate antigens in a wide range of tissues (eg, bursa of Fabricius, feather follicles, spleen, esophagus, and crop)[53] T: Specific treatment not available. However, individuals within many species may make full recoveries. For example, lorikeets (*Trichoglossus* sp.) and Eclectus parrots (*Eclectus* sp.) often develop protective hemagglutination inhibition antibody (HI) titers alongside cessation of virus excretion[53] P: Apparently resistant to extreme temperatures and various chemical disinfectants. Disinfection using peroxide compounds (Virkon S - Lanxess aktiengesellschaft, Cologne, Germany) has been recommended for use in captive breeding programs. No commercially available vaccine but an experimental inactivated vaccine using inactivated virus or recombinant proteins was effective[53]
Parrot bornaviruses 1–8 (PaBV-1 to PaBV-8) are genetically highly divergent and belong to 2 separate viral species, Orthobornavirus alphapsittaciforme (PaBV-1 to PaBV-4, PaBV-7, and PaBV-8) and Orthobornavirus betapsittaciforme (PaBV-5 and -6).[54]	E: PaBV-2 and, especially PaBV-4 are most commonly diagnosed in captive psittacines. The transmission is poorly understood. Horizontal transmission (fecal/urinary-oral) is considered rather inefficient in subadult and adult birds (eg, individuals cohoused with persistently infected birds can remain free of detectable virus for even years). Experimental parenteral (IM, SC, IV, or intracerebral) inoculation of avian bornaviruses provoked that nearly all birds developed persistent infection. Contrarily, mucosal inoculation of cockatiels with similar doses of PaBV-2 or PaBV-4 via peroral, IN, or oculo-nasal routes did not result in detectable persistent infection, even

(continued on next page)

| Table 3 |
| (continued) |

Selected Infecto-Contagious Diseases with Epidemiologic Impact for Neonate and Juvenile Psittacines

when mucosal lesions had been induced before inoculation.[54] Vertical transmission of avian bornavirus-RNA to the embryo has been reported but viable virus could not be isolated and negative chicks can be obtained after correctly disinfecting the shells and foster-rearing the chicks[55]

CS: Parrot bornaviruses provoke lymphoplasmocytic ganglioneuritis. The nerves of the proventriculus and ventriculus are the most commonly affected, resulting in nerve dysfunction and consequent proventricular dilatation (also known as proventricular dilatation disease [PDD]). However, other diseases may present with similar gastrointestinal signs and nondigestive bornavirosis also occur. PDD may manifest as weight loss despite normal appetite, lethargy, weakness, regurgitation, crop impaction, defecation of undigested seeds or other foods, or even sudden death. Nondigestive bornaviral infections can affect the central nervous system (may manifest as ataxia), the choroid and the optic nerve (may manifesting as blindness), the autonomic nerves of the heart and the adrenals, among others[54]

AD: PDD can be diagnosed based on clinical signs, diagnostic imaging techniques (dilated proventriculus) and histopathological examination of biopsies of affected areas (eg, proventriculus [full thickness], ventriculus, or crop). Occasionally, mild anemia, hypoproteinemia, or elevated creatine kinase may be seen. Bornaviral confirmation can be achieved by viral isolation (detects viable virus) or by detection of viral RNA by reverse transcription-PCR methods. Cloacal swabs usually contain higher amounts of viral RNA than pharyngeal swabs and whole blood samples. Viral RNA is also detectable in urine samples and feather calami. Detection of avian bornavirus (ABV)-specific antibodies in serologic assays confirms exposure to the virus but future negativizations of low-titer positive individuals are possible[54]

PD: Macroscopic: Low body condition, distended proventriculus, and undigested food in feces in case of PDD. Microscopic: Lymphoplasmocytic ganglioneuritis. The highest loads of viral RNA and antigen are mainly detected in brain, eye, and adrenal gland but lower loads can be found in liver, spleen, and skeletal muscle[54]

T: Specific treatment not available. Supportive care

P: No vaccines are commercially available. Avian bornaviruses are very unstable in the environment. Prevention is based on testing during quarantines in isolation. Some infected birds may be negative for

(continued on next page)

Table 3 *(continued)*	
Selected Infecto-Contagious Diseases with Epidemiologic Impact for Neonate and Juvenile Psittacines	
	viral shedding and seroconversion, resulting in false-negative results. Eradication programs are generally long. Testing the parents, isolating positive individuals, and preventing horizontal transmission by disinfecting (eg, 3% hydrogen peroxide) and artificial incubating the eggs is recommended if positive tested birds are part of the collection[54]
Psittacine poxvirus	E: Reported in several psittacine species. Virulence varies depending on the host.[56] Infections are more common in juveniles kept outdoors in neotropical locations.[22] Transmission occurs through contact of open wounds with infected tissues or aerosols (rare), by insect bites (mosquitoes), and by exposure to contaminated food or fomites (eg, perches or feeding bowls)
	CS: Three forms of disease have been traditionally reported: Cutaneous or dry, diptheric or wet, and systemic. At early stages, serous ocular discharge, rhinitis, and conjunctivitis (which may progress to ulceration and dry crusty lesions on the eyelid margins) can be observed. Amazon parrots may also develop a severe upper respiratory tract disease. Small to large raised and proliferative lesions are more common on the nonfeathered areas around the face, cere, and feet. Mortality rates are highest when diphtheritic lesions cause defects in the mucosal barrier of the alimentary and respiratory tract, allowing secondary infections. The systemic form carries the gravest prognosis with birds often dying acutely (24–48 h) from infection[56]
	AD: The clinical changes associated with the cutaneous form of psittacine poxvirus are often suggestive. Histopathological PCR[56]
	PD: Macroscopic: The clinical changes associated with the cutaneous form of psittacine poxvirus are often suggestive. Microscopic: Cardiac and hepatic necrosis, air sacculitis, pneumonia, celomitis, and accumulation of necrotic debris on the surface of the alimentary tract. Intracytoplasmic inclusion bodies (Bollinger bodies) may be found in the mucosa of the sinuses, trachea, crop, esophagus, or pharynx[56]
	T: Specific treatment not available. Topical disinfection of the lesions and supportive care until the immune system is able to control the infection. Antimicrobials may be required to control secondary opportunistic infections. Surgical removal of proliferative lesions may be useful in severe cases in which they impair feeding, respiration or vision[56]
	P: Poxviruses are very resistant virus able to survive on perches and in dried scabs for months to years. Isolate infected individuals. Poxviruses can withstand 1%

(continued on next page)

Table 3 (continued)	
Selected Infecto-Contagious Diseases with Epidemiologic Impact for Neonate and Juvenile Psittacines	
	phenol and 1:1000 formalin for 9 d but 1% potassium hydroxide, heating to 50°C for 30 min or 60°C for 8 min will inactivate them.[57] Prevent transmission by fomites, vectors, and contact with infected individuals
Chlamydia psittaci (intracellular, gram-negative bacterium)	E: Zoonotic. The infectious elementary bodies can survive out of the host (protected by organic material), and inside the host cells, for several weeks. Infection can occur either by inhalation or by ingestion of infectious particles. *C psittaci* can replicate in the lungs, air sacs, and pericardium of infected birds, as soon as 24 h after infection and hematogenously spread within 48 h. After 72 h, the infected birds are able to shed *C psittaci* in the environment. A large number of elementary bodies can be shed continuously or intermittently in feces, urine, ocular and nasal discharge, and oropharyngeal mucus. *C psittaci* can be detected in feces 10 d before the onset of clinical signs. Respiratory infections spread through the lungs and air sacs to other organs, resulting in a symptomatic disease, whereas oral–intestinal infections are less likely to cause symptoms, often leading to chronic, nonsymptomatic forms of the disease. Vertical transmission has been demonstrated in budgerigars. Cockatiels can shed *C psittaci* through their feces for more than 1 y after an active infection[58]
	CS: Respiratory signs (eg, sneezing, dyspnea, and/or oculo-nasal discharge), conjunctivitis, lethargy, anorexia, regurgitation, vomiting, green diarrhea, tremors, torticollis, low reproductive rate, and death. The usual incubation period ranges from 3 d to several weeks[58]
	AD: Based on suggestive clinical signs (if present) and diagnostic test findings (eg, hematology [anemia, marked leukocytosis or leukopenia, and heterophilia]), blood biochemistry (increased levels of aspartate aminotransferase, lactate dehydrogenase, creatine phosphokinase, and bile acids), diagnostic imaging (eg, suggestive of pneumonia, air sacculitis, splenomegaly, and/or hepatomegaly), endoscopy, antigen enzyme-linked immunosorbent assay and PCR, and serology positive titers. Clear definitions of suspected and confirmed cases in birds and humans have been reported[59]
	PD: Gross and histologic lesions (eg, hepatitis, splenitis, and pneumonia) are not pathognomonic. Giemsa, Giménez, Ziehl-Neelsen, Stamp, and Macchiavello stains are normally used to stain *C psittaci* in tissue samples. Chlamydial isolation remains the gold standard for its diagnosis.

(continued on next page)

Table 3 (continued)	
Selected Infecto-Contagious Diseases with Epidemiologic Impact for Neonate and Juvenile Psittacines	
	T: Doxycycline is the drug of choice for oral administration (dosage recommendations are as follows: 25–35 mg/kg every 24 h for cockatiels; 25–50 mg/kg for Senegal parrots and blue-fronted and orange-winged Amazon parrots; and 25 mg/kg every 24 h for African gray parrots, Goffin's cockatoos, blue and gold macaws, and green-winged macaws. A starting dosage of 25–30 mg/kg every 24 h is recommended for cockatoos and macaws, and 25–50 mg/kg every 24 h is recommended for other psittacine species.[59] Treatment duration may vary from 21 to 45 d depending on the species.[59,60] Azithromycin: Cockatiels treated with azithromycin at 40 mg/kg PO were free of infection after treatment for 21 d. It is not known if this treatment regimen is effective in other species. Injectable doxycycline administered at doses of 75–100 mg/kg IM every 5–7 d for the first 4 wk and subsequently every 5 d for the duration of treatment. This formulation can cause irritation at the injection site[59]
	P: Based on testing, isolating, and treating positive individuals
Ectoparasites and endoparasites	E: More common in chicks kept on outdoor facilities. Ectoparasite (red mites [*Dermanyssus gallinae*], Northern fowl mites [*Ornithonyssus sylviarum*], fire ants, and ticks) may vary depending on the geographic location
	CS: Ectoparasites (eg, paleness, pruritus and erythema, or hemorrhages…)/Endoparasites (eg, weight loss, diarrhea, hematochezia, and melena)
	AD: Macroscopic or microscopic visualization of parasitic forms. The elimination of some endoparasites can be intermittent
	PD: Sometimes not specific. Pale organs. Macroscopic or microscopic visualization of parasitic forms
	T: Specific antiparasitic treatments
	P: Control intermediary hosts for parasites with indirect life cycles. Environmental ectoparasite treatment

Abbreviations: AD, antemortem diagnosis; CS, clinical signs; E, epidemiology; PD, postmortem diagnosis; T, treatment; and P, prophylaxis.

(eg, *E coli*, *Klebsiella* sp, or *Enterobacter* sp) may vary in their pathogenicity. Furthermore, some clinicians would treat if there is an excessive proportion of gram-negative bacteria, if the white blood cell count is elevated, and/or if clinical signs are present, whereas others will treat elevated gram-negative numbers independently of the white blood cell count. Therefore, bacterial and fungal cultures and sensitivities should be performed, when possible, in order to minimize the risk of antimicrobial resistance in breeding collections; however, obtaining results may require days. Anaerobic bacteria are considered pathogenic. Cost reduction in next-generation sequencing technologies is starting to make this technology accessible to clinical laboratories.

Hematology and blood biochemistry

The right jugular vein is the optimal venipuncture site. Unless severe anemia is suspected, 1% of body weight (1 mL/100 g) can be safely collected from this site. Toenail clipping has been reported as adequate for packed cell volume but it is considered painful and unreliable for total white blood cell count and inorganic phosphorus evaluation. The sample often contains tissue fluid, cellular debris and macrophages, cells not normally seen in peripheral blood (eg, osteoblasts and osteoclasts) or may be contaminated with urates or microorganisms.[61,62] Nestling psittacines have lower packed cell volumes (20%–30%), which may increase to adult ranges by 9 to 11 weeks of age in most species. Total white blood cell count is higher (20,000–40000 cells/μL) in neonates. A transition from heterophilia to lymphocytosis has been reported in some species of juvenile psittacines. The levels of total protein (1–3 mg/dL) and uric acid in serum are lower in chicks than in adults, whereas alkaline phosphatase and creatine kinase are higher.[35] Exsanguination by decapitation immediately after humane euthanasia of chicks is a useful method to collect large volumes of blood for diagnostic procedures.

Molecular laboratory techniques

Viral and bacterial polymerase chain reaction (PCR), serology, and viral isolation are molecular laboratory techniques useful when attempting to create a free of contagious disease colony.

Additionally, DNA sexing using PCR technology available commercially from diagnostic laboratories using eggshell, whole blood, or freshly plucked feathers (down feathers or otherwise) is a relatively less-invasive technique when compared with sexing via endoscopy. Please note that diagnostic imaging techniques may be also useful if the chick is large enough to allow visualization of the gonads.

Parasitology

Parasitologic examination of samples includes cheap and fast diagnostic techniques, which may be part of every initial medical examination in chicks removed from nests.

Diagnostic imaging

Radiography, ultrasonography, endoscopy, fluoroscopy, magnetic resonance imaging (MRI), and computed tomography (CT) have similar indications independent of the age of the bird. Physiologic variations observed in chicks include but are not restricted to enlarged proventriculus and ventriculus, dilated intestinal loops, reduced air sac space due to dilatation of the gastrointestinal tract, open growth plates of the long bones, and reduced general muscle mass.[35] Ultrasonography in chicks has the diagnostic advantage of providing better echographic windows than in adults due to their more compressed air sacs and their less-calcified skeleton. Micro-CT-scan and micro-MRI provide higher definition than standard CT-scan and MRI but these technologies still remain nonaccessible to most clinicians.

Endoscopy

This technique is useful for diagnostic and therapeutic minimally to noninvasive procedures (eg, assessment of eyes, otic canals, oral cavity, crop, and cloaca) but its safety is reduced when performing more invasive procedures, such as celioscopy, in very young and small birds due to their smaller size and their more compressed air sacs due to the proportionally enlarged intracelomic (ICe) organs when compared with older individuals.

Necropsy

Gross postmortem examination, cytology, and histopathology are extremely useful in the management of collections. Egg and fetal necropsies are very useful to detect contagious, environmental, congenital, developmental, and hereditary disorders and to monitor the health status of a collection (**Fig. 13**). The embryo's general condition and position must be assessed. Abnormal tissues and fluids must be cultured and examined histopathologically. The shell is examined for color, texture, shape, thickness, and the presence or absence of stress lines.[22] Embryonal malposition and inadequate moisture loss are among the most common causes of embryonic mortality before hatching. Embryonal malpositions have not been studied exhaustively in Psittaciformes. The normal psittacine embryo assumes the hatching position with its head below the air cell just before hatching. Psittacines have shorter and thicker necks when compared with chicken embryos and do not normally tuck their heads under their right wing. Instead, they barely tuck their head and typically lay it close to the right-wing tip. Hatching occurs in stages (draw down, internal pip, external pip, and emergence from the egg) and is the time of highest mortality in embryonic development.[22] Malpositions commonly occur secondary to hyperthermia or elevated temperatures, which also cause premature pipping. Two of the most common psittacine malpositions are when the head is located at the small end of the egg and when the beak is rotated away from the air cell. Eggs incubated below optimum temperatures develop more slowly and typically have more problems with hatching. Excessive humidity results in the development of "wet chicks." These chicks drown at pipping, due to remaining albumin, and are often edematous. Eggs exposed to low humidity may dry out, causing adherence of the shell membrane to the chick, preventing normal pipping.[22]

Therapeutics

Common routes of drug administration in psittacines include intramuscular (IM), SC, ICe, intravenous (IV), intraosseous (IO), intranasal (IN), per os (PO), and per cloacal. When IV catheterization is not possible, an IO catheter may be used instead. Drug dilution is commonly used to facilitate administration of correct dosages to small birds.

Supportive care (ie, to maintain hydration and a positive energy balance) must be provided until an accurate diagnosis is achieved. Medications used in pediatric psittacines include antibiotics (eg, trimetoprim-sulfametoxazole, amoxicillin-clavulanate, enrofloxacin, doxycycline, and so forth), antifungals (eg, nystatin, voriconazole, terbinafine, itraconazole, amphotericin B), antiparasitics (eg, fenbendazole, metronidazole, trimethoprim-sulfametoxazole), and miscellaneous drugs (eg, metoclopramide, cisapride, calcium, silymarin (milk thistle), furosemide, enalapril, probiotics, and prebiotics [although frequently used, their utility remains controversial]). Quinolones must be avoided in growing chicks due to their effects on cartilage development. Drugs such as trimethoprim-sulfa, doxycycline, and nystatin may cause regurgitation and, if still needed, parenteral formulations of trimethoprim-sulfa or doxycycline [N.B.,

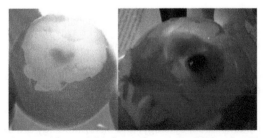

Fig. 13. Egg necropsies provide useful information to establish a healthy population.

both drugs given parentally are painful] may be used until regurgitation is controlled. It also must be remembered that oral absorption of nystatin is almost null. Therefore, alternatives such as terbinafine, itraconazole, or fluconazole may be better systemic alternatives. Fenbendazole may result in aplastic anemia in very weak birds.

Anesthesia and Monitoring

Due to length limitations, this section will only focus in the differences between neonate and adult psittacine sedation and anesthesia and monitoring. The author would invite the reader to read a more extensive review about these topics in psittacines elsewhere.[63]

Psittacine chicks are altricial and, therefore, more prone to develop hypothermia than feathered individuals. The low-energetic reserves of chicks make them more prone to develop hypoglycemia. Additionally, very young individuals present a higher anesthetic risk because of potentially altered responses to drugs caused by impairment or immaturity of the cardiovascular, respiratory, hepatic, renal, and nervous systems. Airway intubation and vascular access are recommended but may not be easy in very small individuals. IO catheterization may be easier than obtaining a vascular access in some individuals. Anesthetic face masks may be used when tracheal intubation is not feasible. Air sac intubation will only be useful in larger individuals as the air sacs of very young psittacine chicks are relatively smaller in proportion than adult ones due to the relative ICe organomegaly characteristic of their age. Because of the small size of parrots, nonrebreathing circuits, such as lightweight T-pieces, are preferred to reduce resistance to airflow to minimize dead space, and therefore rebreathing of carbon dioxide. The standard anesthetic bags can be replaced for balloons of volumes proportional to the size of the chick.

In relation to anesthetic monitoring, pulsating flow detection by placing a Doppler probe in an artery or the keel of very young (which is not completely calcified) individuals can be used to monitor heart rate. Electrocardiography can be used to monitor heart rate and rhythm independently of the size of the chick. If the electrocardiograph forceps are too traumatic for their delicate skin are too large, they can be attached to the metallic part of hypodermic needles placed through the skin. Esophageal stethoscopes allow heart rate monitoring with minimal external physical contact with the bird. Assessment of the respiratory function relies on continuous monitoring of respiratory rate and, with some limitations, of end-tidal CO_2. The use of microstream capnography, a type of side-stream technology, which allows sampling of very low gas flows (eg, up to 50 mL/min), is recommended in avian species because of their small size. The use of pulse oximetry in psittacines remains controversial. Arterial blood gas analyses may be a complementary tool to assess breathing function, especially in case of respiratory impairment. Temperature can be measured in the esophagus or, less reliably, the cloaca (less reliable) with a thermometer or with infrared technology.

SUMMARY

Psittacine neonate and pediatric care has markedly improved within the last decades due to a better understanding of the nutritional, environmental, and behavioral requirements of multiple species. Medical advances in diagnostic techniques and increased related knowledge have changed the way breeding collections are managed. The application of concepts such as the closed aviary and new diagnostic, preventive, and therapeutic protocols have resulted in healthier breeding and juvenile populations. This article reviews the most important concepts and protocols to provide the best possible care to psittacine neonatal and pediatric patients, as well as to set the basis for a healthy psittacine breeding collection.

CLINICS CARE POINTS

- There are advantages and disadvantages to various neonatal rearing techniques.
- Psittacine collections, including their nurseries, benefit from having well-designed facilities and from adhering to he closed aviary concept.
- Neonatal and pediatric psittacine patients present anatomic and physiologic similarities but also differences when compared with adults of the same species. A good understanding of both is paramount for the correct prevention and management of medical disorders.
- Infecto-contagious diseases may affect neonates and adults in different ways and so may require different diagnostic and therapeutic approaches.

ACKNOWLEDGMENTS

The author would like to thank Loro Parque Fundación for the years of contribution to research in psittacine breeding and population management as well as for sharing their great facilities (some of them shown in this article) with the rest of the world.

DISCLOSURE

The author has no conflict of interest and has nothing to disclose.

REFERENCES

1. Styles DK. An overview of psittacine reproductive behavior and infertility problems. AFA Watchbird 2009;36(3):38–49.
2. Kramer J, Klauke N, Bauert M, et al. No evidence for enforced alloparental care in a cooperative breeding parrot. Ethology 2016;122:1–10.
3. Navarro A, Castanon I. Comparative study of the growth rates of hand-raised and parent-raised psittacids in Loro Parque Fundación. Cyanopsitta 2001;60:12–6.
4. Myers SA, Millam JR, Roudybush TE, et al. Reproductive success of hand-reared versus parent-reared cockatiels (*Nymphicus hollandicus*). Auk 1988;105:536–42.
5. Kenedy ED. Determinate and indeterminate egg-laying patterns: A review. Condor 1991;93:106–24.
6. Low R. Fostering parrot eggs: practicalities and ethics. Available at: http://www.avianrearingresource.co.uk/species/documents/277.pdf. Accessed 01.06.2023.
7. Millam JR. Neonatal handling, behavior, and reproduction in orange-winged Amazons and cockatiels Amazona amazonica and Nymphicus hollandicus at the Department of Animal Science, University of California. Davis. Int. Zoo Yearbook 2000;37:220-231.
8. Aengus WL, Millam JR. Taming parent-reared orange-winged Amazon parrots by neonatal handling. Zoo Biol 1999;18:177–87.
9. Fox RA, Millam JR. The effect of early environment on neophobia in orange-winged Amazon parrots (*Amazona amazonica*). Appl Anim Behav Sci 2004;89:117–29.
10. Collete JC, Millam JR, Klasing KC, et al. Neonatal handling of Amazon parrots alters the stress response and immune function. Appl Anim Behav Sci 2000;66:335–49.

11. Schmid R, Doherr MG, Steiger A. The influence of the breeding method on the behaviour of adult African grey parrots (*Psittacus erithacus*). Appl Anim Behav Sci 2006;98(3–4):293–307.

12. Berg KS, Delgado S, Cortopassi KA, et al. Vertical transmission of learned signatures in a wild parrot. Proc R Soc A B 2012;279:585–91.

13. Masin S, Massa R, Bottoni L. Evidence of tutoring in the development of subsong in newly-fledged Meyer's parrots *Poicephalus meyeri*. Anais da Academia Brasileira de Ciencias 2004;76(2):231–6.

14. Fox R. Chapter 10. Hand-rearing: Behavioral impacts and implications for captive parrot welfare. In: Luescher UA. Manual parrot behavior. USA: Blackwell Publishing. Iowa; 2006. p. 83–91.

15. Rowley I, Chapman G. Cross-fostering, imprinting, and learning in two sympatric species of cockatoo. Behaviour 1986;96:1–16.

16. Klinghammer E. Factors influencing choice of mate in altricial birds. In: Stevenson HW. Early behavior: cooperative and developmental approaches. New York Wiley; 1967. p. 5–42.

17. Renton K, Salinas-Melgoza A, De Labra-Hernández MA, et al. Resource requirements of parrots: Nest site selectivity and dietary plasticity of Psittaciformes. J Ornithol 2015;156:73–90.

18. Juniper T, Parr M. Parrots. Natural history of the parrots. In: Juniper T, Parr M, editors. A guide to the parrots of the World. Christopher Helm Publishers; 2010. p. 19–25.

19. Martin SG, Romagnano A. Chapter 9: Nest box preferences. In: Luescher AU. Manual of parrot behavior. USA: Blackwell Publishing. Iowa; 2006. p. 79–82.

20. Demlong MJ, Bohmke B. A temperature-controlled nest box for thick-billed parrots. Int Zoo Yearbook 2000;37:191–5.

21. Monaco E, Hoppes S, Guo J, et al. The detection of avian bornavirus within psittacine eggs. J Avian Med Surg 2012;26(3):144–8.

22. Romagnano A. Psittacine incubation and pediatrics. Vet Clin Exot Anim 2012;15: 163–82.

23. Meehan CL, Mench JA. Environmental enrichment affects the fear and exploratory responses to novelty of young Amazon parrots. Appl Anim Behav Sci 2002;79:75–88.

24. Fox RA, Millam JR. Novelty and individual differences influence neophobia in orange-winged Amazon parrots (*Amazona amazonica*). Appl Anim Behav Sci 2007;104:107–15.

25. Luescher AU, Sheehan K. Rearing environment and behavioral development of psittacine birds. Current issues and research in veterinary behavioral medicine. Papers presented at the fifth international veterinary behavior meeting. Purdue University Press; 2005. p. 35–41.

26. Leger St. J. Nondomestic avian pediatric pathology. Vet Clin Exot Anim 2012;15: 233–50.

27. Cornejo J, Dierenfeld ES, Bailey CA, et al. Nutritional and physical characteristics of commercial hand-feeding formulas for parrots. Zoo Biol 2013;32(5):469–75.

28. Cornejo J, Dierenfeld ES, Renton K, et al. Fatty acid profiles of crop contents of free-living psittacine nestlings and of commercial hand-feeding formulas. J Anim Physiol Anim Nutr 2021;105(2):394–405.

29. Groffen H, Watson R, Hammer S, et al. Analysis of growth rate variables and post-feeding regurgitation in hand-reared Spix's macaw (*Cyanopsitta spixii*) chicks. J Avian Med Surg 2008;22(3):189–98.

30. Groffen H, Watson R, Raidal S. A critical analysis into the captive management variables surrounding the occurrences of regurgitation in hand reared spix's macaws *Cyanopsitta spixii* at al Wabra wildlife preservation. Proc. of AAVAC Annual Conference Adelaide 2009;165–78.

31. Sánchez-Migallón Guzmán D, Beaufrére H, Welle KR, et al. Birds. In: Carpenter JW, Harms CA, editors. Carpenter's exotic animal formulary. Sixth edition. Elsevier; 2022. p. 223–444.

32. Clubb KJ, Skidmore D, Schubot RM, et al. Growth rates of hand fed psittacine chicks. In: Schubot RM, Clubb SL, Clubb KJ, editors. Psittacine aviculture: perspectives, techniques, and research. Loxahatchee (FL): Avicultural Breeding and Research Center; 1992. 14.1-19.1.

33. Williams DR, Brainard DH, McMahon MJ, et al. Double-pass and interferometric measures of the optical quality of the eye. J Opt Soc Am 1994;11:3123–35.

34. Buyukmihci NC, Murphy CJ, Paul-Murphy J, et al. Eyelid malformation in four cockatiels. J Am Vet Med Assoc 1990;183:1305–6.

35. Flammer K, Clubb S. Neonatology. In: Ritchie BW, Harrison GJ, Harrison LR, editors. Avian medicine: principles and application. Lake Worth (FL): Wingers; 1994. p. 805–38.

36. Reinschmidt M. Kunstbrut und Handaufzucht von Papageien und Sittichen. Bretten: Arndt-Verlag; 2000.

37. Harcourt-Brown N. Development of the skeleton and feathers of dusky parrots (*Pionus fuscus*) in relation to their behavior. Vet Rec 2004;154:42–8.

38. Calvo Carrasco D. Fracture management in avian species. Vet Clin North Am Exot Anim Pract 2019;22(2):223–38.

39. Sabater González M. Avian articular orthopedics. Vet Clin North Am Exot Anim Pract 2019;22(2):239–51.

40. Bennet RA, Gilson SD. Surgical management of bifid sternum in two African grey parrots. Am Vet Med Assoc 1999;214(3). 372-352.

41. Evans DE, Tully TN, Strickland KN, et al. Congenital cardiovascular anomalies, including ventricular septal defects, in 2 cockatoos. J Avian Med Surg 2001; 15(2):101–6.

42. Greenacre CB, Watson E, Ritchie BW. Choanal atresia in an African grey parrot and an umbrella cockatoo. J Assoc Avian Vets 1993;7(1):19–22.

43. Bowles HL. Surgical resolution of soft tissue disorders. In: Harrison GJ, editor. Lightfoot TL. Clinical avian medicine. Spix Publishing; 2006. p. 775–89.

44. Doneley RJT. Transsiuns pinning to correct lateral deviation of the upper beak in juvenile macaws. J Avian Med Surg 2021;35(1):68–74.

45. Gelis S. Evaluating and treating the gastrointestinal system. In: Harrison G-J, Lightfoot T, editors. Clinical avian medicine. Spix Publishing; 2006. p. 411–40.

46. Huynh M, Sabater González M, Beaufrére H. Avian skull orthopedics. Vet Clin Exot Anim 2019;22:253–83.

47. Tschudin A, Rettmer H, Watson R, et al. Evaluation of hand-rearing records for Spix's macaw *Cyanopsitta spixii* at the Al Wabra Wildlife Preservation from 2005 to 2007. Int Zoo Yearbk 2010;44:201–11.

48. Clubb SL. Psittacine pediatric husbandry and medicine. In: Altman R, Clubb SL, Dorrestein GM, et al, editors. Avian medicine and surgery. W. B. Saunders Company; 1997. p. 73–100.

49. Waite DW, Eason DK, Taylor MW. Influence of hand rearing and bird age on the fecal microbiota of the critically endangered kakapo. Appl Environ Microbiol 2014;80(15):4650–8.

50. Kenny D, Cambre RC. Indications and technique for the surgical removal of the avian yolk sac. J Zoo Wildl Med 1992;23(1):55–61.
51. Rideout BA. Investigating embryo deaths and hatching failure. Vet Clin Exot Anim Pract 2012;15(2):155–62.
52. Ritchie BW, Niagro FD, Latimer KS, et al. An inactivated avian polyomavirus vaccine is safe and immunogenic in various Psittaciformes. Vaccine 1996;14:1103–7.
53. Pendl H, Tizard I. Chapter 11: Immunology. In: Speer BL, editor. Current therapy in avian medicine and surgery. First edition. St. Louis, Missouri, USA: Elsevier; 2016. p. 400–32.
54. Raidal S. Psittacine beak and feather disease. In: Speer BL, editor. Current therapy in avian medicine and surgery. First edition. St. Louis, Missouri, USA: Elsevier; 2016. p. 51–9.
55. Rubbenstroth D. Avian bornavirus research - A comprehensive review. Viruses 2022;14:1513, 30 pp.
56. Lierz M. Avian bornavirus and proventricular dilation disease. In: Speer BL, editor. Current therapy in avian medicine and surgery. First edition. St. Louis, Missouri, USA: Elsevier; 2016. p. 28–46.
57. Katoh H, Ogawa H, Ohya K, et al. A review of DNA viral infections in psittacine birds. J Vet Med Sci 2010;72(9):1099–106.
58. Van Riper C, Forrester DJ. Avian pox. In: Thomas NJ, Hunter DB, Atkinson CT, editors. Infectious disease of wild birds. Ames: Blackwell Publishing; 2007. p. 131–76.
59. Crosta L, Melillo A, Schnitzer P. Chlamydiosis (Psittacosis). In: Speer BL. Current therapy in avian medicine and surgery. First edition. St. Louis, Missouri, USA: Elsevier; 2016. p. 82–93.
60. Balsamo G, Maxted AM, Midla JW, et al. Compendium of measures to control Chlamydia psittaci infection among humans (psittacosis) and pet birds (avian chlamydiosis), 2017. J Avian Med Surg 2017;31(3):262-282.
61. Sánchez-Migallón Guzmán D, Díaz-Figueroa O, Tully T, et al. Evaluating 21-day doxycycline and azithromycin treatments for experimental Chlamydophila psittaci infection in cockatiels (Nymphicus hollandicus). J Avian Med Surg 2010;24(1): 35–45.
62. Bennet TD, Lejnieks DV, Koepke H, et al. Comparison of hematologic and biochemical test results in blood samples obtained by jugular venipuncture versus nail clip in Moluccan cockatoos (Cacatua moluccensis). J Avian Med Surg 2015;29(4):303–12.
63. Sabater González M, Adami C. Psittacine sedation and anesthesia. Vet Clin Exot Anim Pract 2022;25(1):113–34.

Pediatric Medicine of Galliformes

Rebecca Pacheco, DVM*, Miranda J. Sadar, DVM, DACZM

KEYWORDS

- Chicken pediatrics • Chick diseases • Nutritional deficiency • Chick orthopedics

KEY POINTS

- Obtain chicks from reputable sources and implement excellent brooding and biosecurity measures for the flock.
- Disease prevention is preferred over reactive management.
- Early detection of clinical disease is imperative to prevent further loss of chicks.
- Necropsies are recommended in any cases of sudden death or euthanasia due to disease.

NATURAL HISTORY

Domestic chickens (*Gallus gallus domesticus*) are thought to have originated from domestication of wild red junglefowl (*G gallus*) in Southeast Asia. Domestication resulted in rapid dissemination of fowl across the world for meat and egg use.[1] Currently, chickens are used globally in massive numbers on a commercial basis as well as in small backyard flocks. The wild red junglefowl remains and is found ubiquitously throughout their native range, including cities and urban areas, as well as in deciduous rainforests.[1,2]

Chickens are hardy and adapt well to a range of living conditions. They are prolific egg producers and lay clutches of 8 to 12 eggs, though they are indeterminate layers and will continue to lay as many eggs as necessary to fill their clutch numbers, even when eggs are removed.[3] This lends well to long periods of egg production, which commercial egg producers have capitalized on. Chickens have also been domesticated into breeds, which are prolific growers for use as meat. Their utility in both egg laying and meat production is, in part, what has led to the domestic chicken being established as the most commercially produced animal in the world.[2] Outside of these larger production facilities, chickens have always had a place on a smaller scale for hobby and subsistence farmers and as pets for urban households.[4] Chickens used for these purposes can be purebred, outdoor hybrids, or heritage breeds as opposed

Department of Clinical Sciences, Colorado State University's College of Veterinary Medicine and Biomedical Sciences, 300 West Drake Road, Fort Collins, CO 80523, USA
* Corresponding author.
E-mail address: b.pacheco@colostate.edu

Vet Clin Exot Anim 27 (2024) 295–311
https://doi.org/10.1016/j.cvex.2023.11.009
1094-9194/24/© 2023 Elsevier Inc. All rights reserved.

to the commercial breeds developed for large-scale farming. Chicks can be obtained from various sources including commercial, online, and private hatcheries, farm and feed stores, and hobby farms.

Nevertheless, backyard and small-scale flocks are susceptible to the same diseases of commercial chickens and are subject to the same veterinary legal regulations that commercial operations abide by. Other gallinaceous birds grouped generally into "poultry," "Galliformes," and "chicks" in this article include turkeys, pheasant, guineafowls, peafowl, and other exotic game bird species.

The topic of incubation and hatching could span an entire book itself, and most backyard chicken hobbyists will be purchasing day-old chicks and not incubating eggs on their own. Therefore, coverage in this article will be brief. It is important that a veterinarian understand that problems with parents, as well as problems during the incubation period itself, can significantly affect the health of chicks. During incubation, the effects of humidity, temperature, ventilation, rotation, incubator hygiene, and human handling can all affect the robustness and health of chicks after hatching.[5] A chick that dies during hatching, or within days of hatching, likely experienced abnormalities during incubation or was affected by a vertically transmitted disease.[4,6]

Breeding practices also greatly affect chick outcome. Factors to consider are selection of the hen and cock, the environment that chickens are kept in, what the disease prevalence and risk are, and diet. It is advisable to use hens that are in prime breeding age and not too old; in general, optimal egg production and fertility is up to 4 years of age.[4] The hen should have been proven to produce eggs with good shell quality, consistently sized and shaped eggs, and no abnormally formed eggs. Cock fertility is influenced by nutrition, orthopedic health, inbreeding and genetics, cock to hen ratios, and age. Egg-laying chickens in general live between 6 and 8 years, with hen fertility dropping at 3 to 4 years of age and cocks maintaining fertility for longer, although exact reproductive lifespan varies.[4,7] Breeding animals should be kept in sanitary and disease-free conditions. General coop maintenance recommendations include weekly removal of feces and soiled bedding and cleaning of food and water containers with a 1:1 ratio of vinegar and water solution. The removal of deeper layers of substrate and freshening with new bedding should be completed monthly, and a full cleanout with floor sanitation should be performed twice yearly. Many products are available to reduce ammonia buildup in substrate, with zeolite and limestone products (Sweet PDZ, Spokane, WA, USA) being safe and inexpensive.[2,8] Layer feeds are inappropriate for use in hens used to produce eggs for incubation and hatching. Breeder rations generally provide a higher protein content, increased calcium with balanced phosphorus, and fortification with select vitamins and minerals to provide a growing embryo with appropriate nutrients.[4]

Good breeding practices also entail the use of clean equipment for incubation, hatching, and brooding, monitoring the development of the embryo during incubation, incubation conditions to ensure proper conditions are maintained, and the chicks closely at hatching. In general, a 25% bleach solution is recommended as a disinfectant for incubators before use and between uses.[9] Disease can be transferred between eggs within an incubator; thus, it is important to remove any abnormally developing eggs in the process of incubation.[4,6] Several brands of incubator are available for purchase at most farm supply stores, including Brinsea (Titusville, FL, USA) and Harris Farms (Nolensville, TN, USA).

Hatching takes place over the course of 3 days, and rotation of the eggs should be discontinued during this time period. Humidity and temperature should be maintained at incubation levels during the hatching process and chicks minimally disrupted during this time. The chick must first begin "pipping" its way through shell membranes at the onset of hatching, and only in the final part of hatching will the chick fully pip through the shell with its egg tooth. The egg tooth is a small horn on the tip of the rhinotheca the chick uses in the process of hatching, which will fall off within the first few days of life. Once chicks are hatched, they will be damp and have a thick, wet urachus, similar to an umbilicus in mammals (**Fig. 1**). They should remain in the incubator until their down is dry and the urachus has shriveled, at which point they can be moved into a brooder. This drying-off process generally takes 12 to 24 hours (**Fig. 2**).[4] During this time, chicks should be evaluated for deformities and abnormalities, and affected chicks should be euthanized.[4,6] Chicks have a yolk supply that is used for nutrition during the first 48 to 72 hours of life; therefore, a lack of eating and drinking immediately after hatching is not abnormal. If a chick does not eat and drink on its own after 72 hours, a thorough examination should be performed and euthanasia or medical intervention considered.[2,4,6]

The brooder is the area in which chicks will be reared until they reach adulthood. Day-old chicks require precise brooding, as they have downy feathering and lack adult plumage that would allow them to regulate their temperature. When allowed to be reared by their parents, the hen will carefully ensure chicks are warm by brooding them in her feathers. When brooding chicks, different ages should not be mixed to avoid bullying behaviors and competition for food and water. Similarly, chicks of different breed sizes (eg, bantams vs Rhode Island red) should not be mixed to avoid similar issues.[4,5]

When raised under human care, artificial brooding is required to ensure proper growth and health of chicks. There are several brooder kits that can be purchased online or from farm and feed stores, and some keepers may choose to make their own. The brooder walls should be tall enough to prevent chicks from escaping as they gain mobility, or the brooder can have a mesh lid that allows for plenty of ventilation. The basic needs for a brooder are a substrate that can be kept clean and dry, supplemental heat, and food and water containers (**Fig. 3**).[4,6]

Substrates commonly used include aspen shavings, corn or walnut pellets, compressed newspaper pellets, or straw. The use of aromatic shavings, including pine and cedar, is discouraged due to respiratory irritation. Care must be taken when sourcing substrates to avoid those that may be contaminated or of poor quality, as straw and wood shavings in particular can carry *Aspergillus fumigatus*, a respiratory fungus that can cause high mortality in chicks.[2,10] Substrate should be thick and

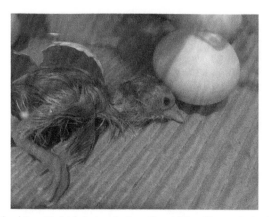

Fig. 1. Newly hatched "wet" chick in incubator. The chick will remain in the incubator until dry, typically 12 to 24 hours. (*Courtesy of* Sarah Seleta Nothnagel, (ASCP)cm.)

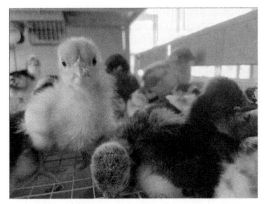

Fig. 2. Day-old chicks dried off in incubator. (*Courtesy of* Heather Reider, Colorado State University.)

provide proper footing for chicks and should be spot-cleaned daily with full removal of bedding performed regularly, before any wet clumps form.

Common heating elements include simple red light bulbs, ceramic bulbs, and heat plates. Red light or ceramic heating bulbs should be suspended over the center of the brooding area, and temperature is controlled by raising and lowering the bulb until optimal temperature is reached (see **Figs. 3** and **4**). In general, for the first week of life, the temperature at the hottest place available in the brooder should be 35°C (95°F). This is decreased by about 2 to 3° C (5° F) each week until about 4 to 5 weeks of age, at which time supplemental heat can be discontinued and chicks maintained at an ambient temperature of about 21°C (70°F).[4,6] Heat bulbs containing polytetrafluoroethylene coating (Teflon, The Chemours Company, Wilmington, DE, USA) could potentially lead to high mortality respiratory toxicity and should be avoided.[11] Heat plates, which often seem as a flat heat element that can be raised and lowered on legs, can be directly temperature controlled via a rheostat. They also can be elevated as chicks grow in height. A general rule to determine if the temperature is adequate is to monitor how chicks distribute themselves in the incubator. Chicks should be evenly spread out in the enclosure if they are comfortable and the temperature is appropriate.

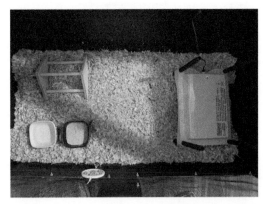

Fig. 3. Example of homemade chick brooder with aspen shaving substrate and plate-style heat source (Brinsea, TM). (*Courtesy of* Sarah Seleta Nothnagel, (ASCP)cm.)

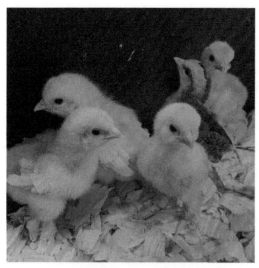

Fig. 4. Chicks in incubator under red lamp heat source. (*Courtesy of* Sarah Seleta Nothnagel, (ASCP)cm.)

Chicks that cluster and amass directly under the heat source are generally too cold, and chicks that distribute away from the heat source at the furthest margins of the enclosure are too hot.[4,6]

Commonly used feeding devices include gravity and trough feeders. Gravity feeders have holes at the bottom, which allow chicks to stick their heads through in order to eat (**Figs. 5** and **6**). Trough feeders have a cover to reduce food wastage. Feeders should be covered to prevent chicks from directly sitting and defecating in them or have small openings to eat from to prevent contamination (**Fig. 7**). Waterers should be shallow to prevent drowning, or small clean stones can be placed in the water trough to prevent drowning (see **Figs. 5, 6,** and **8**). Raising feeders and waterers is another way to reduce contamination.[2,6]

Chicks should be fed a starter crumble. In laying breeds, this should be fed for weeks 0 to 3, and then chicks transitioned to a grower crumble or pellet for weeks 4 to 16. In meat breeds, chicks should be fed starter feed for weeks 0 to 2, then grower

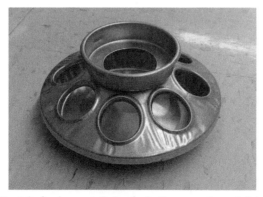

Fig. 5. Metal gravity-style feeder or waterer. A plastic reservoir containing food or water is placed into the top that allows automatic filling of the base.

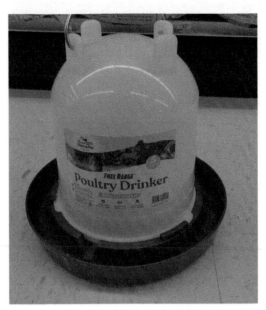

Fig. 6. Plastic gravity-style waterer with a narrow trough to discourage contamination and drowning. (*With permission from* Manna Pro®, Compana Pet Brands.)

feed from 2 to 6 weeks, and then a finisher feed from 6 weeks until slaughter. Laying breeds should be transitioned to an adult layer feed at about 16 weeks of age.[6] For turkeys (*Meleagris gallopavo*) and helmeted guineafowl (*Numida meleagris*), which grow larger overall than chickens, the transition to a maintenance feed can occur at 16 weeks and to a layer feed once they begin to produce eggs.[4,6] There are commercially available turkey-specific feeds, and guineafowl can generally be fed chicken feeds. There are also game bird formulations marketed for turkeys, peafowl, pheasants, quail, and other exotic Galliformes. These formulations generally have a higher protein content due to the slightly more insectivorous diets of wild species. Despite this, it is common to feed chicken products to the majority of gallinaceous birds.[2,6]

Determining vaccination status can be challenging, as online sources may not disclose information, and farm and feed stores may not have information readily available. It is

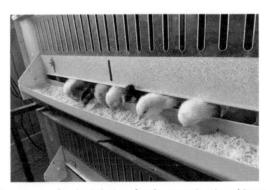

Fig. 7. Trough-style access to food minimizes fecal contamination. (*Courtesy of* Heather Reider, Colorado State University.)

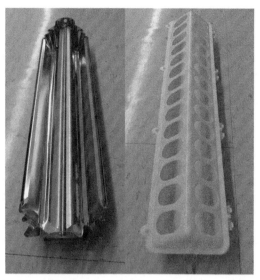

Fig. 8. Metal and plastic trough-style chick feeders. Only the head is able to access the plastic version, reducing contamination.

generally recommended to have chicks vaccinated for Marek's disease (gallid alphaherpesvirus 2), either in ovo or at 1 day of age.[2] Other vaccinations that are commonly administered to commercial layer and broiler chickens depend on production needs and exposure risk.[2] These include infectious bronchitis (a coronavirus), Newcastle disease (avian paramyxovirus type 1), infectious bursal disease (IBD) (a birnavirus), infectious laryngotracheitis (gallid alphaherpesviurs 1), *Mycoplasma gallisepticum*, poxvirus, avian encephalomyelitis (Tremovirus A), infectious coryza (*Avibacterium paragallinarum*), and coccidiosis.[2] However, vaccination for these diseases is uncommon in chicks sold to backyard hobbyists. Vaccination by the client or an avian veterinarian is typically prohibitive or not advised for multiple reasons including vaccine cost, inability to obtain individual or small quantities of vaccine, limitations with storage and administration, and risks of exposure and shedding when dealing with live vaccines for certain diseases. Therefore, when advising owners about vaccination, it is generally recommended they purchase chicks that have already been vaccinated for Marek's disease.[2,6]

DISEASES OF CHICKS

Chicks will commonly be presented to a veterinarian for evaluation of clinical signs related to infectious disease, orthopedic problems, or with a history of chick loss in the group. Many of these presentations can be traced back to infectious organisms, nutritional-related disorders, or abnormalities associated with incubation. Infectious disease in particular can pose a diagnostic challenge; therefore, it is advised to submit deceased or euthanized chicks for necropsy and histopathologic evaluation.[10] Once an infectious disease is present in a flock, it can be difficult to eradicate. Many diseases are transmitted vertically from an infected hen into the egg, which consequently can be spread via horizontal transmission to other chicks during incubation or after hatching.[2,6] Many infectious diseases can exist without causing clinical signs in adults if they survive the disease as chicks, which then establishes asymptomatic carriers within a flock. Thus, chicks from an outwardly "healthy" adult flock can still harbor and introduce disease into a new flock.[2] Considerations for owners should include disease transfer risk from existing flock members to new additions, introduction of disease from new chicks to established flock members, immunity of established flock animals to endemic disease versus poor immunity of new chicks, and biosecurity practices currently in place. Recommendations to owners could include an "all-in, all-out" approach to husbandry, where a group of animals is kept with no new additions from chick to death, or strict biosecurity that keeps growing chicks entirely separate from the established flock until adulthood.

RESPIRATORY

Aspergillosis, colloquially known as "brooder pneumonia," is caused by fungal lesions in the respiratory tract caused by A fumigatus. Aspergillus spp are ubiquitous in the environment; therefore, utmost care must be taken to maintain clean incubator and brooding conditions. Wood shavings, straw, and hay bedding can harbor fungal spores, and wet or moist conditions can lead to fungal proliferation. Chicks inhale the fungus, where it settles and forms plaques in the lungs, trachea, oral cavity, and air sacs. The disease can also spread to visceral organs. A fumigatus infection may present as increased mortality in chicks during weeks 0 to 2, which may or may not be accompanied by respiratory signs including dyspnea, orthopnea, tail bobbing, respiratory secretions, white oral plaques, and sneezing. Treatment is not recommended, as azoles are not labeled in chickens, and meat and egg withdrawal times are for the life of the animal.[2,6,10] Birds in severe respiratory distress should be euthanized and necropsied to confirm a diagnosis, and focus should be on the prevention of disease.

Other respiratory pathogens to be aware of, but that generally typically affect adult chickens, include Mycoplasma spp, Pasteurella multocida (fowl cholera), A paragallinarum (infectious coryza), gallid herpesvirus 1 (infectious laryngotracheitis), coronavirus (infectious bronchitis), poxvirus, and Syngamus trachea (gapeworm).[2,6,10,12] In general, if young poultry are affected by these diseases, the presentation may simply be increased mortality and/or sudden death. Importantly, if clinical signs are seen, they are often similar among infectious agents and the specific causative pathogen cannot be determined based on signs alone. Therefore, in a flock with increased mortality or general respiratory disease, it is critical to recommend necropsies on deceased or euthanized animals.

Chicks should be submitted whole for gross necropsy and full histopathology to obtain the most information, and swabs or frozen tissue samples of the respiratory tract saved before formalin fixation. Alternatively, swabs or fresh tissue samples of the oral cavity, trachea, lungs, and air sacs can be obtained for submission to a laboratory for the above-mentioned viral and bacterial diseases if full necropsy cannot be performed.

GASTROINTESTINAL

Salmonella spp are a common cause of morbidity and mortality in juvenile and adult chicken flocks. The Salmonella genus is a rod-shaped, Gram-negative bacteria with two species: S enterica and S bongori. S enterica has many subspecies of varying infectivity and severity, and for ease of reference, these are shortened without using the enterica designation.[8] These subspecies, also called serovars, of Salmonella also vary in their zoonotic potential. It is important to note that Salmonella spp is a normal organism that is present in the intestinal tract of healthy chickens, and human exposure comes most commonly from contaminated egg and meat products as well as contact with the environment chickens live in.[2,8] Owing to environmental and direct exposure to Salmonella spp, it is always advised to thoroughly wash hands after handling live Galliformes and working in their living spaces.

Salmonella pullorum is the most significant serovar in pediatric chicks, as it causes severe clinical signs in newly hatched and young chicks. The disease was previously known as "white diarrhea disease" and is today sometimes referred to as "pullorum disease." *S pullorum* is a vertically transmitted disease, with an infected hen harboring bacteria in the ovary and passing it into the egg. When the chick hatches, the down feathers are contaminated, and bacteria are easily spread horizontally via aerosolization in the incubator and brooder.[8,13] Affected chicks are weak and obtunded at hatching and may have drooped wings. Chicks may huddle together and lack an appetite. Overall mortality varies up to 100%, and this disease is reportable to the US Department of Agriculture (USDA), National Animal Health and Reporting System.[2,8,13] Owing to this being a reportable disease and the ability for disease survivors to perpetuate the lifecycle, it is advised that groups of chicks where *S pullorum* is identified are euthanized.

Paratyphoid *Salmonella* spp infection describes a set of *S enterica* serovars including, but not limited to, Typhimurium, Enteritidis, and Arizonae. In general, for paratyphoid *Salmonella* spp, adult chickens act as carriers and shedders (shedding through feces and carrying the organism in the ovary); however, severe clinical disease and mortality are seen in chicks 3 weeks of age and younger.[6,8,13] Clinical signs in chicks are nonspecific and include lethargy, fluffed appearance, huddling together, and white or yellow pasty diarrhea. Control of paratyphoid *Salmonella* can be difficult due to carrier status and the ability for living fomites such as rats, mice, and humans to horizontally spread this disease. Control is aimed at coop biosecurity, vermin control, vaccination if possible, and depopulation of affected flocks as opposed to treatment of affected individuals.[2,6,8]

Salmonella gallinarum is a serovar that can affect poultry of any age and is transmitted both vertically and horizontally through asymptomatic shedders. In chicks that are affected at hatching, signs include decreased hatch rate and fluffed and lethargic chicks with dyspnea and/or white to yellow diarrhea. In general, this serovar affects chicks greater than 12 weeks of age and causes higher mortality in adults than in young chickens. This serovar is also reportable in the United States, thus if individuals are diagnosed based on bacterial culture, further flock recommendations can be made based on recommendations from the USDA Animal Plant and Health Inspection Service.[2,6,8]

Coccidiosis is an important disease that affects all ages of poultry and is ubiquitously present within flocks under human care. The protozoal parasite responsible for disease, *Eimeria* spp, has many individual species that are host-specific and not transmissible between poultry species. Coccidiosis does not have maternal immunity instead immunity is based on chronic exposure to the organism in the environment. Other factors such as exposure dose, previous exposure to the same species, previous treatment with anticoccidial medication, vaccination status, and even genetic immunity can play a role in disease severity.[8,12,14] *Eimeria* spp cannot be fully eradicated from an environment, and some exposure to the organism is necessary for poultry to maintain immunity against clinical disease. The life cycle includes a noninfective oocyst shed into the environment via feces, where the infectious stage, a sporulated oocyst, develops when exposed to warm, moist, and oxygen-rich conditions. Thus, the burden of infectious coccidian organisms in the environment can be reduced by maintaining dry, clean, and well-ventilated substrate. This should be a focus of management of coccidiosis for backyard poultry flocks. Other management techniques include deep bedding to dilute the concentration of feces, the addition of rock salt at 60 to 80 pounds/100 square feet as a base layer, and reducing stock density so each bird has greater than 5 square feet (>1.5 m^2) of space.[2,8,15] With regard to young chicks, because there is no maternal immunity passed, it is important to be cautious when introducing nonimmune chicks that have been raised separately from other flock members into the general population. This critical period is typically between 3 and 6 weeks of age; however, older chicks can still have clinical disease if they have not developed immunity or are exposed to a species to which they have not been previously exposed. Common management strategies to prevent clinical disease from coccidiosis in young chicks include biannual treatment of the adult flock with feed-based anticoccidial medication, feed-based treatment of chicks at 14 days of age or later, and replacement of the top layer of substrate before introduction of chicks into the established flock.[2,15] Affected chicks can present with lethargy, pale comb and wattles, fluffed appearance, frank blood in the droppings, poor growth, and heat-seeking behavior.[2,8] Definitive diagnosis can be made on fecal floatation or on necropsy of deceased chicks.[2,14] Supportive treatment with subcutaneous fluid therapy, heat support, antibiotics for secondary bacterial infection, and amprolium in water (Corid, Huvepharma, Peachtree City, GA, USA) can be implemented for affected individuals. Feed-based anticoccidial medications such as amprolium, clopidol, and diclazuril are typically not helpful in acute disease, and instead should be used as a prophylactic treatment to reduce overall coccidia numbers in an established flock.[8,14] Surviving chicks develop excellent immunity and can be integrated into the general population with regular feed-based coccidial treatment. Combination vaccines are available for some common species of chicken coccidia; however, these are more commonly used in large-scale chicken operations with known heavy coccidial burdens. It is uncommon to see chicks destined for purchase as backyard chickens to be vaccinated against coccidia.[8]

IBD, also known as Gumboro disease, is caused by IBD virus (IBDV) in the genus Birnavirus. The viral agent exhibits tropism for immature B-lymphocytes and therefore targets the bursa of Fabricius in young poultry. Destruction of immature lymphocytes within the bursa combined with waning maternal immunity causes significant immunosuppression in affected chicks aged 3 to 6 weeks, and earlier infection tends to result in subclinical disease. Clinical signs are nonspecific and include lethargy, fluffed appearance, diarrhea, and in severe cases anorexia, tremors, and death. Morbidity for many strains can reach up to 100%; however, mortality varies based on strain.[2,6] Subclinically affected individuals may exhibit immunosuppression and increased susceptibility to other infectious diseases such as *Escherichia coli*, coccidiosis, and necrotic enteritis.[2] There is no treatment available for IBDV aside from supportive cares. Practically, IBD is a disease problem of commercial flocks and large-operation farms. The IBD virus is highly stable and resistant in the environment and can contaminate living spaces for months, facilitating spread via fecal–oral, fomite, and live vector routes. Owing to the resistant nature of the virus, sanitation and cleaning regimens can be unsuccessful, and successful management of IBD comes from strict vaccination protocols and all-in-all-out management. It is uncommon to see vaccination protocols in place for small-scale chicken operations.

Intestinal nematodes are another parasite contributing to clinical disease in young poultry. The most significant agents include *Ascaridia* spp, *Capillaria* spp, and *Heterakis* spp, which can be termed roundworms, threadworms, and cecal worms, respectively. *Ascaridia galli* is the most common disease agent for ascariasis and has a direct life cycle, causing intestinal mucosal damage and potential obstruction of the intestinal lumen. Birds less than 3 months of age are most susceptible and show signs of poor growth, lethargy, diarrhea with or without blood, and weakness. Diagnosis of ascariasis can be made based on zinc sulfate or sodium nitrate fecal floatation.[2] *Capillaria obsignata* is the most problematic species of threadworm, using a direct lifecycle.

This parasite can affect multiple regions of the small intestine, burrowing into the mucosal layer to cause hemorrhagic enteritis, mucosal thickening, and, at times, intestinal obstruction. Clinical signs include diarrhea, weight loss, poor growth, and thin body condition. Diagnosis can be made based on intestinal mucosal scrapings viewed under a microscope; however, for individuals with a lighter worm burden, intestinal mucosal washing may be required for diagnosis. It is important to consider several factors when treating poultry for helminths, as there is increasing resistance to many common antiparasitic drugs and drugs available for use in poultry are limited. Current recommendations include treating only groups that are severely affected by helminthic disease and using environmental control measures such as rotating grazing areas, ensuring that substrate is cleaned regularly, and maintaining good coop sanitation measures.[16] The only treatment currently approved for treatment of helminthiasis in poultry is fenbendazole; dosing can vary but in general a common protocol is feed-based at 50 to 80 mg/kg of feed for 5 to 7 days.[17,18] Interestingly, *Heterakis* spp do not commonly cause direct clinical disease in poultry, although in high numbers they can induce typhlitis. *Heterakis* spp are vectors for the protozoal parasite *Histomonas meleagridis*, which causes blackhead disease in turkeys. *Heterakis* spp can also use an intermediate host, the earthworm, to further transmit *H meleagridis* to other species that ingest an infected earthworm. Treatment for *Heterakis* spp is similar to management of ascariasis. Histomoniasis itself is a disease most recognized in turkeys; however, it can affect other game bird species and has been seen in backyard chicken flocks. This protozoal parasite uses poultry hosts to replicate in the cecum, where it then infects *Heterakis* spp worms and is shed in roundworm eggs into the environment. This is the stage where earthworms can ingest roundworm eggs and act as paratenic hosts. Subsequently, birds that ingest contaminated feed or fomites, or ingest an infected paratenic host become infected. Clinical signs include dull mentation and lethargy, drooped wings, and watery to yellow diarrhea. Young birds can be more severely affected and can die within days of exhibiting disease. In turkeys, mortality can reach 70% to 100%.[19] No treatment is available for histomoniasis infection. In general, intestinal nematode management plans should include good coop management, in addition to treatment with anthelmintics. Many nematode species eggs remain infective in the environment for extended periods of time (eg, 160 weeks for *A galli*), and many are spread via insect and annelid vectors and intermediate hosts.[2] Managing coop substrates in a similar fashion to managing coccidiosis, and implementing control of invertebrates in the coop area can reduce infective doses of nematodes.

NEUROLOGIC

Chicks can hatch with congenital neurologic diseases, including hydrocephalus, anophthalmia, and calvarium malformations. Some congenital malformations occur with increased frequencies in certain breeds, such as an increased incidence of cranial malformation (vaulted skull) in crested phenotype chickens, notably Polish and Silkie chickens.[20] A vaulted skull is commonly associated with brain malformation or herniation and associated neurologic signs. In general, with the above congenital malformations, treatment decisions can be made based on the severity and type of clinical signs. A bird with a mildly vaulted skull may not exhibit significant neurologic abnormalities, although another individual may exhibit severe torticollis resulting in difficulty eating and drinking. Signs may also worsen or abate as the chick grows in size, so time with monitoring and supportive care can be advised in some cases.[2] Torticollis, or "wry neck," is another general term that encompasses multiple etiologic causes. It may be due to congenital malformation, nutritional deficiency, infectious central neurologic system (CNS) disease, or trauma. History of onset, progression, severity, and the presence of other clinical signs can help to discern between these causes, and treatment recommendations made based on how the torticollis affects the individual and suspected etiology. See "other infectious" for information on Marek's disease.

Avian encephalomyelitis, or "epidemic tremor," is a viral disease (Tremovirus A) seen in chicks aged 1 to 3 weeks. The virus is transmitted vertically from the hen or horizontally via oral ingestion and spread to the CNS. Incubation via horizontal transmission is typically ≥11 days, and vertical transmission results in clinical signs within 7 days. The classic clinical signs are ataxia with head and neck tremors, sometimes preceded by general lethargy. Treatment is supportive care, and in general, mortality is about 25% to 50%, with morbidity up to 60%. Recovered chicks can display permanent ataxia and may develop cataracts within weeks after infection; therefore, euthanasia may need to be considered. Infected chicks shed for 2 weeks after infection, although birds greater than 4 weeks of age are typically resistant to clinical infection.[2,6,12]

Enterococcus spp is a genus of Gram-positive, facultative anaerobic bacteria that has been reported to cause neurologic disease and mortality in poultry. The organism causes encephalomalacia, resulting in clinical disease in chicks aged 3 to 12 days. Disease can include neurologic signs including torticollis, head tremors, and decreased mentation. Other signs include evidence of sepsis including diarrhea, weight loss, pale comb, and acute death. In one study, *Enterococcus* spp was attributed to 22% of histologically diagnosed brain disorders in broiler chickens.[8,12]

OTHER INFECTIOUS

Omphalitis, or "mushy chick disease," is a general term used to refer to a variety of bacterial infections that affect the urachus of young chicks. The urachal region typically is swollen, red, and potentially oozing or wet. Owing to the urachus connecting the yolk sac internally, it is common for infection to ascend and cause yolk sacculitis, which can lead to sepsis. Affected chicks may present with acute death or "ill thrift" with a ruffled appearance, lethargy, fecal staining around the vent, dyspnea, and inappropriate positioning in the brooder. By the time chicks exhibit clinical signs, treatment is generally ineffective, and euthanasia should be considered. Despite being caused by a bacterial infection, the disease is typically not contagious to other birds and instead is acquired through unsanitary brooder conditions, which allows opportunistic bacteria to infect the urachus. The disease is most commonly seen in the first 2 weeks of life, when the urachus is still healing and the yolk sac is being reabsorbed. Common pathogens leading to omphalitis include E coli (termed colibacillosis), *Staphylococcus* spp, *Pseudomonas* spp, *Proteus* spp, or a combination of bacteria. The prevention of disease is the best course to avoid morbidity and mortality due to omphalitis. This starts with sanitary incubating conditions, followed by maintaining a clean brooding environment for chicks.[2,21]

Marek's disease, or "range paralysis," is perhaps one of the most recognized diseases of domestic chickens and to a lesser extent other Gallinaceous species. Marek's disease is caused by an alphaherpesvirus of the *Mardivirus* genus and is found ubiquitously around the world affecting domestic poultry. Three serotypes are commonly recognized: serotype 1 (oncogenic), serotype 2 (non-oncogenic), and serotype 3 (herpesvirus of turkeys), with varying virulence existing due to multiple factors. Marek's can be a frustrating disease, as individual birds may be asymptomatic shedders due to a confluence of genetic resistance, vaccination, virus virulence, and latent infection. The virus replicates and is shed in feather follicle epithelium; thus, airborne exposure to feathers and dander is the route of transmission. It is recognized that the virus can remain infectious in feather material for several months and potentially years in colder environments. There is also a recognition that chickens can shed from the skin for up to 18 months and that insect vectors may also play a role as mechanical vectors.[2,10,12]

Chicks should be vaccinated in ovo or at 1 day of age. Vaccination helps provide immunity by reducing viral replication and reducing chances of latent infection but does not prevent disease. Marek's disease virus is considered a lymphoproliferative virus, and clinical infection results in deposition of lymphoid cells into various tissues in the body.[2,8,12] Various clinical manifestations may develop depending on the tissues infected. Chicks will most commonly be presented with lymphoid lesions of nerves and ganglia, resulting in the inability to walk, with one pelvic limb frequently posted forward and the other back. A lymphodegenerative syndrome can also affect chicks, resulting in immunosuppression and early mortality. This can be difficult to discern from other causes of mortality in young chicks. Chicks can start showing signs of disease at 9 days of age, and morbidity generally increases within the flock and persists for 4 to 10 weeks. Other Marek's disease manifestations include deposition of lymphoid aggregates in the iris, leading to an ocular form visualized as a pale change in iris color and dyscoria. More commonly seen in latent affected and adult birds would be visceral deposition of lymphoid tissue, seen as tumors on the reproductive organs, liver, heart, spleen, and kidneys. The development of lymphoid deposits in the skin alone is known as skin leukosis.[2,6,10,12] There is no treatment for Marek's disease, although supportive care for affected chicks including hydration, feeding, management to prevent recumbency ulcers, and keeping the vent clean can be attempted. Mortality can be up to 100%, but in chicks that recover can have varying degrees of permanent neurologic dysfunction. It is important to necropsy deceased chicks, even if they do not exhibit classic signs of Marek's disease, because not all forms cause outward neurologic disease.[2,10]

ORTHOPEDIC

Perosis, commonly known as slipped tendon, is an orthopedic disease where the extensor tendon of the tarsus (gastrocnemius tendon) luxates, and as the pelvic limb develops, the tibiotarsal and tarsometatarsal bones may improperly form. This is thought to be multifactorial, with manganese, choline, and/or biotin deficiencies considered to be contributing factors. Other predisposing factors include heavy-bodied breeds (particularly broiler breeds) and environmental factors, such as slick/slippery flooring.[2,6,22,23] Clinical signs may affect one or both pelvic limbs and include valgus or hyperextension of the intertarsal joint, inability to stand and walk, visible bony malformation, abnormal joint rotation, thickening of bones above/below the intertarsal joint, thickening of the tarsal region, and pododermatitis. Treatment has been attempted with supplementation of the aforementioned nutrients and various tendon stabilizing/tacking surgeries with bandaging.[2,6,23] Prognosis is generally considered poor, especially as the chick ages. It is important to inform clients that if this condition is left untreated that it leads to a nonmobile bird. Harnesses, slings, wheelchairs, and maintaining a chicken as a "down" animal can have serious welfare implications. Therefore, in advanced cases or those where treatment does not lead to complete ambulation, euthanasia should be recommended.[2,4,22,23]

Splay leg, also known as spraddle leg, is a condition resulting in abduction of both pelvic limbs. In severe cases, the chick is unable to ambulate; however, in less affected cases, attempts to ambulate may be made with varying success. Many causes have been proposed, including genetic factors, nutrition, hyperthermia during incubation or brooding, and inappropriately slick substrates during brooding, but it is likely that this condition is multifactorial in etiology.[2,4,12] It is vital to initiate treatment as soon as possible in the disease process, otherwise changes can be permanent. Treatment options include hobbles of the tarsometatarsi to correct the abduction, and in younger chicks, placement in a shot glass or other small cup for prolonged periods of time. Even with treatment, the disease can still be intractable and euthanasia should be considered if it is unsuccessful or if the defect is so severe that it limits ambulation.[2]

Some chicks can hatch with crooked or bent digits or may develop abnormalities over time. If crooked digits are noticed, application of tape splints to the feet as soon as possible is often the best course of treatment. Tape splints can be made using multiple layers of overlapped white athletic tape (Zonas tape, Johnson & Johnson, New Brunswick, NJ, USA) and placed on the plantar and dorsal surfaces of the foot, encompassing all toes with digit 1 facing caudally and digits 2 to 4 facing cranially and evenly spread. The tape splint should be kept clean and dry, and replaced if it becomes dirty. The splint should be removed 5 to 7 days later for evaluation of the digits. If adequate correction of the deformity has not been achieved, the splints should be replaced and rechecks should continue at 5 to 7 day intervals until adequate correction is achieved.

NUTRITIONAL DISEASES

Most vitamin and mineral deficiencies are easily avoided by providing age-appropriate commercial chick feeds. Some nutritional deficiencies occur due to poor diet of the parents, an imbalance caused by providing other sources of food (nutrient dilution), and improper storage of feed. It is important that parents, particularly the hen, are on a breeder-specific feed as opposed to layer or flock maintenance, because layer feeds are inadequate to provide hens with nutrients necessary to lay healthy eggs intended for hatching chicks. The quality of some vitamin and mineral additives degrades over time and degradation can be affected by storage conditions; therefore, it is important for chick owners to check expiration dates and ensure food has been stored properly.[6,8]

Vitamin A deficiency leads to poor growth. Chicks are presented thin, weak, and fluffed. It also induces squamous metaplasia of epithelial cells in many tissues, including glands and mucosal surfaces.[6] This can induce respiratory signs, intestinal malabsorption, and general unthriftiness.[2,6] It can be difficult to distinguish from many other infectious and noninfectious diseases; therefore, an assumption of vitamin A deficiency should be made if other infectious diseases have been ruled out. Supplementation with vitamin A should be implemented, although treatment outcomes vary and are often poor. Supplementation in drinking water with a poultry-specific multivitamin can be used when attempting to treat a vitamin A disorder (Durvet Vitamins and Electrolytes for Poultry, Durvet, Blue Springs, MO, USA), as most of the injectable vitamin A products are in too high of a concentration to safely supplement vitamin A parenterally. If attempting to use injectable protocols, a dose of 20,000 U/kg intramuscularly once weekly is an adequate dosage.[17]

Chicks with vitamin B1 (thiamine) deficiency, also termed "polyneuritis," are typically presented with a poor appetite with weight loss and subsequent lethargy, weakness, and potentially neurologic signs. In advanced stages, chicks will hock-sit and stargaze. If suspicious of thiamine deficiency, the feed should be evaluated as some deficiencies are induced by thiaminase-heavy fish meal-based diets, which are currently uncommon in commercial diets.[24] Exogenous thiamine supplementation can reverse clinical signs in mildly affected chicks, but neurologically affected chicks may not respond to treatment.[4] Exogenous supplementation with a water-based multivitamin can be used, and injectable or oral vitamin B preparations can be dosed at 1 to 2 mg/kg by mouth or intramuscularly once daily.

Vitamin B2 (riboflavin) deficiency, known as "curly toe disease," causes poor myelination of nerves, which causes clenching of the feet with the chick walking on the dorsolateral surface of the foot at the time of hatching.[2,6] Chicks may use their wings to attempt to ambulate, resulting in abrasions on the wingtips. Disease can spontaneously resolve after hatching, as the body's demand for riboflavin decreases and dietary riboflavin becomes sufficient to meet the body's needs. Treatment is with vitamin B complex supplementation as recommended for thiamine deficiency.

Vitamin D_3 deficiency, termed "rubber legs" or "Rickets," is an uncommon deficiency seen in chicks raised outdoors on a commercial diet. Vitamin D_3 is commonly supplemented in feed as cholecalciferol and is balanced with calcium and phosphorus in the diet. Vitamin D_3 requires ultraviolet-B light to be synthesized by the body; therefore, chicks raised solely indoors can have a deficiency of vitamin D. Vitamin D is required to synthesize proteins that bind calcium and control absorption of dietary calcium from the intestines as well as translocating blood calcium for bodily use. Therefore, deficiency can result in inadequate calcium absorption or can contribute to an imbalance of calcium and phosphorus in the body. Clinical signs of vitamin D deficiency are typically related to calcium deficiency including hard, painful joint swellings commonly in the pelvic limbs, poorly mineralized and flexible bones, tibial chondrodysplasia, swelling of rib cartilages, soft beak, and malformed or stunted pelvic limbs.[6,8,24] Treatment in cases due to the lack of ultraviolet exposure includes at least 30 minutes of ultraviolet light exposure daily. In severe cases, 1000 U/300 g of injectable vitamin D3 intramuscularly once weekly can be used. Care in vitamin D_3 injectable formulation selection should be taken as many products are highly concentrated, and overdose induces toxicity.

Vitamin E deficiency induces an encephalomalacia, known as "crazy chick disease" colloquially, and can also produce an exudative diathesis and muscular dystrophy type disease in young chicks. The preferred form of vitamin E used by poultry is α-tocopherol, which is a fat-soluble vitamin naturally available in plants and seed oils.[2,6,8] Vitamin E acts as an antioxidant in body tissues, and deficiency results in cell membrane damage and, of particular clinical importance, damage to blood vessels and capillary permeability.[8] Encephalomalacia is seen in young chicks aged 2 to 3 weeks and up to 5 weeks and results in ataxia, torticollis, paresis, and abnormal coordination. Most chicks will die, and treatment after clinical signs are apparent is ineffective. Exudative diathesis is a result of increased capillary permeability in tissues and results in subcutaneous plasma and blood leakage seen as blue, green, or black discoloration over the breast muscles and wing regions. This can be seen in conjunction with muscular dystrophy, thought to be induced by concurrent amino acid deficiency and resulting in muscle necrosis and weakness due to capillary obstruction. Treatment can be attempted via vitamin E in drinking water; however, the condition is typically fatal and clinically affected chicks should be euthanized.[6,8] Prevention is key for avoiding vitamin E deficiencies and can be performed by ensuring a commercial chick diet is provided during growth. An oral dose of vitamin E (Durvet Vitamin E and Selenium Gel, Durvet, Blue Springs, MO, USA) can be administered to affected chicks at 300 U per bird.[24] An injectable dose for chickens has not been established, but 0.06 mg/kg intramuscularly has been used in psittacines and ratites.[17]

OTHER

The equivalent of an umbilical hernia, or omphalocele, can be seen in chicks, which is due to an unretracted yolk sac. The yolk sac is present at hatching and should normally involute on day 1 or 2. The yolk sac provides nutrition and maternal antibodies to the chick in this critical post-hatching period. If a yolk sac does not retract, this leaves the chick susceptible to omphalitis and an open body wall. It is thought that improper incubation parameters or problems during the hatching period can predispose a chick to this condition. Treatment includes good sanitation and cleaning of the region followed by surgical omphalectomy and supportive care. Subcutaneous fluids, pain management, antibiotic therapy, anti-inflammatory therapy, and nutritional support are all considered components of treatment. Even with surgery and supportive care, the body wall may not close and the chick is predisposed to omphalitis; therefore, prognosis can be guarded.[2,10]

SUMMARY

Galliform pediatric medicine can be an intimidating branch of veterinary medicine for practitioners. Obtaining a thorough clinical history, diet review, and husbandry details are key components in establishing potential disease etiologies. Understanding of basic pediatric galliform feeding and rearing is crucial in being able to direct owners in optimizing husbandry practices at home. Likewise, being able to recognize potential pitfalls in chick management is important so that a preventative care program, quarantine protocol, and coop biosecurity plan can be implemented before clinical problems arise in a flock. If clinical disease is present in a chick group, it is important to be able to treat individual animals if needed, as well as the entire group if the problem is of infectious or nutritional origin. When disease is discovered, it is vital to recommend correct sample collection and submission, as well as recommending necropsy if available, to determine the ultimate cause of morbidity and mortality. As a practitioner establishing a veterinary-client-patient relationship with gallinaceous bird owners, it is your responsibility to understand governmental regulations set regarding use of medications in these species, as misuse of drugs in food-producing species can have licensure implications. Government resources are readily available online outlining rules and regulations as well as providing consultation resources regarding poultry species.

DISCLOSURE

No conflict of interest exists between the authors and any commercial or financial individual or institution. No funding was required for the production of this manuscript.

REFERENCES

1. Eda M. Origin of the domestic chicken from modern biological and zooarchaeological approaches. Anim Front 2021;11(3):52–61.
2. Greenacre CB, Morishita TY. Backyard poultry medicine and surgery: a guide for veterinary practitioners. Ames, IA: Wiley-Blackwell; 2021.
3. Harrison GJ, Lightfoot T, editors. Clinical avian medicine. Palm Beach, FL: Spix Publishing; 2006.
4. Damerow G. Chicken health handbook. North Adams, MA: Garden Way Publishing, Storey Communications, Inc; 1994.
5. Archer GS, Cartwright L. Incubating and Hatching Eggs. Texas A&M University AgriLife Extension. April 2022. https://cdn-de.agrilife.org/extension/departments/posc/posc-pu-018/publications/files/incubating-and-hatching-eggs.pdf.

6. Poland G, Raftery A, editors. BSAVA manual of backyard poultry medicine and surgery. Quedgeley, Gloucester, UK: British Small Animal Veterinary Association; 2019.

7. Stuttgen S. Life cycle of a laying hen. University of Wisconsin-Madison, Livestock Division of Extension. 2023. https://livestock.extension.wisc.edu/articles/life-cycle-of-a-laying-hen/.

8. Pattison M, McMullin PF, Bradbury JM, et al, editors. Poultry diseases. 6th edition. Philadelphia, PA: Elsevier; 2008.

9. Sanitation of incubator and equipment. PennState Extension - Pennsylvania 4-H. https://extension.psu.edu/programs/4-h/get-involved/teachers/embryology/teacher-resources/supporting-subject-matter/incubation/sanitation-of-incubator-and-equipment#:~:text=Clean%20the%20incubator%20immediately%20after,-bleach%20or%20disinfectant%2C%20if%20necessary.

10. MSD Animal Health. Important poultry diseases. Boxmeer, The Netherlands: Intervet International bv, subsidiary of Merck & Co; 2012.

11. Shuster KA, Brock KL, Dysko RC, et al. Polytetrafluoroethylene toxicosis in recently hatched chickens (Gallus domesticus). Comp Med 2012;62(1):49–52.

12. Swayne DE, Boulianne M, Logue CM, editors. Diseases of poultry. 11th ed. Ames, IA: Wiley-Blackwell; 2020. Vol 1-2. vols 1–2.

13. Yeakel SD. Pullorum Disease in Poultry. In: Merck manual - veterinary manual. Whitehouse Station, NJ: Merck & Co, Inc; 2022.

14. Gerhold RW. Coccidiosis in Poultry. In: Merck manual - veterinary manual. Whitehouse Station, NJ: Merck & Co, Inc; 2023.

15. Lorenzoni G. Managing chicken coccidiosis in small flocks during summer. Penn State Extension. March 27, 2023. https://extension.psu.edu/managing-chicken-coccidiosis-in-small-flocks-during-summer.

16. Macklin KS, Hauck R. Helminthiasis in Poultry. In: Merck manual - veterinary manual. Whitehouse Station, NJ: Merck & Co, Inc; 2022.

17. Carpenter JW, Harms CA, editors. Carpenter's exotic animal formulary. Philadelphia, PA: Elsevier; 2023.

18. Lighty, M. Deworming Backyard Poultry. Penn State Extension. 2023. https://extension.psu.edu/deworming-backyard-poultry.

19. Blackhead disease in Poultry. U.S. Food and Drug Administration. December 13, 2019. https://www.fda.gov/animal-veterinary/resources-you/blackhead-disease-poultry#:~:text=Blackhead%20disease%20(histomoniasis)%20is%20an,by%20the%20roundworm%20Heterakis%20gallinarum.

20. Wang Y, Gao Y, Imsland F, et al. The crest phenotype in chicken is associated with ectopic expression of HOXC8 in cranial skin. PLoS One 2012;7(4). https://doi.org/10.1371/journal.pone.0034012.

21. Sander JE. Omphalitis in Poultry. In: Merck manual - veterinary manual. Whitehouse Station, NJ: Merck & Co, Inc; 2022.

22. Olgun O. Manganese in poultry nutrition and its effect on performance and eggshell quality. World's Poult Sci J 2017;73(1):45–56. https://doi.org/10.1017/s0043933916000891.

23. Nka P, Sharma S, Chaudhary RN, et al. Surgical correction of perosis/slipped tendon in a white Pekin duck- case report. International Journal of Current Microbiology and Applied Sciences 2018;7(12):389–92. https://doi.org/10.20546/ijcmas.2018.712.048.

24. Korver D. Vitamin Deficiencies in Poultry. In: Merck manual - veterinary manual. Whitehouse Station, NJ: Merck & Co, Inc; 2023.

Neonatal Care of Anseriformes

Michele Goodman, VMD[a],*, Christine T. Higbie, DVM, DACZM[b]

KEYWORDS

- Duckling • Gosling • Cygnet • Drip-feeding

KEY POINTS

- Neonatal waterfowl benefit from swimming in water from a young age to maintain feather condition and for good welfare.
- Food presentation based on the species' natural history stimulates self-feeding behavior.
- Parent-rearing promotes natural behaviors.
- Developmental disorders often result from poor nutrition, overcrowding, and lack of exercise; disorders can often be corrected if detected early.

 Video content accompanies this article at http://www.vetexotic.theclinics.com.

NATURAL HISTORY

Members of the order Anseriformes consist of 3 families: the Anhimidae or screamers native to South America, the Anseranatidae or Magpie goose (*Anseranas semipalmata*) native to Australia, and the diverse Anatidae, which is composed of ducks, geese, and swans that reside across the globe. The focus of this article will be on the Anatidae with taxonomic classification following Livezey[1] with an emphasis on relevant nesting and rearing strategies that may influence neonatal care. Species that are not well represented in managed care are excluded. For detailed global species accounts, see Kear.[2]

Time from hatching to fledging can vary greatly within individual tribes. Along with individual species differences, this variation relates to day length, native geographic range, and food abundance with arctic nesting species fledging earlier than temperate or tropical species.[3,4] In general, species that achieve reproductive capacity at an older age have longer parental care periods extending months and sometimes up until almost a year of age.[2] Parental care strategies, incubation lengths, and age at fledging and reproduction for various tribes of Anseriformes are summarized in **Table 1**.

a Elmwood Park Zoo, 1661 Harding Boulevard, Norristown, PA 19002, USA; b The Philadelphia Zoo, 3400 W. Girard Avenue, Philadelphia, PA 19104, USA
* Corresponding author.
E-mail address: mgoodman@elmwoodparkzoo.org

Vet Clin Exot Anim 27 (2024) 313–339
https://doi.org/10.1016/j.cvex.2023.11.010
1094-9194/24/© 2023 Elsevier Inc. All rights reserved.

Table 1
Taxonomy of anseriformes[1,2]

Tribe	Common Name	Sexual Dimorphism	Parental Care	Incubation Length	Age at Fledging	Age at Reproduction
Dendrocygnini	Whistling ducks	No	Parents share incubation and rearing	22–31 d	50–70 d	1 y
Anserini and similar	True geese	No	Female incubation, rearing by both parents	20–30 d	35–60 d	2–3 y
Ceropsini and Tadorninae	Cape barren goose, sheldgeese, spur-winged geese	No	Female incubation, rearing by both parents	22–33 d	84–96 d	2–3 y
Cygnini	Swans	No	Parents share incubation and rearing	31–42 d	65–140 d	3 y minimum
Anatini and similar	Dabbling ducks, perching ducks	Varies by species	Varies by species, female solely responsible for incubation	21–35 d	42–80 d	1 y
Aythyini	Diving ducks	Yes	Female incubation and rearing	23–32 d	45–70 d	2 y
Mergini	Sea ducks	Yes	Female incubation and rearing	22–30 d	56–70 d	2–3 y
Oxyurini and Thalassornithini	Stiff-tailed ducks, white-backed duck	Yes (Oxyurini); no (Thalassornithini)	Female incubation and rearing	22–33 d	Around 60 d	1–2 y

REGULATIONS AND FLIGHT RESTRICTION

In the United States, native waterfowl species are protected under the US Fish and Wildlife Service Migratory Bird Treaty Act (MBTA) of 1918. Species covered by the MBTA are regulated species and require state and federal permits to maintain and breed in managed care. Clinicians should become familiar with the laws and regulations for the area in which they practice. Effective in August 2023, the US Department of Agriculture Animal Welfare Act includes birds and licenses may be required.

Captive-bred waterfowl covered under the MBTA must be properly marked or identified before 6 weeks of age in order to distinguish these birds from wild-caught waterfowl. Acceptable marking methods include the following:

> removal of the hind toe from the right foot, pinioning of a wing by removing the metacarpal bones of one wing or a portion of the metacarpal bones thereby rendering the bird permanently incapable of flight, banding of one metatarsus with a seamless metal band or tattooing a readily discernible number of letter or combination thereof on the web of one foot.[5]

The amputation of the metacarpal bones, a procedure known as pinioning, is restricted or illegal in several countries.[6] This marking technique is more commonly used as a method of flight restriction, which permits birds to be housed in open-top enclosures without the risk of escape. Historically, this procedure is performed on very young birds at 2 to 3 days of age and is generally not performed under anesthesia by a veterinarian. As the focus on animal well-being continues to increase, this procedure is being performed less frequently in the United States in general and is being performed more frequently by veterinarians with some level of analgesia and anesthesia. Ultimately, it may be restricted or prohibited. Although alternative methods for flight restriction have been developed including tendonectomy[4] and feather follicle extirpation,[7] the focus should be on creative facility design that allows birds to safely maintain flight and express their full range of natural behaviors.

NESTING, INCUBATION, AND HATCH

Although waterfowl lay a clutch of eggs during a short timeframe, often laying 1 egg every 24 to 48 hours, they incubate eggs synchronously such that all neonates hatch within a relatively short period.[8] In managed care, incubation can be performed underneath the parent bird(s), underneath a surrogate bird, or in an incubator. A higher hatch success is often achieved when incubation is at least started under a parent or surrogate bird as opposed to solely relying on an incubator.[9]

Artificial incubation requires strict attention to hygiene to reduce cases of omphalitis. Infections are often caused by gram-negative bacteria, most commonly *Salmonella* spp or *Escherichia coli*.[10,11] On external pip, eggs should be transferred to a hatcher that can maintain a higher humidity to prevent desiccation of egg membranes. From the time of external pip, full hatching generally occurs within 48 hours. Waterfowl are highly precocial and will often leave the nest within 24 to 48 hours of hatching and will start to feed within 24 to 48 hours of nest departure. All bird species begin the dynamic process of yolk sac resorption after hatch and waterfowl resorb their yolk sac during the first 7 days of life.[12]

Although assisted hatching can be performed with Anseriformes, particularly in cases of malpositioning, neonates that require assistance have a high rate of complications and a higher mortality rate associated with exhaustion or incomplete resorption of yolk sacs, particularly if intervention is delayed.[10]

INITIAL CARE

The umbilicus of neonates hatched in an incubator or hatcher should be monitored for signs of inflammation and infection, and may benefit from daily application of iodine to the umbilicus for 1 to 5 days until healed.[10,11] Individuals that have undergone any sort of assisted hatching are at increased risk of omphalitis, likely due to incompletely absorbed yolk sacs.[10] Antimicrobial therapy, isotonic fluid supplementation, and probiotics are reported to improve outcomes in a small number of cases where assistance was provided.[13]

IDENTIFICATION AND SEX DETERMINATION

Identification of individual birds can be accomplished by the application of color-coded cable ties for neonates and of seamless or seamed bands for older juveniles and adults. All bands require monitoring (daily for neonates) for correct positioning and for an appropriate fit particularly in growing birds. Bands should reside solely over the tarsometatarsus and should be unable to flip up over the hock joint or down over the foot joint.

Male Anseriformes possess an erectile phallus that allows for sex to be determined at only a few days of age by gentle eversion of the cloaca.[4] With some practice, this procedure, known as vent sexing, allows direct visualization of either the phallus or the distal oviduct by cloacal examination such that neonatal sex can be determined accurately (**Fig. 1**). When vent sexing young neonates, gentle pressure must be used so as not to rupture the yolk sac.[14]

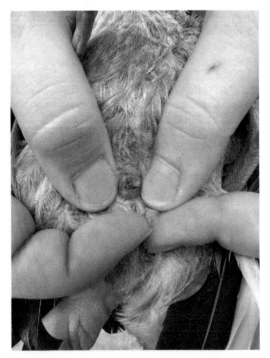

Fig. 1. Vent sexing an immature Brazilian teal (*Amazonetta brasiliensis*) shows eversion of the cloaca and the protrusion of a small phallus.

RESTRAINT AND HANDLING

Neonatal waterfowl are easily restrained using 2 hands around the body, keeping the wings tight to the body (**Fig. 2**). The body should be supported at all times but the legs can be supported or left to hang depending on what seems comfortable to the bird. A wing hold, where the thumb and middle finger restrain each humerus and the pointer finger separates the 2 wings, should not be performed in growing birds because this can strain the shoulder girdle. A towel can be used for larger juveniles. Care should be taken when handling young waterfowl when growing primary feathers because they will bleed if bent or broken, which requires prompt removal. As with any bird, handlers should refrain from tightly gripping around the sternum because this can restrict respiration.

Assemble all necessary supplies including potential therapies before patient handling, including examination tools, fluids, gavage-formulas, or medications. Neonates should be monitored for signs of stress associated with handling (**Fig. 3**). Handling should be minimized to what is clinically necessary particularly in debilitated individuals. Parent-reared waterfowl may be less tolerant of handling than hand-reared individuals. Open mouth breathing can be a sign of stress or overheating; if this behavior is observed, the examination may have to be discontinued or performed over multiple shorter handling sessions.

CLINICALLY RELEVANT HUSBANDRY

Once hatched and dry, neonatal waterfowl should be moved into a brooder and placed under a heat source with an item to provide comfort to the birds that simulates being brooded (a feather duster, stuffed animal, or hide pocket). The heat source should provide a localized warm temperature of approximately 32°C (90°F) that can be decreased gradually during the first 1 to 2 weeks by a few degrees every few days depending on species and ambient temperatures.[15] Neonates should be monitored for signs of suboptimal environmental temperatures. Birds that huddle underneath the warmest part of the brooder and refuse to move may be too cold, whereas birds that avoid the comfort item and exhibit open mouth breathing may be too warm. Food and water should be offered immediately because this can help to stimulate the growth and development of the gastrointestinal tract.[16,17] There are several types of brooder designs that are useful for rearing waterfowl.

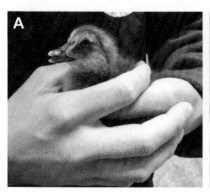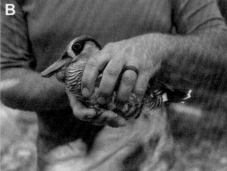

Fig. 2. Restraint approach for neonatal and juvenile waterfowl. (*A*) Duckling restraint. (Photo courtesy of Ian Gereg, Ambler, PA). (*B*) Restraint technique for juvenile waterfowl where the bottom hand supports the body and the top hand contains the wings.

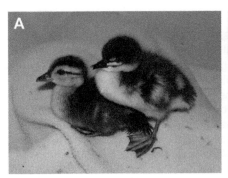
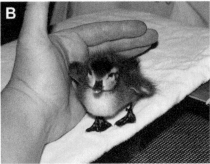

Fig. 3. Monitor neonates for signs of stress during handling. (*A*) Stable ducklings with bright eyes and normal wing position. (*B*) Unstable wood duckling with sunken eyes, fluffed appearance, and outstretched wings.

The Dry Brooder

A dry brooder is a box with a solid or screen bottom that is generally covered with towels or rubber matting to promote foot health. A heat source is set up on one side of the brooder in the form of a heating pad or heat lamp along with a comfort item (**Fig. 4**). Use caution when using a heat lamp to prevent comfort items from being directly heated up. Mortalities have been reported in commercial poultry with the use of polytetrafluoroethylene-coated heat lamps; these should be avoided in all avian species.[18] Halogen infrared heat bulbs provide adequate warmth and are both shock and water resistant. Food and water are provided on the side of the brooder away from the heat source. A wet brooder can often be converted into a dry brooder by using 2 perforated floors, 1 over each pool (**Fig. 5**). A dry brooder can be used for all species but is generally limited to short-term use as waterfowl benefit from immediate access to swimming water. A dry brooder can also be used intermittently for neonatal waterfowl that are struggling to establish waterproofing until their feather condition improves.

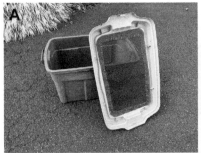
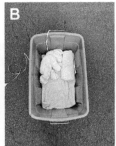
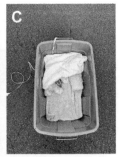

Fig. 4. Dry brooder configured with a heating pad and a hide pocket. (*A*) Lidded plastic tubs of various sizes can be converted to dry brooders. A section of the lid is removed and replaced with heavy-duty mesh screening secured with cable ties (the head of the cable tie should be fastened on the outside of the lid). (*B*) A heating pad covers half of the bottom of the brooder and is set to low. Rolled towels and/or stuffed animals are used around the edges of the warm side of the tub. (*C*) A towel is then placed on top of the towels and stuffed animals to create a hide pocket that simulates parental brooding. Food and water are provided on the nonheated side of the tub.

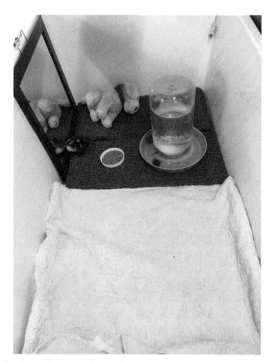

Fig. 5. An aquatic bird-rearing cubicle can be converted to a dry brooder by adding an additional perforated floor. For small neonates, the floors can be covered with unbacked PCV coiled matting and / or towels.

The Wet Brooder

A wet brooder can be created from a converted shipping tote or can be a specifically designed product for brooding with a dedicated land portion along with a ramped in-ground swimming pool (**Fig. 6**). A heat source is set up on the dry side of the brooder. The in-ground swimming pool is equipped with an overflow mechanism, which allows for the constant provision of clean surface water. The dry side of the brooder is covered with unbacked polyvinyl chloride (PVC) coiled matting to provide traction and foot protection. This is unnecessary when using an aquatic bird-rearing cubicle because the perforated floors maintain adequate foot health. Food can be provided on the dry side of the brooder in a dish or can be floated or sunk in the pool. The constant fresh water reduces concerns over food items fouling the water and causing issues with feather condition. The audible dripping and water movement provides a more natural environment conducive to self-feeding behavior.

Wet brooders for highly aquatic species (eg, Mergini, Oxyurini, and so forth) are made from converted shipping totes and tend to have a greatly reduced land space in favor of a larger swimming area (**Fig. 7**). A land portion is often constructed of PVC-coated wire in the center of the brooder with gradually sloped smooth edges into the water. The standpipe with overflow is often in the middle of the pool directly underneath the land area.

A Note on Swimming and Waterproofing

Waterproofing is maintained primarily by feather structural alignment because of regular preening with the uropygial or preen gland serving as a conditioning agent to

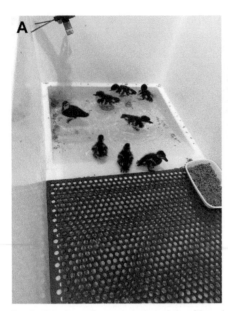
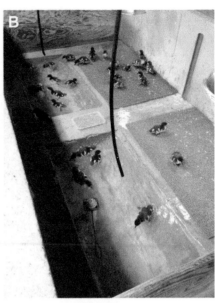

Fig. 6. Wet brooders can be modular fiberglass tanks or can be built-in with ramped concrete pools. All styles should feature an overflow. (*A*) An aquatic bird-rearing cubicle shown with a variety of food items placed in the pool and in a dish on the dry side of the brooder. (*B*) An interconnected series of built-in wet-brooders with removable partitions allow for large numbers of neonates to have access to in-ground pools with gradual ramps for easy exit. (Photo courtesy of Ian Gereg, Ambler, PA.)

decrease the rate of feather wear and deterioration.[19] Waterfowl are equipped to swim shortly after hatching regardless of whether or not they have been brooded by a parent.[20] Some waterfowl species, namely those with heavily aquatic lifestyles, preen and defecate more efficiently in water and are predisposed to cloacal impactions in managed care, which may relate to them having fewer opportunities to swim.[21] Neonates hatched in an incubator and placed directly in the water are able to stay dry and

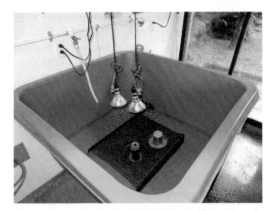

Fig. 7. Heavily aquatic species can be housed in a wet brooder with only a small central land area. Courtesy of Debbie Schouten, Dry Creek Waterfowl, Port Angeles, WA.

maintain buoyancy (see Video 1). Recommendations not to provide swimming water until birds are fully feathered are detrimental to animal well-being and likely stem from misconceptions about waterproofing coming from the preen gland of the adult during brooding.

Birds can have access to constant clean and overflowing ambient temperature swimming water provided that they have access to a land portion or haul-out where they can warm up, preen, and rest. If these strict husbandry guidelines are not followed, feathers may become soiled with food or feces and feather quality may be poor. In these cases, birds may quickly become wet and hypothermic if given access to swimming water. In order to reestablish feather condition, birds should be given frequent access to swimming water for short periods until they become wet (**Fig. 8**). Once wet, they should be dried off with a towel and moved to a dry brooder (or the second perforated floor installed over the pool in an aquatic bird-rearing cubicle). Birds should be encouraged to preen and brood in a hide pocket or under a feather duster until dry. Preening can be stimulated by increasing airflow using, for example, a low-powered fan, pet dryer, or hair-dryer. Once dry, place them in the water again. This process can be repeated 4 to 6 times daily until waterproofing is reestablished.

Special Considerations for Parent Rearing

Parent rearing allows for birds to be maintained in larger, more naturalistic enclosures and promotes natural behavior. Enclosures should mimic natural history and should be quiet and comfortable to encourage parental care (**Fig. 9**). Parent-reared birds should not be handled unless necessary to rule out injury or illness because this can result in abandonment particularly for inexperienced parents. Young should be provided with an appropriate starter diet (offered in close proximity to the adult diet)

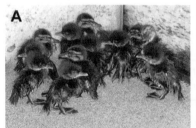
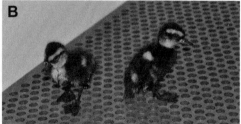
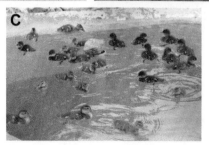

Fig. 8. Establishing waterproofing in neonatal waterfowl. (*A*) Ducklings with poor waterproofing will seem wet shortly after swimming. Ducklings should be removed from a wet brooder and allowed to brood until dry. (*B*) As waterproofing improves through frequent short access to swimming water, only small areas on the chest and ventrum will seem wet and swimming times can be increased. (*C*) Several days after waterproofing procedure was established, ducklings from A are fully waterproof and have unlimited access to swimming water. (Photo courtesy of Ian Gereg, Ambler, PA.).

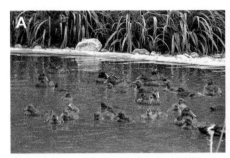
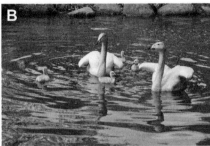

Fig. 9. Parent-reared birds can often remain in large enclosures. (A) Common eider (*Somateria mollissima*) ducklings benefit from being parent reared by a group of adults in a crèche. Photo courtesy of Ian Gereg, Ambler, PA. (B) Whooper swans (*Cygnus cygnus*) displaying protective behavior with wings out while tending to their cygnets. Photo courtesy of Ian Gereg, Ambler, PA.

and precautions should be taken to ensure that birds cannot fall down drainpipes or squeeze through gaps in fencing. Neonates must easily be able to get into and out of any swimming water.

For inexperienced parents, indoor or outdoor enclosures can be set up for parent rearing with shallow feeding dishes and swimming pools with rocks or ramps for easy access (**Fig. 10**). Rubber matting should cover smooth or slippery floor surfaces. Supplementary heat can be provided by low-powered lamps to guard against inefficient brooding behavior by adults. Families should be closely monitored for signs of parental care because intervention must be timely in the event a problem develops. Caregivers should use caution when entering and exiting enclosures because parents of certain species (namely swans and geese) may display aggression, which can result in accidental injury to offspring by trampling.

Growth and Enclosure Progression

Enclosure sizes should increase with neonatal growth. Continuous supplemental heat is required for less than 2 weeks (generally 1 week for grazing species), after which

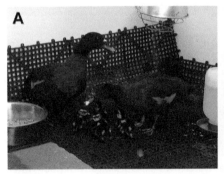
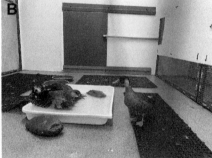

Fig. 10. Indoor enclosures can be set up for duck or goose families featuring shallow pools with rocks, heat lamps, and shallow food dishes. This enclosure will allow for more careful monitoring of neonates for 1 to 2 weeks after which time they are moved into larger outdoor enclosures. (A) Hartlaub's ducks (*Pteronetta hartlaubii*) tending young. Photo courtesy of Ian Gereg, Ambler, PA. (B) Brazilian teal (*Amazonetta brasiliensis*) hen showing defensive posture with bill open with brood behind her.

time birds should be shifted or moved outside during the day to benefit from natural light and foraging opportunities. A day pen can be constructed of lightweight materials with a hinged lid that can be moved to fresh lawn daily to promote grazing (**Fig. 11**). These pens offer limited protection against predators and should always be located inside a secure area with birds brought indoors overnight.

As soon as ambient temperatures allow, birds should be housed outside in aviaries that feature in-ground swimming pools with overflow pipes (**Fig. 12**). Overflow pipes should be covered with a rock or screened to prevent access by smaller birds. Outdoor enclosures should exclude wildlife and domestic animals that can predate neonatal waterfowl. Predator exclusion barriers and electric fencing can aid in deterrence. Substrates should be varied for foot health and should include river stones of various sizes, natural grass, or groundcover.

CONSPECIFICS ARE CRITICAL

Waterfowl are social animals and require conspecifics during growth and development. Singly raised waterfowl are prone to imprinting on people and can develop behavioral abnormalities at sexual maturity. Neonatal waterfowl of different species can often be housed together successfully provided that they are approximately the same size and/or life stage. When an individual bird must be housed alone either due to lack of available conspecifics or due to medical concerns, a mirror should be provided in addition to a comfort item. Removing a single bird from an established clutch to provide company to a solitary bird undergoing medical treatment can be beneficial for recovery.

NEONATAL WATERFOWL NUTRITION

Natural history provides valuable insight into appropriate diet and feeding methods. Food presentation in managed care should be informed by natural behaviors and should include natural food items. Food should be presented in ways that are easily recognizable for the species in care; for example, grazing species should have opportunities to graze, surface-water feeding species should be able to dabble, and diving species should be encouraged to up-end and dive to obtain food (**Fig. 13**). A base diet specifically designed for wild waterfowl should also be provided (**Table 2**). At the time of publication, Mazuri (St. Louis, MO) provides the only commercially available product line designed for wild waterfowl available in the United States with products

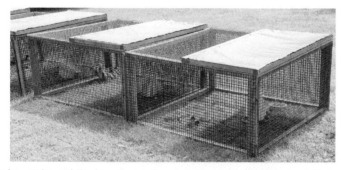

Fig. 11. Lightweight mobile day pen can be placed over fresh substrate daily to encourage grazing and provides access to sunlight while a partially enclosed hinge roof provides shade. Photo courtesy of Ian Gereg, Ambler, PA.

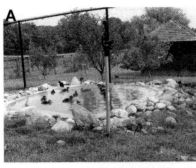
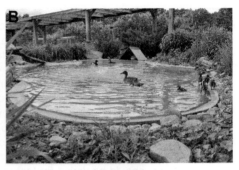
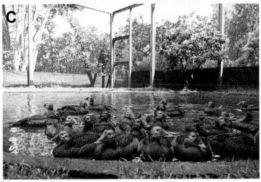

Fig. 12. Outdoor enclosures should provide adequate predator exclusion, abundant swimming water with overflow piping, and varied substrates. Live plants provide enrichment and shelter. (*A*) Small in-ground pool with covered overflow provides suitable housing for juvenile waterfowl. Photo courtesy of Ian Gereg, Ambler, PA. (*B*) Moderately sized in-ground pool with covered overflow provides appropriate housing for older juveniles, larger numbers of birds or for parent-reared groups. Photo courtesy of Ian Gereg, Ambler, PA. (*C*) This large in-ground pool provides juvenile sea ducks with deeper swimming water and consistent fresh water flow to maintain feather condition. Photo courtesy of Debbie Schouten, Dry Creek Waterfowl, Port Angeles, WA.

suitable for both neonatal and adult waterfowl. Other commercial products designed for domestic waterfowl may be appropriate (namely for domestic waterfowl); however, medicated feeds should be avoided as well as feeds marketed as "all flock" products for various taxa. Although all Anseriformes are precocial, some may be reluctant to

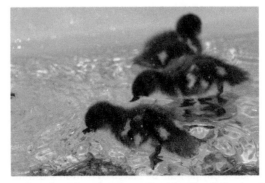

Fig. 13. Food presentation should encourage natural feeding behavior. Scaly-sided mergansers (*Mergus squamatus*) along with other diving ducks will look below the surface for food.

Table 2
Base diets and presentation for various tribes of Anseriformes

Food Item	Species	Developmental Stage	Presentation
Mazuri Waterfowl Starter #5641	All	Hatch until sufficient size for larger pellet or until primary feathers are in sheath	Offer in dish dry or float in water (See Video 2)
Mazuri Waterfowl Maintenance #5642	All	Goslings and Cygnets can start to consume at 3–4 wk of age, can mix with Purina Duck Grower or can be fed alone	Offer in dish dry or float in water
Purina Duck Grower/Purina Duck Feed	Dendrocygnini, Anserini and similar, Cygnini, Anatini and similar	Goslings and cygnets can start to consume at 3–4 wk of age, other species at 4 wk and older based on body size, mix with Mazuri Waterfowl Maintenance	Only offer in dish dry, pellet will not float and if wet, can form paste, which is difficult to consume and can lead to impactions
Mazuri Sea Duck Diet #5681	Aythyini, Mergini, and Oxyurini	Ducklings at 3–5 wk of age depending on body size	Offer in dish dry or float in water

self-feed particularly if singly housed, injured, debilitated, or in cases of wild orphans admitted for rehabilitation. These individuals may require supplemental nutrition provided either by gavage-feeding or by drip-feeding.[22,23] Supplemental feeding is only required for the first 5 to 7 days of life until birds are eating sufficiently to maintain and gain weight and is then discontinued. Whenever possible, food items should be placed on shallow white lids or floated in white pans or trays for maximum visual contrast to facilitate self-feeding behavior. Live prey and other food items can be used to top off base diets to encourage consumption (**Table 3**).

CLINICAL PRESENTATIONS FOR NEONATAL WATERFOWL

Waterfowl bills are adapted to facilitate eating and, unlike in some other avian species, do not continue to grow their bill nails over time except for some scoters and eiders. Bill injuries, often secondary to trauma, can hinder their ability to obtain food or to maintain feather condition and waterproofing appropriately. Euthanasia should be considered for bill injuries that result in loss of waterproofing or inability to remove ectoparasites.[23]

Waterfowl are prone to several developmental abnormalities that can result from improper diet (often excessive protein and deficiencies in B-vitamins and other nutrients), lack of exercise, and overcrowding.[4,24,25]

Angel Wing and Droop Wing

Both disorders affect the carpal joint of growing waterfowl and will render a bird flightless if not corrected during development while there is still active blood supply to the feathers.[26] These conditions manifest during the development of primary feathers, which place strain on the carpal joint causing an outward or downward deviation of the distal wing (**Figs. 14** and **15**).

For cases of droop wing (ie, no outward deviation at the carpal joint), the distal 3 to 5 primary blood feathers can be carefully plucked. An oral analgesic can be provided for

Table 3
Additional food items for Anseriformes

Food Item	Species	Presentation
Mazuri Nestling Handfeeding Formula #5S90	All	Add hot water and mix into gavage feeding consistency. Feed 0.1 mL per 10 g bird for neonatal supplemental feeding. Feed every 2–4 h to maintain weight
Chopped greens (high-calcium greens preferred)	All species; less appropriate for Mergini	Finely chop for all species; goslings and cygnets capable of tearing from whole leaves or whole heads
Duckweed	All species of ducks except for Mergini, cygnets	Harvest fresh from natural ponds, contains live aquatic invertebrates which may harbor intermediate life stages of various parasites, which is not generally of clinical concern
Live mealworms	All species of ducks, particularly Aythyini, Mergini and Oxyurini	Sprinkle on top of dry diet or float in water
Krill (frozen)	Aythyini, Mergini, and Oxyurini	Chop
Fish (live or frozen)	Mergini	Silversides, smelt, and minnows (See Video 3)
Aquatic invertebrates (frozen preferred but freeze-dried can be used)	Aythyini, Mergini, and Oxyurini	Provide in water only. (See Videos 4 and 5.) If providing in standing water without an overflow, water should be changed every 3–6 h Frozen invertebrates thawed in water can be sucked up into a syringe and used to drip feeding (See Video 6)

1 to 3 days following feather removal. The reduction in weight alone often leads to clinical resolution; however, encouraging exercise and use of the wings is also beneficial. In severe cases, affected wings may need to be bandaged as described in the following paragraph for angel wing.

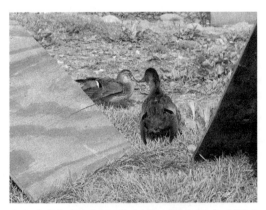

Fig. 14. The falcated duck (*Mareca falcata*) on the right displays bilateral drooped wings and is unable to pick up the wings due to carpal joint weakness.

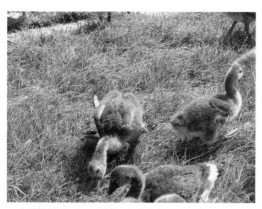

Fig. 15. Bilateral angel wing in a Canada goose (*Branta canadensis*) featuring an outward deviation of primary feathers at the carpal joint.

For cases of angel wing, when an outward deviation at the carpal joint is present, a bandage with or without a splint must be applied to correct the position of the carpal joint. Bandaging is generally successful if the condition is addressed quickly (within 3–5 days of onset). Once primary feathers are fully developed and no longer contain a blood supply, bandaging attempts will not resolve the condition, and it should be considered permanent. A figure-of-8 or modified figure-of-8 wrap is applied to the affected wing with paper tape, which generally has an appropriate level of stickiness while not compromising feather condition (**Fig. 16**A). A modified figure-of-8 uses only a single loop of tape to immobilize the carpus and elbow joints and is easier to apply to smaller neonates (see **Fig. 16**B). Depending on the size and age of the bird, the splint may have to be replaced daily to allow for growth and should generally be left in place for 2 to 4 days. A lightweight waterproof splint (eg, porous thermoplastic material, craft foam, and padded aluminum splint) can be applied to the dorsal surface of the wing and incorporated into a figure-of-8 splint to provide additional stability for larger birds. If after 4 days of splinting the condition is not resolved, provide 1 to 2 days of rest and then replace the splint for an additional 2 to 4 days.

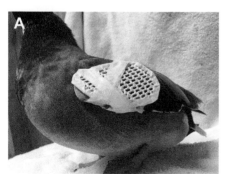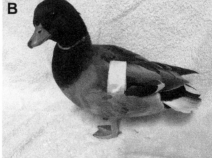

Fig. 16. Splinting approaches for developmental wing abnormalities. (*A*) Figure-of-8 wrap applied with paper tape. A splint can be used for additional stability in larger neonates. (*B*) Modified figure-of-8 wrap applied with paper tape. This minimal bandage can be sufficient to correct angel wing in most neonates.

Perosis or Slipped Tendon

Cases of perosis are often presented acutely with non–weight-bearing either unilaterally or bilaterally. Presentation generally aligns with periods of rapid growth where the weight of the bird cannot be supported by weak tendons, ligaments, and other soft tissue structures.[4,26] Either a medial or lateral luxation of the gastrocnemius tendon from the condylar groove of the hock joint can be present (**Fig. 17**).

Treatment should only be attempted in unilateral presentations that are promptly recognized where the tendon can manually be repositioned. Otherwise, euthanasia should be elected. Although surgical repair techniques have been described for this condition, the procedure is rarely successful and highly invasive.[4,27,28] The goal of treatment is to immobilize the hock joint in a partially flexed position that allows the bird to ambulate on the affected leg (see Video 7). Affected birds should be placed on a nonsteroidal anti-inflammatory medication. An antibiotic may be indicated if the hock joint is ulcerated. The selection of material for splinting is dictated by the size of the bird. Thin craft foam should be used for birds weighing less than 150 g, whereas larger birds can benefit from padded aluminum splinting material such as SAM Splint (SAM Medical, OR, USA) that is carefully cut to size with sharp edges taped (**Fig. 18**). Once cut to size, the splint is applied to the dorsal surface of the leg, which permits ongoing monitoring of tendon position. The proximal and distal tabs on either side of the central hinge are folded caudally making sure to leave a gap along the caudal aspect of the leg for tendon monitoring. The central hinge is then folded to keep the leg in a natural standing position such that the bird can walk relatively normally while splinted (**Fig. 19**). Healing is generally achieved within 7 to 10 days of corrective splinting; however, the splint may need to be replaced in fast-growing birds every 48 to 72 hours to prevent constriction injuries.

Angular Limb Deformities

Angular limb deformities, most commonly affecting the tibiotarsus in neonatal waterfowl, can occur because of unresolved perosis or may contribute to the development of perosis. Other injuries or nutritional imbalances may also lead to this disease. Once the deformity is present, treatment is often not possible and euthanasia is recommended.

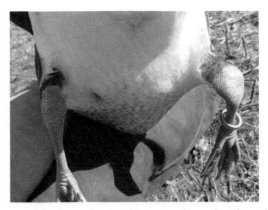

Fig. 17. Juvenile lesser white-fronted goose (*Anser erythropus*) with medial luxation of the right gastrocnemius tendon. The tendon position of the left leg is normal.

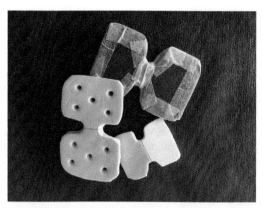

Fig. 18. Splint used to address perosis. When using foam products, a scalpel blade can be used to score the hinge point where the splint will rest on the dorsal aspect of the hock joint. When using a padded aluminum splint, all cut edges should be covered with tape.

Traumatic Conditions

Neonatal waterfowl can be presented with various forms of trauma secondary to predator attack, entanglement, and so forth and are managed similarly to adult waterfowl and other avian species. See Goodman 2017[26] for detailed orthopedic management techniques for Anseriformes.

Presentations of knuckling or walking on the dorsal surface of the foot manifest in neonatal waterfowl because of various distal leg injuries. Injuries require that the affected bone or joint be maintained in a normal position pending resolution of inflammation. For injuries affecting the hock joint, the splint described above for perosis can be used. For injuries affecting the foot joint or phalanges, a sandal should be constructed of thin craft foam and applied to the plantar surface of the foot. When using craft foam, a semicircular hole should be cut into the foam at the location of the central pad to reduce buoyancy and allow the birds to swim normally while splinted. The sandal should cover the entire plantar surface of the foot with the toes spread and the nails slightly overhanging the edge of the sandal. Attach the sandal to the foot in an interdigitating fashion using paper tape. For smaller neonates less than 150 g, 0.5-inch paper tape can encircle the tarsometatarsus and can then

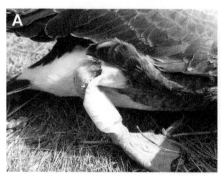
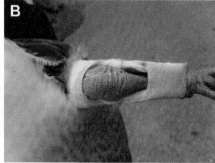

Fig. 19. Perosis splint application. (*A*) Lateral view of applied splint. (*B*) Caudal view of applied splint with visibility of gastrocnemius tendon for ongoing monitoring during healing.

connect to the sandal keeping the foot joint in a normal flexed position. For larger neonates, the traditional sandal includes a flap for the tarsometatarsus where there is a notch cut out for the foot joint (**Fig. 20**). This splint is then applied to the plantar surface of the foot and secured in the same way as the sandal. The upper portion of the splint is then applied to the caudal tarsometatarsus and secured. If this approach fails to yield a normal foot position, 2 pieces of cloth tape are applied (which will hold suture, whereas paper tape will not). One piece will encircle the tarsometatarsus and the other the widest portion of the foot with toes spread. A tension line can then be sewn, taking care only to sew through the tape to keep the foot in a normal flexed position. Birds will walk normally with this splint and the condition normally resolves within a week. This splint should be changed every 2 to 3 days or as needed to account for growth.

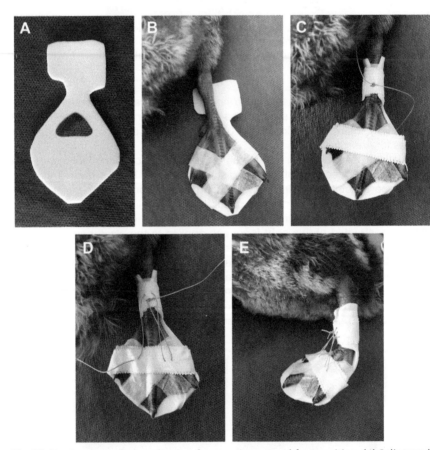

Fig. 20. Tension-line splint application for ensuring normal foot position. (*A*) Splint made of foam with opening cut at the location of the central pad. (*B*) Paper tape applied in an interdigitating pattern to secure the splint to the foot. (*C*) Cloth tape is applied around the tarsometatarsus and around the widest portion of the foot to hold the tension line. Tension line starts midtarsometatarsus and is secured only through the layer of cloth tape. (*D*) Pattern for tension line running from tarsometatarsus to the lateral interdigital webbing, back up to the tarsometatarsus, then to the medial interdigital webbing and back up to the tarsometatarsus. Tension is placed on the line until the foot is maintained in a normal flexed position. (*E*) Completed splint.

Pododermatitis

Pododermatitis is a captivity-associated condition that is routinely observed in neonatal waterfowl. It is often attributed to poor husbandry with inadequate swimming water and hard smooth substrates. Mild-to-moderate cases often respond to changes in husbandry practices, antimicrobial and anti-inflammatory therapy along with low-level laser.[29] If practical, topical therapy with 5% dimethicone mixed with arnica gel and panthenol in equal ratios can be applied up to twice daily. Topical products should be free of petroleum-based ingredients to preserve feather condition and water-proofing. Severe or chronic cases often require systemic antimicrobial therapy. The localized application of antimicrobial therapy via regional limb perfusion may augment systemic therapy and promote more rapid healing.[30–32] Potentially nephrotoxic drugs can be administered safely to euhydrated animals via regional limb perfusion.[33] Un-treated cases will continue to progress and result in osteomyelitis. Underlying podo-dermatitis may contribute to the incidence of amyloidosis, which is common in waterfowl species.[29,34] Given the avascular nature of the affected site, surgical tech-niques are rarely successful in Anseriformes and often results in significant scar tissue formation that prevents complete healing.

Infectious Diseases

Select infectious diseases commonly seen in juvenile waterfowl are summarized in **Table 4**.

PREVENTATIVE HEALTH RECOMMENDATIONS
Routine Diagnostic Testing

Routine fecal testing can be performed on neonatal and juvenile waterfowl and should include at least a direct smear and fecal flotation evaluation. For birds housed in a nat-ural enclosure, fecal sedimentation can be added into surveillance practices to improve detection of trematode ova.[35] Although routine hematology can be performed and may be helpful for the detection of hemoparasites, the stress of frequent capture, particularly in large naturalistic enclosures, rarely outweighs the benefits of blood evaluation.

Prophylactic Medication Administration

Because of concerns with anthelmintic resistance, routine deworming in the absence of a confirmed parasite infection is not recommended. There are certain cases, partic-ularly in large-scale avicultural, research or zoologic facilities, where prophylactic treatment may be indicated. When hemoparasites are known to cause clinical disease in susceptible species, the routine prophylactic administration of antimalarial medica-tions in juvenile waterfowl where contact with vectors cannot be prevented is appro-priate and can be performed as in Sphenisciformes.[36] Affected facilities should additionally take measures to reduce environmental mosquito burden through the strategic use of insecticides, fans, and mosquito traps. Species susceptibility is often facility dependent by collection composition; however, common eider (*Somateria mol-lissima*) and other *Somateria* species tend to be highly susceptible to hemoparasites, particularly *Plasmodium* spp.[37,38]

Sterilization

Although a reduction or elimination of egg-laying may be desirable in some cases, particularly in domestic waterfowl, surgical sterilization is not recommended unless a medical emergency necessitates that surgery be performed such as dystocia,

Table 4
Selected infectious diseases of neonatal and juvenile Anseriformes, including species predilection, epizootiology, clinical signs, diagnosis, and treatment and control

Disease Agent		Species Affected	Epizootiology	Clinical Signs	Diagnosis	Treatment and Control
Bacterial						
Avian tuberculosis[4,11,34,50]	*Mycobacterium avium*	All; white-winged wood ducks highly susceptible	Bacteria is persistent in the environment, which can lead to significant burden in captive facilities	Progressive weight loss; neonates can be infected at young ages but often do not show signs of disease for months or years	Acid-fast stain	No treatment currently recommended. Occurrence may be higher in facilities with overcrowding and poor water quality
New Duck Disease/ Infectious Serositis[11,34]	*Riemerella anatipestifer*	All	Highly contagious pathogen likely acquired through the respiratory tract or by entry through foot lesions. Acute form common in domestic ducklings <6 wk of age	Listlessness, ocular and nasal discharge, mild coughing and sneezing, tremors of the head and neck, incoordination, and diarrhea. Postmortem lesions include fibrinous visceral membranes, pericarditis, air sacculitis and meningitis	Bacterial isolation from aerobic culture	Antibiotics if given in the early stages of disease and as directed by sensitivity results. Resistance is becoming increasingly common. Vaccine not widely available
Viral						
Duck Viral enteritis/Duck Plague[4,11,34]	Anatid-herpesvirus-1	All; muscovy ducks and wood ducks highly susceptible	Mass mortality events can be seen in captive facilities	Often present acutely dead. Clinical signs before death include lethargy, serosanguinous nasal discharge, and hematochezia	Polymerase chain reaction (PCR), virus isolation	No treatment. Prevent interaction between wild waterfowl and captive individuals. Reportable disease
West Nile Virus[41]	Flavivirus	All	Transmitted by *Culex* mosquitoes	Neurologic signs consistent with meningoencephalitis	Immunohistochemistry	Vector control; commercially available equine vaccine
Highly Pathogenic Avian Influenza[4,41]	Orthomyxovirus	All	Susceptibility often strain and species dependent; many waterfowl species act as asymptomatic carriers	Wide range of clinical signs from mild sinusitis to severe neurologic disease and acute death		Treatment not indicated for high-path strains; reportable disease
Avian Pox[4,11,34]	Avipoxvirus	All; Aythyini, Oxyurini, and Mergini more susceptible	Transmitted by arthropod vectors	Wart-like lesions on feet, pharynx, around mouth, and eyes (where skin is exposed)	Inclusion (Bollinger) bodies identified on microscopy, PCR, virus isolation	Supportive care. Control insect vectors

Fungal

Aspergillosis[11,51–53]	Aspergillus fumigatus, Aspergillus flavus, Aspergillus niger	All; Mergini more susceptible	Ubiquitous opportunistic pathogen. Disease often triggered by stress or immunosuppression. Predisposing conditions may include malnutrition, corticosteroid use, preexisting disease, poor husbandry (ie, sanitation, ventilation), and heat (especially in thermo-intolerant species). Fungal spores enter the body most commonly through inhalation, although localized disease can occur with contact with broken skin or ingestion. Hematogenous spread can lead to systemic disease	Range from upper and lower respiratory tract disease, nonspecific signs such as wing droop, anorexia, emaciation, change or loss of voice (seen with tracheal granulomas) to sudden death	Definitive diagnosis requires culture and/or histopathology. Hematological findings may show elevated white blood cell count with leukocytosis, monocytosis, and lymphopenia; radiographs may show space-occupying masses or air sac densities. Serology is a helpful tool to aid diagnosis but cannot be used as a sole indicator. Endoscopic examination of air sacs and trachea provides an excellent means for collecting samples while providing an opportunity to directly assess the extent of disease	Treatment rarely successful in advanced cases. Antifungal medications including amphotericin B, itraconazole, voriconazole, and terbinafine can be used systemically, orally, topically via nebulization, or by direct application to air sac lesions. Surgical removal of aspergillomas also may be indicated

Protozoal

Enteric coccidiosis[11,34,53]	Eimeria spp, Tyzzeria spp, Wenyonella spp, Isospora spp Occasionally Cryptosporidium spp	All	All species are susceptible. Lesions are noted in the intestinal mucosa. Many coccidia species are host-species specific	Clinical signs vary from acute death, mucosanguinous diarrhea, or asymptomatic presentations	Fecal flotation, histopathology	Improve hygiene, sulfonamides, and amprolium
Renal coccidiosis[11,53–55]	Eimeria truncata, Eimeria boschadis, Eimeria somateriae	Reported in young geese more than other taxa	Disease can cause high mortality in domestic waterfowl particularly in flocks housed in crowded conditions with poor sanitation	Weakness, anorexia, weight loss, diarrhea. Postmortem lesions include pale, swollen kidneys with multifocal white (urate) lesions	Fecal flotation, renal cytology to look for oocysts, histopathology	Strict sanitation and disinfection, sulfonamides, house juvenile birds separately from adults. Sulfonamides for treatment
Hemosporidiosis[50,56]	Leucocytozoan, Plasmodium, Hemoproteus spp	Eiders highly susceptible but can affect all species	Disease aligns with heavy mosquito burden in summer months	Anemia, weight loss, lethargy, ataxia, and sudden death	Blood smear and PCR testing	Antimalarial medications. Avoid contact with vectors (black flies for Leucocytozoon)

(continued on next page)

Table 4
(continued)

	Disease Agent	Species Affected	Epizootiology	Clinical Signs	Diagnosis	Treatment and Control
Helminths						
Thorny-headed worm[57,58]	Acanthocephala spp	Mortality in cygnets and domestic ducklings; high parasite burdens reported in wild eiders along with other members of Mergini	Indirect life cycle makes infection in captivity uncommon	Anorexia, lethargy, weight loss; rarely causes intestinal perforation	Fecal flotation, histopathology	No effective treatment
Gapeworm[4,11,57]	Syngamus trachea, Cyathostoma bronchialis	Goslings of all species more susceptible than ducks and swans	Parasite has direct life cycle but often uses paratenic hosts, including snails and earthworms	Coughing and lethargy; dyspnea in severe cases	Fecal flotation, direct smear from trachea	Treatment successful with most anthelminthics
Trematodes[50,57]	Multiple species of flukes reported	Presents most commonly in diving species Aythini and Mergini	Consumption of intermediate hosts (snails, crayfish, and so forth), often in dirt-lined ponds	Varies by species of trematode; often weight loss, hemorrhagic enteritis or upper respiratory signs	Eggs can often be detected in feces or in tracheal swabs. Fecal sedimentation may be required	Removal of intermediate hosts can be difficult but should be attempted. Praziquantel often effective but higher doses may be required than what is reported for cestodes
Schistosomes[4,34,59,60]	Multiple genera reported impacting Anseriformes	Presents most commonly in diving species Aythini and Mergini but can be found in all species	Found in arteries; causes granulomatous encephalitis	Sudden death, lameness, lethargy, weight loss, anorexia, and ataxia	Postmortem identification of parasites in arteries; thrombosis commonly identified in caudal mesenteric vein and branches	High doses praziquantel required to control infection in affected birds (up to 200 mg/kg). Control of intermediate hosts (molluscs) if possible to break life cycle
Toxic						
Avian botulism[4,34,50]	Neurotoxin produced by Clostridium botulinum	All	Bacteria ubiquitous in environment; fluctuating water levels in warm temperatures expose toxin-laden organic debris. Carcass-maggot cycle perpetuates outbreaks as maggots serve to concentrate toxin	Ascending paresis and flaccid paralysis	Mouse inoculation test (rarely performed in clinical setting); diagnosis by exclusion and positive response to treatment	Prevent standing water. Administration of active charcoal along with copious fluids to flush toxin from affected bird. Antitoxin available for equids has been used in waterfowl. High recovery rate achievable with treatment

yolk coelomitis, ectopic eggs, or neoplasia.[39] The administration of GnRH agonists such as leuprolide acetate and deslorelin have not resulted in long-term suppression of egg-laying like has been reported in other avian taxa.[39] Castration of male waterfowl is rarely performed, technically difficult and is generally not indicated outside of underlying disease such as neoplasia.[39,40]

Vaccination

Juvenile waterfowl should be vaccinated against West Nile Virus in endemic areas because many species are susceptible to clinical disease and death.[41,42] Vaccination can be performed at as early as 3 weeks of age without adverse effects but should not be performed before 3 weeks of age due to the potential for maternal antibody interference.[43,44] A typical vaccine series consists of 3 doses of an inactivated vaccine spaced 3 weeks apart with subsequent annual boosters.[45] Antibody production following vaccination is inconsistent between avian species; however, numerous studies suggest a benefit to vaccination even if studied birds did not develop antibodies.[46,47] Vaccination of adult birds should take place in the spring for Anseriformes because this precedes egg laying and the eclipse molt, and should give time for an adequate immune response to develop before the start of mosquito season. This schedule may allow for enhanced maternal antibody transfer into the egg and a more robust immune response in the neonate until the vaccine series can be initiated in the neonate.[44] The timing of vaccination may have to be adjusted for individual facilities based on climate or other factors including alterations made to breeding seasons through the use of artificial lighting.

The widely accepted dose volume for waterfowl is 1 mL per bird per dose; however, smaller volumes may be used successfully that are scaled by animal weight.[45,47] The Innovator West Nile Virus equine vaccine (Zoetis Animal Health, MI, USA) has been used extensively across avian taxa with few adverse events observed; however, recent studies suggest that other vaccine types are also effective and safe.[43,45,46] It is worth noting that the canarypox vectored West Nile Virus equine vaccine Recombitek (Merial, GA, USA) resulted in a reduction in body mass and caused significant local inflammation and, in some cases, necrosis in immunized falcons (*Falco* spp) and scrub jays (*Aphelocoma californica*).[48,49]

CLINICS CARE POINTS

- Neonatal Anseriformes require specialized care for successful development. Knowledge of natural history is essential for successful rearing.

- Early and regular access to water for swimming promotes normal physical and mental development, feather health, and normal feeding behaviors.

- Corrective splinting can be performed to rectify many developmental disorders—the use of lightweight, waterproof materials when splinting allows birds to ambulate normally and continue to swim.

- Captivity-associated diseases can be minimized through proper husbandry and hygiene.

- Anseriformes are susceptible to a variety of bacterial, viral, fungal, and parasitic diseases, some of which are reportable to state health agencies.

DISCLOSURE

Michele Goodman is the co-owner of Leucopsis products, manufacturer of the Aquatic Bird Rearing Cubicle, located in Ambler, PA.

SUPPLEMENTARY DATA

Supplementary data to this article can be found online at https://doi.org/10.1016/j.cvex.2023.11.010.

REFERENCES

1. Livezey BC. A phylogenetic analysis of basal Anseriformes, the fossil *Presbyornis*, and the interordinal relationships of waterfowl. Zool J Linn Soc 1997;121: 361–428.
2. Ducks Kear J. Geese and swans. Oxford: Oxford University Press; 2005.
3. Shekkerman H, Tulp I, Piersma T, et al. Mechanisms promoting higher growth rate in arctic than in temperate shorebirds. Oceologica 2003;134:332–42.
4. Olsen JH. Anseriformes. In: Ritchie BW, Harrison GJ, Harrison LR, editors. Avian medicine: principles and application. Florida: Wingers Publishing; 1994. p. 1238–75.
5. US Fish and Wildlife Service. Frequently asked questions about a federal Migratory Bird Waterfowl Sale and Disposal permit. https://www.fws.gov/sites/default/files/documents/3-200-9FAQ.pdf. Accessed September 16, 2023.
6. Tyson E. For an end to pinioning: The case against the legal mutilation of birds in captivity. J Ethics 2014;4:1–4.
7. Krawinkel P. Feather follicle extirpation: operative techniques to prevent zoo birds from flying. In: Miller RE, Fowler ME, editors. Fowler's zoo and wild animal medicine, ume 7. Missouri: Elsevier Saunders; 2012. p. 275–80.
8. Flint PL, Lindberg MS, MacCluskie MC, et al. The adaptive significance of hatching synchrony of waterfowl eggs. Wildfowl 1994;45:248–54.
9. Klimstra JD, Stebbins KR, Heinz GH, et al. Factors related to the artificial incubation of wild bird eggs. Avian Biol Res 2009;2:121–31.
10. Bailey T, Magno MN. Reproduction, neonatology. In: Samour J, editor. Avian medicine. 3rd edition. Missouri: Elsevier Limited; 2016. p. 549–58.
11. Routh A, Sanderson S. Waterfowl. In: Tully TN, Dorrestein GM, Jones AK, editors. Avian medicine. 2nd edition. Philadelphia: Elsevier Saunders; 2009. p. 275–308.
12. Jamroz D, Wertelecki T, Wiliczkiewicz A, et al. Dynamics of yolk sac resorption and post-hatching development of the gastrointestinal tract in chickens, ducks and geese. J Anim Physiol Anim Nutr 2004;88:239–50.
13. Kasielke S. When Good Eggs Go Bad: Hatching Assistance and Necropsy. In: Proceedings American Association of Zoo Veterinarians Conference, 2010. Available at: https://www.vin.com/apputil/content/defaultadv1.aspx?pId=11321&catId=156099&id=9966859&ind=145&objTypeID=17&print=1. Accessed August 22, 2023.
14. Hochbaum A. Sex and age determination of waterfowl by cloacal examination. In: Hyde DO, editor. Raising wild ducks in captivity. New York: E.P. Dutton and Co; 1974. p. 254–64.
15. Gereg I. An introduction to hand-rearing waterfowl, 44. Chandler, AZ: American Association of Zookeepers, Inc. Animal Keepers Forum; 2017. p. 342–3.
16. Williams MA, Lallo CHO, Sundaram V. The effect of early post hatch feeding times on the growth and development of the gastrointestinal tract of mule ducklings to five days of age. Braz J Poul Sci 2020;23:1–10.
17. Mikec M, Bidin Z, Valentić A, et al. Influence of environmental and nutritional stressors on yolk sac utilization, development of chicken gastrointestinal system and its immune status. World's Poult Sci J 2006;62:31–40.

18. Boucher M, Ehmler TJ, Bermudez AJ. Polytetrafluoroethylene gas intoxication in broiler chickens. Avian Dis 2000;44:449–53.
19. Terrill RS, Schultz AJ. Feather function and the evolution of birds. Biol Rev 2023; 98:540–66.
20. Anderson DL. Waterfowl rehabilitation: a primer for veterinarians. Seminars Avian Exot Pet Med 2004;13:213–22.
21. Pokras MA. Captive management of aquatic birds. AAV Today 1988;2:24–33.
22. Goodman M. Sea ducks. In: Duerr RS, Gage LJ, editors. Hand-rearing birds. 2nd edition. New Jersey: Wiley and Sons; 2020. p. 107–17.
23. Goodman M. Natural history and medical management of waterfowl. In: Hernandez SM, Barron HW, Miller EA, et al, editors. Medical management of wildlife species: a guide for practitioners. New Jersey: Wiley and Sons; 2020. p. 229–47.
24. Goodman M. Ducks, geese and swans: an introduction to waterfowl medicine. Proc Assoc Avian Vet Annual Conference 2017;55–67.
25. Kear J. Notes on the nutrition of young waterfowl, with special reference to slipped-wing. Int Zoo Yearbk 1973;13:97–100.
26. Goodman M, Schott R, Duerr RS. Waterfowl (Ducks, Geese, and swans). In: Duerr RS, Purdin GJ, editors. Topics in wildlife medicine: orthopedics. Minnesota: National Wildlife Rehabilitators Association; 2017. p. 99–119.
27. Arora N, Yadav P, Chaudhary R, et al. Surgical correction of perosis/slipped tendon in a white pekin duck-case report. Int J Curr Microbiol App Sci 2018;7: 389–92.
28. Wolfe DA. Surgical correction of perosis in a 3-week-old mallard duck. Vet Med Small An Clin 1978;73:1567–70.
29. Bumblefoot Blair J. A Comparison of Clinical Presentation and Treatment of Pododermatitis in Rabbits, Rodents and Birds. Vet Clin North Am Exot An Pract 2013; 16:715–35.
30. Fiorello CV. Intravenous regional antibiotic perfusion therapy as an adjunctive treatment for digital lesions in seabirds. J Zoo Wildl Med 2017;48:189–95.
31. Knafo SE, Graham JE, Barton BA. Intravenous and intraosseous regional limb perfusion of ceftiofur sodium in an avian model. Am J Vet Res 2019;80: 539–46.
32. Huckens GL, Sim RR, Hartup B. Adjunctive Use of Intravenous Antibiotic Regional Limb Perfusion in Three Cranes with Distal Limb Infections. Animals 2021;11:1–6.
33. Clarke LL, Ratliff C, Mans C. Clinicopathologic findings in chickens *(Gallus gallus domesticus)* administered amikacin through intravenous regional limb perfusion. J Avian Med Surg 2022;36:187–91.
34. Fenton H, McManamon R, Howerth EW. Anseriformes, ciconiiformes, charadriformes, and gruiforms. In: Terio KA, McAloose D, et al, editors. Pathology of wildlife and zoo animals. UK: Academic Press; 2018. p. 693–716.
35. Assis JCA, López-Hernández D, Favoretto S, et al. Identification of the avian tracheal trematode *Typhlocoelum cucumerinum* (Trematoda: Cyclocoelidae) in a host-parasite-environment system: diagnosis, life cycle, and molecular phylogeny. Parasitology 2021;148:1383–91.
36. Grilo ML, Vanstreels RET, Wallace R, et al. Malaria in penguins – current perceptions. Avian Pathol 2016;45:393–407.
37. Spottiswoode N, Bartlett S, Conley K, et al. Analysis of *Plasmodium* lineages identified in captive penguins (*Spheniciformes* spp.), Eiders (*Somateria* spp.),

and Inca Terns (*Larosterna inca*) in a North American zoological collection. J Zoo Wildl Med 2020;5:140–9.

38. Hollmén TE, Franson JC. Infectious diseases, parasites and biological toxins in sea ducks. In: Savard J-PL, Derksen DV, Esler D, et al, editors. Ecology and conservation of north American sea ducks. Boca Raton: CRC Press; 2015. p. 97–124.

39. Echols MS. Anseriforme husbandry and management. In: Greenacre CB, Morishita TY, editors. Backyard poultry medicine and surgery: a guide for veterinary practitioners. 2nd edition. New Jersey: Wiley Blackwell; 2021. p. 56–106.

40. Chitty J. Behavioral disorders. In: Poland G, Raftery A, editors. BSAVA manual of backyard poultry medicine and surgery. Gloucester: British Small Animal Veterinary Association; 2019. p. 228–32.

41. Hess JC, Pare JA. Viruses of waterfowl. Sem Avian Exot Med 2004;13:176--83.

42. Cox SL, Campbell DG, Nemeth NM. Outbreaks of West Nile virus in captive waterfowl in Ontario, Canada. Avian Pathol 2015;42:135–41.

43. Jarvi SI, Lieberman MM, Hofmeister E, et al. Protective efficacy of a recombinant subunit West Nile virus vaccine in domestic geese (*Anser anser*). Vaccine 2008;1–7.

44. Tizard I. The avian antibody response. Seminars Avian Exot Pet Med 2002; 11:2–14.

45. Bergmann F, Fischer D, Fischer L, et al. Vaccination of zoo birds against west nile virus – a field study. Vaccines 2023;11:652.

46. Jiménez de Oya N, Escribano-Romero E, Blázquez AB, et al. Current progress of avian vaccines against west nile virus. Vaccines 2019;7:126.

47. Okeson DM, Llizo SY, Miller CL, et al. Antibody response of five bird species after vaccination with a killed West Nile Virus vaccine. J Zoo Wildl Med 2007;38: 240–4.

48. Angenvoort J, Fischer D, Fast C, et al. Limited efficacy of West Nile virus vaccines in large falcons (*Falco* spp.). Vet Res 2014;45:41.

49. Wheeler SS, Langevin S, Woods L, et al. Efficacy of three vaccines in protecting Western scrub-jays (*Aphelocoma californica*) from experimental infection with West Nile virus: Implications for vaccination of Island scrub-jays (*Aphelocoma insularis*). Vector Borne Zoonotic Dis 2011;11:1069–80.

50. Olsen GH. Bacterial and parasitic diseases of anseriformes. Vet Clin N Am 2009; 12:475–90.

51. Pollock C. Fungal diseases of columbiformes and anseriformes. Vet Clin Exot Anim 2003;6:351–61.

52. Pollock C. Waterfowl diseases: A "cheat sheet". In: Lafebervet website, 2012. Available at: https://lafeber.com/vet/waterfowl-diseases-a-cheat-sheet/. Accessed August 20, 2023.

53. Backues KA. Anseriformes. In: Miller RE, Fowler ME, editors. Zoo and wild animal medicine, ume 8. Missouri: Elsevier Saunders; 2015. p. 116–26.

54. Gomis S, Didiuk AB, Neufeld J, et al. Renal coccidiosis and other parasitologic conditions in lesser snow goose goslings at Tha-anne River, west coast Hudson Bay. J Wildl Dis 1996;32:498–504.

55. Oksanen A. Mortality associated with renal coccidiosis in juvenile greylag geese (*Anser anser anser*). J Wildl Dis 1994;30:554–6.

56. Atkinson CT. Hemosporidiosis. In: Friend M, Franson JC, editors. Field manual of wildlife diseases: general field procedures and diseases of birds. Wisconsin: USGS; 1999. p. 193–9.

57. Ballweber AR. Waterfowl Parasites. Sem Avian Exot Med 2004;13:197–205.
58. Cole RA. Acanthocephaliasis. In: Friend M, Franson JC, editors. Field manual of wildlife diseases: general field procedures and diseases of birds. Wisconsin: USGS; 1999. p. 241–3.
59. Wojcinski ZW, Barker IK, Bruce HD, et al. An outbreak of schistosomiasis in atlantic brant geese, *Branta bernicola hrota*. J Wildl Dis 1987;23:248–55.
60. Blankespoor CL, Reimink RL, Blankespoor HD. Efficacy of praziquantel in treating natural schistosome infections in common mergansers. J Parasitol 2001;87: 424–6.

Columbiform Pediatrics

Nicolas Schoonheere, DMV[a],
Graham Zoller, DMV, IPSAV (Zoological Medicine), Dip ECZM (Avian)[b],*

KEYWORDS

- Pediatrics • Pigeons • Circovirus • Rotavirus • Preventive medicine • Trichomonas
- *Streptococcus* • Vaccination

KEY POINTS

- Pigeons have been bred since antiquity as a source of food and as messengers. In recent history, they have also been bred for their beauty and for racing competitions. Preventive aspects of pediatrics have risen in importance given the interests at stake during international competitions.
- Nutritional intake and immunity of pigeons from their development in the egg to their first days after hatching depend directly on the nutritional and immune status of the parents. Therefore, vaccination and appropriate nutrition of the parents are crucial to the health of the chicks.
- Squabs are fed with a liquid called "crop milk" by the parents during their first week of life. This fluid, composed of desquamated epithelial cells of the crop, is rich in lipid and proteins which allow for the very high growth rate observed in pigeons. Crop milk is also rich in antibodies.
- Multiple changes occur in the life of young pigeons during weaning including separation from the parents, changes in feeding, and contact with other birds. These changes are stressful and concurrent to the decrease of passive immunity. As a consequence, some benign infectious diseases in adult birds can have more serious consequences in younger animals.
- Numerous vaccines have been developed against an increasing number of viral and bacterial diseases. The vaccination schedule can be designed according to health history of the loft, endemic diseases in the area, and future activity of the pigeons.

INTRODUCTION

Columbidae is the only extant family in the order Columbiformes and includes about 310 species of pigeons and doves divided into approximately 50 genera. The subfamily Columbinae is the most important one and is composed of 181 species including the genera *Columba* and *Streptopelia*. The birds in this family are distributed

[a] Centre Vétérinaire Exclusif NAC VTNac Hingeon, 1 Grand Route, 5380 Hingeon, Belgium;
[b] Centre Hospitalier Vétérinaire OnlyVet – Exotic Pet Department, 7 Rue Jean Zay, 69800 Saint-Priest, France
* Corresponding author.
E-mail address: graham.zoller@gmail.com

Vet Clin Exot Anim 27 (2024) 341–357
https://doi.org/10.1016/j.cvex.2023.11.011
vetexotic.theclinics.com

worldwide with the exception of Arctic and Antarctic regions and they primarily feed on seeds, fruits, and plants. They greatly vary in size and color, ranging from the small common ground dove (*Columba passerina*) weighing approximately 30 g to the Victoria crowned pigeon (*Goura victoria*) weighing 2.4 kg on average. This article focuses on pigeons (*Columba livia*) due to the importance of pediatrics in this species. Many of the diseases discussed here can also affect other species of Columbiformes.

Pigeons have been bred by humans since antiquity. The Egyptians, Greeks, and Romans used them as a source of meat and feathers and had already used them as messengers. Afterward, pigeons have followed human history and have been bred for multiple reasons including food production (ie, meat, eggs), transmission of messages, ornament, and since the nineteenth century, for sport. Over the centuries, numerous breeds have been specifically developed for these different uses, which have led to the large number of breeds described today.

Today, pigeons remain very popular birds. They are still used for their production of meat, for their beauty, or for the simple pleasure of their company, but they are increasingly bred for pigeon racing, especially in developing countries. Pigeon racing aims at releasing birds at the same location with the objective that each pigeon returns back to its home as fast as possible. Competitions can involve up to several tens of thousands of pigeons, which can be released more than a 1000 km (620 miles) from their home. The increasing craze generated by this sport has led some pigeons to reach a star status with market values occasionally hitting up to 2 million USD.

One loft racing is a modern form of pigeon racing developed as a direct consequence of globalization. This type of race is currently a big trend where all the pigeons entered in the race are housed in one gigantic loft that can accommodate up to several thousand racing pigeons from all over the world. The pigeons' breeders send the racing pigeons they have produced by the age of 6 weeks to one of these gigantic lofts located all over the world and where the birds will establish domicile. From there, pigeons will be trained together, transported to the same location and involved in common competition. This phenomenon has become popular since the beginning of the twenty-first century.

Pediatric medicine, and more specifically the preventive aspects of it, represents an increasingly important aspect of veterinary practice given the interest at stake with these new breeding techniques and to a lesser extent in more traditional breeding systems as well.

NATURAL HISTORY
Mating

Courtship ritual of pigeons is short and is rapidly followed by mating, which is initiated by the female. The female moves into a crouched position as an invitation for the male to position on top of her. At the same time, the female flips her tail over her back so that the male can adjust his position to allow juxtaposition of their cloacas. The pigeons will remain in this position for few seconds and ejaculation happens quickly.

Incubation

In rock doves (*C livia*), the female lays the first egg 9 to 10 days after mating and generally late in the evening. The second egg is laid approximately 44 hours later and incubation starts at that time. Both parents take turns incubating the eggs. Incubation lasts on average 18 days and starts after the laying of the second egg. Wild pigeons breed mostly during spring and summer, but captive pigeons can breed all year long using artificial lighting and techniques such as uncoupling. Uncoupling is a technique where the male and the female of a breeding pair are separated for a minimum period of 1 month. The couple will mate when reunited.

Parental Care

In all Columbidae species, the chicks (or squabs) are fed by both parents during their first days of life. Parents regurgitate the content of their crop directly into the beak of the squabs. The composition of this content changes over time and two periods can be recognized.

- The squabs are unable to digest whole seed during their first week of life. Parents will feed them with a liquid called "crop milk," which is composed of desquamated epithelial cells of the crop. The production of crop milk, as well as the behavioral modifications ensuring parental care, is induced by increased secretion of prolactin. Crop milk is especially rich in lipid and proteins. It is the only food the squabs will consume during their first week of life[1] (**Table 1**).
- The crop milk is progressively replaced by regurgitation of moistened grains after the first week.

Squabs raised in optimal conditions are ready for weaning by the age of 23 days and can be separated from their parents. Without human intervention, they will naturally leave the nest at 30 to 35 days old.

DEVELOPMENT OF THE PIGEON
Physical Development

The age at which pigeons are considered adults is variable according to the selected criteria. Squabs are able to feed themselves by 23 days of age, are able to fly by 5 to 6 weeks, and are able to breed when they are 5 months old on average. Their immune system is considered mature shortly thereafter and pigeons are generally considered "fully" adult by the age of 7 to 8 months.

Weight

The growth rate of pigeons during their first days of life is very important and possibly unique among birds. The weight of domestic pigeons at birth is approximately 15 g and is multiplied by 2 during the first 48 hours of life and by 20 during the first month of life. The composition of crop milk is one of the reasons explaining this very high growth speed (**Fig. 1**). The growth rate progressively slows down afterward to reach the adult weight by the age of 4 to 5 months.

Table 1 Chemical composition of crop milk	
Nutrient	**Concentration (% as is)**
Moisture	64–84
Crude protein	11–18.8
Ether extract	4.5–12.7
Ash	0.8–1.8
Carbohydrate	0–6.4

From Sales J, Janssens GPJ. Nutrition of the domestic pigeon (Columba livia domestica). Worlds Poult Sci J 2003;59:221-232.

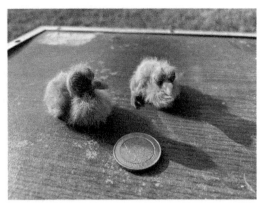

Fig. 1. Squabs just after hatchling.

Feathers

Pigeons hatch covered in a feathery yellowish down. The first feathers start to grow approximately 8 to 10 days after hatching (**Fig. 2**). The size of the pigeons at that age is ideal for banding. Bands carrying an individual number are used to identify specific individuals. Pigeons are fully feathered by the age of 16 to 18 days. Pigeons hatched early during the year (from January to March) have their first molt by the age of 2 months during which they change all the feathers of the mantle (ie, all the feathers with the exception of flight feathers). Pigeons hatched later during the breeding season will not have this molt, but they will develop the flight feathers at a younger age instead. Primary remiges are replaced successively, beginning with the most proximal ones. A steady and normal replacement of the remiges is a sign of a healthy pigeon. In late August or early September, pigeons will go through a so-called "big molt" during which all the feathers of the mantle are replaced. Many pigeon fanciers keep young pigeons in semidarkness for a few hours a day to delay this molt and allow pigeons to compete for a longer period of time.

Flight

Pigeons attempt to fly for the first time when they are approximately 1 month old. They are able to take off and reach perches placed at a height of a few centimeters from the

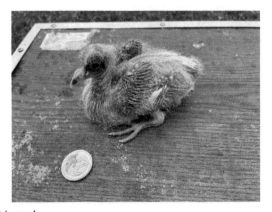

Fig. 2. Ten-day-old squab.

ground at this time. The first true flight usually happens by 5 weeks of age, and pigeons are fully able to remain in the air 1 week later.

Sexing

Sexual dimorphism is almost nonexistent in young pigeons. It is therefore nearly impossible to differentiate males from females with certainty based on their physical appearance. Sexing pigeons under the age of 4 months with certainty relies on DNA analysis or endoscopic examination to directly visualize the gonads. After 4 months, males progressively develop larger caruncles, bigger heads and bodies, and more colorful iridescent feathers on the side of the neck. The dimorphism is usually obvious at the age of 1 year.

Development of the Immune System

Squabs are mainly protected by passive immunity transmitted from the hen during their first days of life. This immunity is acquired in the eggs and is directly dependent on the immunity of the hen. Crop milk is very rich in antibodies, but these can pass through the intestinal barrier only during the first hours after hatching.[2] As a consequence, these antibodies mostly provide local protection limited to the digestive tract. The passive immunity transmitted from the hen progressively declines afterward and young pigeons develop their own active immunity. The bursa of Fabricius is the primary lymphoid organ and develops during the first 7 to 75 days of the pigeon's life and begins to involute by the age of 3 to 4 months.[3] These features of the development of the immune system are responsible for the late onset of full immunity in pigeons and have direct implications on the occurrence of certain pediatric diseases.

Behavioral Development

The main behavioral changes occur on the development of secondary sex characteristics between the ages of 3 and 5 months. The greatest changes are observed in males and include the development of new behaviors such as defense of a territory, aggression, and courtship rituals. Pair formation usually takes place afterward and pigeons form lifelong couples, except in cases where one of the partners disappear.

Practical Aspects: Clinical Examination of the Young Pigeon

General examination of the young pigeon is relatively similar to that performed in adults, with some exceptions.

Growth curve
The general appearance of the pigeon should be evaluated first from a distance by visual examination. Growth retardation is a nonspecific sign of disease in very young pigeons and can occasionally be very pronounced (**Fig. 3**).

Body condition score
Body condition score is estimated as in other avian species by evaluation of the keel (breast bone), pectoral musculature, and fat deposits (over the sternum and the abdomen). A low body condition is mainly characterized by a sharp keel. An excessively high body condition score is characterized by a plumped and rounded appearance of the chest and by the presence of excessive subcutaneous and intracelomic fat deposits.

Hydration status
Evaluation of hydration status relies on skin elasticity, appearance of the eyes, and characteristics of the mucous membranes.

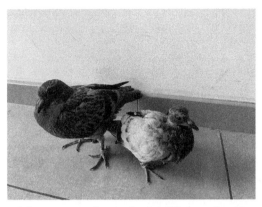

Fig. 3. Two pigeons of the same age (approximately 23 days of age).

Integument

The skin covering the pectoral muscles is evaluated on both sides of the keel where the feathers are easily spread to appreciate the color and texture of the cutaneous surface. The skin of a healthy young pigeon is normally bright pink, which indicates appropriate oxygenation of tissue as well as adequate nutritional intake. Dark-colored skin or excessive amounts of dandruff can indicate health issues.

Healthy birds should have smooth feathers of good quality. Any deterioration of the general condition will induce a decrease in feather quality. Some major pathogens can induce malformation of the growing remiges. Identification of misshapen remiges can therefore lead to a suspicion of a pathologic event at the time when the feather was growing. The feathers and, more particularly, the remiges and contour feathers of the neck will be evaluated for external parasites.

Beak, choana, and throat

The external features of the beak should be evaluated first. The nares are normally dry and clean. The cere should generally be as white as possible in pigeons but individuals younger than 1 month of age normally have a darker cere. The beak is then opened and the oral cavity is inspected. The mucous membranes are normally pink. A red color indicates inflammation, an excessively pale color is consistent with anemia, and a purplish color can be observed in cases of dehydration or respiratory disorders. The choana should be inspected and should be free of material. Abnormal findings in young pigeons may include choanal discharge as well as abscesses or pseudomembranous lesions involving the hard palate or extending deeper in the throat.

Crop

Screening for *Trichomonas* sp or yeasts is a routine procedure in Columbidae. Identification of *Trichomonas* sp relies on a crop wet mount, which is a test wherein a swab of the crop is observed by wet mount microscopy using sterile saline. The sample is ideally analyzed immediately after collection and can be analyzed up to 10 minutes after collection. Microscopically, the parasitic load can be quantified. Some clinicians use home-made scales ranging from 1 to 10 as there are no published scales. Identification of yeasts (eg, *Candida* sp) relies on a cytologic evaluation of a crop smear using a fast stain kit or a Gram stain. The head and the neck of the pigeon are extended, and a swab with a shaft long enough to sample the crop is inserted through the oral cavity down the cervical esophagus.

Droppings and coprology

A thorough macroscopic examination of the droppings is important to identify and differentiate diarrhea from polyuria. Coprological examination should be routinely used when evaluating Columbidae patients. The McMaster method is a simple and frequently used fecal egg count technique. It is a flotation technique using saturated NaCl solution and a McMaster counting chamber for direct microscopic examination. This procedure can reveal oocysts of *Coccidia* sp as well as nematode ova.

HUSBANDRY

Nutritional deficiencies in parents will systematically lead to nutritional deficiencies in young pigeons during their development in the egg and their first days of life after hatching. Moreover, the quality of active immunity of young pigeons is also directly dependent on the nutritional status of the hen.[4] The quality of passive immunity is directly dependent on the immunity of the hen and impacts the humoral immune response of the young pigeons up to 1 year of age.[5] As a consequence, the physical and immunologic development of squabs is directly related to nutrition and immunity (eg, vaccination) of the parents.

Males and females are usually separated in two distinct groups without visual contact for a minimum period of 1 month before mating. This separation will allow synchronization and optimization of mating as well as hatchings.

From Hatching to Weaning (23 days)

Recently hatched squabs are directly dependent on their parents. Their nutritional intake relies successively on egg yolk remnants during their first hours of life, crop milk during their first week, and food material regurgitated by the parents until weaning. Parents are generally fed a mix of grains specifically designed for breeding. The optimal diet for breeding pigeons contains 16% protein and 7% to 8% fat. A balanced proportion of the different grains in the mix is necessary to obtain a formulated ration with an optimal composition. It is recommended to supplement this mix with grit, minerals, trace elements, and vitamins. Few breeders will provide pelleted diets.[1] Hand rearing is not a common practice for breeding of Columbidae.

Weaning

Weaning is a key period in the life of pigeons during which multiple changes happen including the separation from parents and the need for feeding by themselves. For individuals living in a breeding center, grouping with other pigeons of the same or different age can also occur during this period. Grouping can put pigeons in contact with potential pathogens to which they have not yet been exposed. All of these changes are stressful and occur at a period where passive immunity transferred from the hen begins to decline and while active immunity is still weak. The endemic presence of pigeon circovirus (PiCV) in most breeding centers can alter the function of the bursa of Fabricius and worsen immune suppression which can make this period even more complicated. Grouping young pigeons together based on their age with a maximum of 10 days within a group is a way to keep pigeons with identical immune status together and helps to limit the development of some infectious diseases. Weaned pigeons will be initially fed with the same grain mix as the one provided to the parents. A nutritional transition will be performed rapidly to a mix of grain designed for young pigeons with less protein and fat content compared with mixes designed for breeding.

From Weaning to Fledgling

Racing and ornamental pigeons are always fed a mix of grains containing 13% to 14% protein and 6% to 7% fat, which is lower compared with breeding diets. Pigeons raised for human consumption are fed a diet with higher levels of protein and fat. Pigeons intended to free-range or race will need to be provided with access to an outside aviary just a few days after weaning so they become familiar with their environment. Pigeons accustomed to their surroundings will be able to find their way home regardless of the location where they are released.

COMMON DISEASES OF JUVENILE

This review is intended to describe the most common disorders of young pigeons. These will include the main diseases specific to young pigeons as well as diseases affecting pigeons of any age with special implications on younger birds. The immune system of young pigeons is not as efficient as that of adults and some diseases that are benign in adult birds can have more serious consequences in younger animals. This review is not intended to be exhaustive and the reader is referred to other publications for further details.[6]

Nutritional Disorders

Young pigeons undergo particularly rapid growth and require high nutritional provision from their parents, which must meet their own needs in addition to those of the chicks before and during the breeding period. Pigeons in the wild can relatively easily find the various nutrients (eg, mineral and trace elements) required from their environment through their varied and balanced diet. Captive pigeons depend on the feed provided by the breeders or the owners, which increases the risk of deficiencies.

Rickets
Calcium and vitamin D deficiencies are relatively frequent and can manifest with different degrees of severity. One of the first clinical signs in young pigeons is a deviation of the keel bone. The severity of the deviation increases in cases where the nest is not well prepared by the parents or appropriate nesting material has not been provided by the breeder and the young pigeons lay on a hard surface. Provision of additional nesting material and addition of a soft material at the bottom of the nest will help to reduce the deviation. More advanced stages of the disease can manifest as growth retardation, lameness, soft beak, or swollen joints. In the latter cases, the prognosis is guarded to poor.

Polyuria/Polydipsia
Polyuria and polydipsia of nutritional origin in squabs is poorly described in the literature but relatively common in the experience of one author (NS). This syndrome usually occurs 8 to 10 days after hatching because of a water imbalance at the time the pigeons switch from crop milk to regurgitated grains. Parents may suddenly start drinking very large quantities of water which lead to changes in the water to feed ratio of the material that is regurgitated to the young pigeons. The cause is mainly attributed to deficiencies in minerals and trace elements and must be differentiated from infectious disorders (eg, paratyphoid). Such deficiencies induce polyuria in young animals in addition to the parents. In severe cases, the imbalance is such that young pigeons are fed almost exclusively with water which induces significant growth retardation as well as weakness. Milder cases can be self-resolving at the time of weaning. Young pigeons able to feed themselves stop consuming excessive quantities of water from

their parents. Polydipsia resolves also in parents a few days after removal of their offspring. Removal of the young pigeons from their parents can be required to resolve more serious cases. Young pigeons can be moved to a foster pair or be hand raised in cases where fostering is not possible. On resolution of the polyuria/polydipsia, adult pigeons will require supplementation with minerals, vitamins, and trace elements for a minimum of 1 to 2 months before breeding activity resumes.

Trauma

The most frequent traumatic injuries affecting young pigeons occur by the time they start accessing the outdoors and begin to fly. Young pigeons are exposed to different risks. As for other species, traumatic injuries are likely to cause pain and analgesia should be provided appropriately. This topic is outside of the scope of this publication and additional information can be found elsewhere.[7] The same dosages can be used as in adults; however, many analgesic drugs are considered a form of "doping" in racing pigeons.[8]

Crop Injury

It is not unusual for young pigeons to fly against obstacles such as electric cables. This type of collision can cause skin laceration of the neck and occasionally crop perforation. In the latter case, it is frequent to observe water flowing out of the wound when the pigeon drinks. Treatment involves cleaning and disinfection of the lesions followed by suture of the wound.

The crop and skin are closed in separate layers. The prognosis is generally good.

Fractures

Mid-air collision is a common cause of limb fracture. The treatment of choice depends on the type of fracture and generally relies on external skeletal fixator-intramedullary pin tie-in techniques. The prognosis for return to flight is always guarded in cases of wing fracture. The prognosis for recovery is very good in cases of leg fracture.

Wounds Secondary to Predator Attacks (eg, Raptors)

Raptors are the main predators of pigeons. Young pigeons are poorly experienced and represent easy targets for raptors on their first flights. Attacks by raptors are frequent and generally associated with numerous and deep wounds when the pigeon survives. Treatment involves cleaning and disinfection of the wound and suture of the skin is occasionally necessary. The wounds are considered infected and justify the use of antibiotics.

Infectious Diseases

Viral diseases

Rotavirus. Infection of pigeons by rotaviruses has been described for many years.[9] These viruses usually induce mild clinical signs. A new strain of type A rotavirus (G18P) was identified in Australia in 2016 and has since been identified in multiple areas worldwide.[10] This strain can infect pigeons of all ages but morbidity and mortality are higher in young birds. This strain is unique because it is able to disseminate systemically and is not limited to the gastrointestinal tract.[11] Clinical signs include regurgitation, green diarrhea, anorexia, lethargy, and high mortality (ranging between 10% and 40%). Postmortem examination generally reveals hepatic and splenic congestion, mottling, and hypertrophy of variable severity.[12] The diagnosis relies on a polymerase chain reaction (PCR) test performed on a fecal sample. The G18P strain is currently epizootic in many parts of the world and has become enzootic in some locations (eg, Australia). Studies performed in multiple lofts in Germany revealed a high prevalence of this virus in the pigeon population. There is no effective treatment against rotaviruses to date. Supportive care including vitamins and rehydration is generally indicated and can be associated with antibiotic therapy to decrease secondary bacterial infections. A bivalent vaccine against Pigeon Paramyxovirus type 1 (PPMV-1, now called avian avulavirus type 1) and rotaviruses has been available in Europe for several years (RP Vacc, Pharmagal bio) and provides effective protection. Immunization schedule requires two doses administered at 4 and 7 weeks followed by annual booster.

Paramyxovirus (newcastle disease). Newcastle disease is caused by avian avulavirus type 1 (AAvV-1, formerly known as Pigeon Paramyxovirus 1 [PPMV-1]) described in pigeons for the first time in 1971.[13] This disease can affect pigeons of any age. Incubation period can range from 3 days to 3 weeks in pigeons and shedding of the virus can start as soon as 3 days post-infection. The clinical signs and severity of the disease depend on the virus strain. Lentogenic, mesogenic, and velogenic strains are recognized by increasing order of pathogenicity. Clinical signs can include respiratory, digestive, neurologic, and renal disorders. The main clinical signs currently observed in Europe are severe polyuria/polydipsia occasionally associated with neurologic disorders such as torticollis or vestibular disorder. The virus can persist up to 6 weeks in the organism. After 6 weeks, the pigeon is no longer considered contagious. Surviving pigeons can occasionally recover completely following a 2- to 6-month convalescence, even in cases with severe neurologic signs. Pigeons with severe neurologic disorders may be unable to feed themselves and will require to be handfed until they recover. Diagnosis relies mostly on PCR testing of a cloacal swab. There is no specific treatment, and supportive care is usually recommended. Numerous inactivated vaccines are effective against the disease. Newcastle disease is considered a minor zoonosis and can cause a mild and self-limiting conjunctivitis in humans.

Herpesvirus. Columbid herpesvirus-1 (CoHV-1) infection is mainly a respiratory disease, although digestive and other systems can seldomly be involved. The main clinical signs include conjunctivitis and rhinitis, as well as focal mucosal necrosis of the oral cavity, larynx, and pharynx. Pigeons usually scratch their cere, which can turn gray or yellowish. CoHV-1 can establish a latent infection that may be reactivated later similarly to many other viruses belonging to the Herpesviridae family. There is no effective treatment against the virus.[14] Identification and treatment of secondary bacterial (eg, β-hemolytic *Staphylococcus*, *Pasteurella multocida*, *Bordetella bronchiseptica*, *Escherichia coli*, *Mycoplasma* spp) and parasitic infections (eg, *Trichomonas* spp) are important because these co-pathogens can induce reactivation of latent infections. A trivalent vaccine against AAvV-1 (formerly PPMV-1), herpesvirus and a strain of adenovirus is currently available in Europe (Pharmavac PHA, Pharmagal bio).

Circovirus. PiCV infection is responsible for clinical disease affecting mostly young pigeons. Studies identified PiCV in numerous lofts, and this virus is considered widespread among pigeons.[15] Both vertical and horizontal transmission have been described.[16] The pathogenic role of this virus is linked to its tropism for lymphoid tissue and it can induce immunosuppression leading to secondary infections.[17] This virus is often mentioned as one of the main causes of "Young Pigeon Disease Syndrome" (YPDS). Pathogenicity of this virus in the development of YPDS remains controversial because PiCV has been isolated from healthy pigeons, and some pigeons suffering from YPDS are not infected by PiCV. PiCV can lead to weight loss, lethargy, weakness, diarrhea, and vomiting. Subclinical infections without clinical signs have also been described.[18] There is no available vaccine against PiCV. Studies evaluating injection of the viral capsid protein are underway and are showing promising results.[19]

Poxvirus. Pigeon poxvirus is very resistant in the environment. Transmission occurs mostly through direct contacts between pigeons. Ectoparasites can also play a significant role in transmission of the virus. The incubation period ranges from 4 to 12 days. Pigeon poxvirus infection can lead to two types of clinical disease: a cutaneous or dry pox and a diphtheroid or wet pox. The cutaneous form is characterized by the development of epithelioma most commonly on the head (eg, eyes, oral commissure). The diphtheroid form is characterized by plaque formation in the oral cavity and occasionally in the trachea, esophagus, and/or crop.[20] Morbidity can reach 80% to 90%. Mortality is low and death occurs when oral lesions prevent pigeons from eating or from breathing. Diagnosis is easy and relies mostly on visualization of the typical pox lesions. Definitive diagnosis can be achieved with PCR. Excision and curettage of lesions followed by application of an iodine solution is the mainstay of treatment when lesions are severe. The prognosis is good and lesions usually resolve within 3 weeks. Attenuated vaccines are available and prevent the development of clinical signs of the disease.

Adenovirus. Multiple strains of adenoviruses are described in pigeons. These viruses are generally highly contagious and are characterized by mild enteritis or mild hepatitis. Clinical signs include anorexia, regurgitation, and diarrhea. The disease is usually self-limiting within 4 to 5 days and treatment is usually limited to supportive care. Prophylactic antibiotics are occasionally provided to limit bacterial secondary infection. Sudden death can occur in rare instances in pigeons of any age and has been related to a specific strain of adenovirus (pigeon adenovirus 2).[21]

Bacterial diseases

Salmonella (paratyphoid). Paratyphoid is one of the most severe diseases in pigeons. The causative agent is *Salmonella enterica* subsp Enterica serovar Typhimurium variant Copenhagen.[22] This bacterium is highly resistant in the environment and is able to persist in the host even after treatment which explains why healthy carriers are frequent. Transmission to young pigeons occurs most frequently horizontally through excretion in the parents' droppings, but can also occur vertically through the egg. Clinical signs vary depending on the age of the pigeons. The disease can have a peracute form characterized by bacteremia and shock or an acute form characterized by diarrhea, weight loss, anorexia, and death. In adults, the disease can also have a chronic form. Postmortem examination reveals inflammation and ulceration of the digestive mucosa as well as degenerative changes and necrotic foci in the liver, spleen, and kidneys. Diagnosis relies on clinical signs, fecal culture, and identification of the bacteria or serology. The bacterium is naturally sensitive to tetracyclines, sulfamides, and fluoroquinolones, although different levels of antibiotic resistance have been described. Vaccination with autovaccines is the only preventive measure with proven efficacy.[23] Vaccination of the parents is usually effective in protecting chicks against development of the disease and should be performed in breeding centers where *Salmonella* sp has been identified or suspected.

Mycoplasmosis. Three species of *Mycoplasma* are mainly recognized in pigeons: *Mycoplasma columbinum*, *M columborale*, and *M columbinasale*. A study performed in the Netherlands revealed that more than one-third of tested pigeons were carriers of *Mycoplasma* spp. *Mycoplasma* spp are frequently associated with respiratory disorders. Their role as primary pathogens has not been clearly demonstrated, and they may only be responsible for secondary infections.[24] A study revealed that tiamulin administered for 35 days was effective to eliminate *Mycoplasma* spp in pigeons.[25] Pigeons tested positive 13 weeks after the end of the treatment in the same study.

Colibacillosis. Colibacillosis is caused by the bacterium *Escherichia coli* and is generally considered a secondary infection. *E coli* can normally be found in the digestive tract of pigeons and can take advantage of a primary infection (eg, adenovirus, herpesvirus, and trichomonas) to multiply and act as an opportunistic pathogen. The bacteria can induce bacteremia, ingluvitis, or airsacculitis depending on the primary disease. Diagnosis is based on bacterial culture of the lesions. Sensitivity test is recommended to select an effective antibiotic.

Ornithosis (chlamydiosis). *Chlamydia psittaci* is an intracellular bacterium responsible for disease in numerous species including humans. Epidemiologic studies revealed that a variable percentage of pigeons are carriers of *C psittaci* in multiple countries. Prevalence is greater among breeding pigeons than among feral pigeons.[26,27] Pigeons usually carry serotype B which is considered low pathogenicity and less likely transmissible to humans. As a consequence, pigeons usually do not show signs of disease. On occasion, the infection can cause a clinical disease characterized by rhinitis, conjunctivitis, respiratory distress, weight loss, and diarrhea. Mortality is high. The diagnosis is based on identification of *C psittaci* by PCR. Treatment relies on long-term administration of an antibiotic that is effective against intracellular pathogens (eg, doxycycline, erythromycin).

Streptococcosis. Streptococcosis is caused by *Streptococcus gallolyticus*. *S gallolyticus* can be naturally present in healthy pigeons. This bacterium can grow out of control, cross the intestinal wall, and cause bacteremia. Bacterial excretion increases in this situation and allows for environmental contamination and exposure of other pigeons. The suspected factors triggering the multiplication of *S gallolyticus* include immune suppression or concurrent infections. Clinical signs are highly variable and include green diarrhea, anorexia, polyuria and polydipsia, weight loss, wing drooping, and difficulties flying. Postmortem examination reveals petechiae, hepatitis, and necrotic foci in the pectoral muscle and the myocardium. Diagnosis is postmortem and based on identification of the bacteria by culture of the lesions. Antibiotics (eg, amoxicillin, spiramycin, doxycycline) for 5 to 7 days are the mainstay of treatment. Sensitivity testing is recommended because antimicrobial resistance has been observed.[28]

Parasitic diseases
Trichomoniasis (canker). Trichomoniasis is a disease caused by the flagellate protozoan *Trichomonas gallinae*. Direct vertical transmission from parents to their young occurs during feeding. The parasite is of low pathogenicity for adults but it can induce serious disorders in young birds. The severity of the disease depends on a number of factors including parasitic load, virulence, strain, and presence of other pathogens worsening the clinical picture. Clinical signs include both nonspecific manifestations (eg, lethargy) and specific manifestations such as caseous lesions surrounded by a hyperemic area on the mucosa of the mouth, palate, pharynx, esophagus, and crop. Abscesses can appear in the esophagus and the crop. Generalized infection is possible and can create serious lesions in multiple organs including the liver and the umbilicus. Studies revealed that the presence of *Trichomonas* in very young pigeons can alter the composition of the natural microbiota of the crop and the intestines, which could predispose to the development of other disorders.[29] The diagnosis of trichomoniasis is

based on a crop wet mount. Imidazoles are generally used for the treatment. Ronidazole 10% in drinking water at a dose of 5g/2L for 5 days is usually effective. Resistance to treatments has been described on rare occasions.[30] Effectiveness of garlic extract has been demonstrated both in vivo and in vitro.[31] Acidification of drinking water can be used as a preventive measure to limit parasitic development.

Hexamitiasis. *Hexamita columbae* is a flagellate protozoan responsible of catarrhal inflammation of the proximal portion of the small intestines. Clinical signs are usually limited to diarrhea and lethargy. Diagnosis relies on microscopic identification of the parasite on a cloacal swab or a wet mount of fresh feces. Treatment is similar to that for trichomoniasis.

Coccidiosis. *Eimeria columbarum* and *Eimeria labeana* are causative agents of coccidiosis in pigeons. Young pigeons are much more sensitive compared with adults. Young pigeons can develop a green diarrhea, which is rarely hemorrhagic, growth retardation, weight loss, and death within a few days. The diagnosis is based on identification of oocysts in the feces. Feces are mixed with a saturated NaCl solution to concentrate the oocysts on the surface by flotation, and a McMaster counting chamber is used to quantify the parasitic load. The treatment generally involves administration of sulfamides. Toltrazuril in drinking water at a dose of 125 ppm for 3 to 5 days is also effective.[32]

Helminthiasis. *Ascaridia columbae* and *Capillaria obsignata* are the two main nematodes identified in pigeons. *Ornithostrongylus quadriradiatus*, *Syngamus trachea*, *Dispharynx nasuta*, *Tetramere americana*, and *Oxyspirura mansoni* are much less frequently described. Different treatments with variable effectiveness are reported. Moxidectin in drinking water at an empirical dose of 5 mg/L is an effective and convenient alternative to treat a whole flock. Ivermectin at a dose of 0.2 mg/kg subcutaneously is also effective. Fenbendazole administered at 125 ppm in drinking water for 3 days is effective. Fenbendazole is contraindicated during molting or breeding periods, and toxicity has been reported at a dose of 30 mg/kg PO q24 h × 5 days.[33,34]

Numerous species of cestodes have been described in pigeons (eg, *Hymenolepis* sp, *Aporina* sp, and *Raillietina* sp). Infestation of pigeons requires an intermediate host such as slugs, earthworms, or insects. Most cases are isolated. The diagnosis is based on identification of proglottids in the feces or occasionally by direct visualization of worms coming out of the cloaca. Trematodes can also infest pigeons. *Echinostoma* is the most common genus identified in Europe. Praziquantel can be used against cestodes and trematodes at a dose of 10 mg/kg PO twice at a 10-day interval.

Ectoparasites. Numerous external parasites (insects and mites) can infest pigeons. The severity of clinical signs in young pigeons depends on the type of parasite involved and can range from asymptomatic to life-threatening. Some parasites can cause severe anemia and death. Besides infestation of the chicks, a specific problem of external parasites in pediatrics is that they can infest the parents during brooding and contribute to nest abandonment. Both the pigeons and the loft must be treated in cases of infestation.

Fungal diseases. Candidiasis is a digestive mycosis caused by the yeast *Candida albicans*. Excessive use of antibiotics is a predisposing factor in young pigeons. The main clinical signs include mucosal thickening and ulcerations of the oral cavity, esophagus, and crop. Nonspecific clinical signs such as lethargy can also occur. Diagnosis relies on identification of the yeasts either by cytology of a swab or culture. The treatment is based on antifungals (eg, nystatin) administered in drinking water.

PREVENTIVE CARE

Preventive medicine is becoming an increasingly important part of the veterinary care in pigeons as in other species. A broad range of prophylactic measures can be introduced to prevent the development of numerous diseases including infectious and nutritional ones.

Prenatal Prevention

Prophylactic measures necessary to optimize health of young pigeons start before hatching. Immune and nutritional status of the parents as well as their parasitic load will have a direct impact on the health and growth of the chicks. Couples are separated before the breeding period to synchronize mating and hatching. This management system minimizes the mixing of pigeons with different ages and immune status. This is especially important to limit the consequences of viral infection such as PiCV infection. Vaccination of parents is recommended before breeding to ensure the best immunity of the squabs against Newcastle disease, rotaviruses, and *Salmonella* sp. Parents should be fed a balanced and formulated diet before breeding in order to avoid nutritional deficiencies during the breeding period. Screening for parasites, including *Trichomonas* spp, *Eimeria* spp, gastrointestinal worms, and ectoparasites, is indicated and treatment is initiated if indicated to limit the risk of early contamination of the squabs.

Postnatal Prevention

Introduction of new birds

One of the most important prophylactic measures in a breeding facility is to avoid introduction and mixing of young pigeons as much as possible. This measure seeks to reduce the introduction of pathogens when the immune system of pigeons is generally weak. In cases new birds are to be introduced to the facility, isolation and quarantine of the newcomer is required to ensure they do not develop clinical signs. One week of quarantine is generally performed in practice and up to 3 weeks can be required by legal authorities. Newcomers should be vaccinated before their introduction following the same immunization schedule as the birds in the facility. In situations where new pigeons are required for breeding, a good practice is to recommend the introduction of immunocompetent adults only to the breeding department or to introduce eggs that will be incubated by foster parents. Transmission of many pathogens can be avoided with this type of management.

Antiparasitic treatment

It is important to ensure that the loft is free from ectoparasites which could disturb parents during incubation or young pigeons after hatching. Treatment of the loft is required in cases of infestation. It is usually not necessary to treat young pigeons with internal antiparasitic treatment as long as prophylactic treatments have cleared infestation of the parents. A screening for parasites after weaning is generally preferred compared with systematic treatment of young pigeons.

Vaccination

Numerous vaccines are available and effective against an increasing number of viral and bacterial diseases in Europe. The vaccination schedule can be designed according to health history of the loft, endemic diseases in the area, and future activity of the pigeons (eg, shows and competitions) (**Table 2**). Vaccinations against Newcastle disease and rotaviruses are highly recommended given the severity and the endemicity of these diseases in Europe. It is recommended to vaccine young pigeons in contact with other birds (eg, shows, races) against poxvirus using an attenuated vaccine.

Table 2
Example of vaccination schedule in breeding pigeons

Age	Vaccine
4 wk	Rotavirus/Newcastle disease
5 wk	Paratyphoid
6 wk	Poxvirus
7 wk	Rotavirus/Newcastle disease
8 wk	Paratyphoid
Annually	Rotavirus/Newcastle disease/paratyphoid/poxvirus

Vaccination against paratyphoid could be considered in cases where there is a history of paratyphoid in the loft.

SUMMARY

Pigeon pediatrics has developed strongly with the reproduction of valuable birds for racing. The importance of this sport has medical and regulatory implications for the veterinary practitioner. In particular, the clinician must be able to carry out the necessary vaccination protocols and avoid using doping products. A preventive approach is crucial because juveniles have increased susceptibility to many contagious infectious diseases.

CLINICS CARE POINTS

- The immunity of young pigeons is directly dependent on the immune and nutritional status of the hen. Vaccination of the parents and provision of a balanced diet are preventive measure of paramount important for a healthy development of the squabs.
- Rotaviruses are known for many years as pathogens responsible of benign digestive disorders. A new strain of type A rotavirus (G18P) has been identified in 2016 and has spread worldwide. This strain is able to disseminate systemically and is associated with increased mortality.
- Pigeon circovirus has been associated with "Young Pigeon Disease Syndrome" but its significance is still debated. There is no vaccine against pigeon circovirus at the moment, but recent studies evaluating injection of recombinant capsid protein virus-like particles are showing promising results.
- Multiple strains of adenoviruses are described in pigeons and usually cause mild enteritis or mild hepatitis, which are generally self-resolving. A specific strain of adenovirus (pigeon adenovirus 2) associated with sudden death has been described in pigeons.
- Streptococcosis usually responds well to a 5- to 7-day treatment course with antibiotics. Sensitivity test is recommended because bacterial resistance has been observed.

DISCLOSURE

The authors have no commercial or financial conflicts of interest to declare. This study was not supported by a grant.

REFERENCES

1. Sales J, Janssens GPJ. Nutrition of the domestic pigeon (Columba livia domestica). World's Poult Sci J 2003;59:221–32.

2. Engberg RM, Kaspers B, Schranner I, et al. Quantification of the immunoglobulin classes IgG and IgA in the young and adult pigeon (Columba livia). Avian Pathol 1992;21:409–20.

3. Sanchez-Refusta F, Ciriaco E, Germanà A, et al. Age-related changes in the medullary reticular epithelial cells of the pigeon bursa of Fabricius. Anat Rec 1996; 246:473–80.

4. Ismail A, Jacquin L, Haussy C, et al. Food availability and maternal immunization affect transfer and persistence of maternal antibodies in nestling pigeons. PLoS One 2013;8:e79942.

5. Jacquin L, Blottière L, Haussy C, et al. Prenatal and postnatal parental effects on immunity and growth in 'lactating' pigeons. Funct Ecol 2012;26:866–75.

6. Chitty J, Lierz M. BSAVA manual of raptors, pigeons and passerine birds. UK: British Small Animal Veterinary Association; 2008.

7. Heard D. Galliformes and Columbiformes. In: West G, Heard D, Caulkette N, editors. Zoo animal and wildlife immobilization and anesthesia. 2nd edition. UK: Wiley; 2014. p. 473–80.

8. Marlier D. Doping in racing pigeons (Columba livia domestica): A review and actual situation in Belgium, a leading country in this field. Vet Sci 2022;9(2):42.

9. Harzer M, Heenemann K, Sieg M, et al. Prevalence of pigeon rotavirus infections: animal exhibitions as a risk factor for pigeon flocks. Arch Virol 2021;166:65–72.

10. Schmidt V, Kümpel M, Cramer K, et al. Pigeon rotavirus A genotype G18P[17]-associated disease outbreaks after fancy pigeon shows in Germany - a case series. Tierarztl Prax Ausg K Kleintiere Heimtiere 2021;49:22–7.

11. Meßmer C, Rubbenstroth D, Mohr L, et al. Pigeon Rotavirus A as the cause of systemic infection in juvenile pigeons (young pigeon disease). Tierarztl Prax Ausg K Kleintiere Heimtiere 2022;50:293–301.

12. Blakey J, Crossley B, Rosenberger JK, et al. Rotavirus A associated with clinical disease and hepatic necrosis in California Pigeons (Columba livia domestica). Avian Dis 2019;63:651–8.

13. Marlier D, Vindevogel H. Viral infections in pigeons. Vet J 2006;172:40–51.

14. Vindevogel H, Pastoret PP. Pathogenesis of pigeon herpesvirus infection. J Comp Pathol 1981;91:415–26.

15. Silva BBI, Urzo MLR, Encabo JR, et al. Pigeon circovirus over three decades of research: bibliometrics, scoping review, and perspectives. Viruses 2022;14(7): 1498.

16. Duchatel JP, Todd D, Smyth JA, et al. Observations on detection, excretion and transmission of pigeon circovirus in adult, young and embryonic pigeons. Avian Pathol 2006;35:30–4.

17. Abadie J, Nguyen F, Groizeleau C, et al. Pigeon circovirus infection: pathological observations and suggested pathogenesis. Avian Pathol 2001;30:149–58.

18. Schmidt V, Schlömer J, Lüken C, et al. Experimental infection of domestic pigeons with pigeon circovirus. Avian Dis 2008;52:380–6.

19. Huang HY, Silva BBI, Tsai SP, et al. Immunogenicity and protective activity of pigeon circovirus recombinant capsid protein virus-like particles (PiCV rCap-VLPs) in pigeons (Columba livia) Experimentally Infected with PiCV. Vaccines 2021; 9(2):98.

20. Harlin R, Wade L. Bacterial and parasitic diseases of Columbiformes. Vet Clin North Am Exot Pet Pract 2009;12:453–73.

21. Wan C, Chen C, Cheng L, et al. Detection of novel adenovirus in sick pigeons. J Vet Med Sci 2018;80:1025–8.

22. Pasmans F, Van Immerseel F, Hermans K, et al. Assessment of virulence of pigeon isolates of Salmonella enterica subsp. enterica serovar typhimurium variant copenhagen for humans. J Clin Microbiol 2004;42:2000–2.

23. Proux K, Humbert F, Guittet M, et al. Vaccination du pigeon contre Salmonella typhimurium. Avian Pathol 1998;27:161–7.

24. Hellebuyck T, Göbel S, Pasmans F, et al. Co-occurrence of Mycoplasma species and pigeon Herpesvirus-1 infection in racing pigeons (Columba livia). J Avian Med Surg 2017;31:351–5.

25. Howse JN, Jordan FT. Treatment of racing pigeons naturally infected with Mycoplasma columborale and M columbinum. Vet Rec 1983;112:324–6.

26. Ling Y, Chen H, Chen X, et al. Epidemiology of Chlamydia psittaci infection in racing pigeons and pigeon fanciers in Beijing, China. Zoonoses Public Health 2015; 62:401–6.

27. Geigenfeind I, Vanrompay D, Haag-Wackernagel D. Prevalence of Chlamydia psittaci in the feral pigeon population of Basel, Switzerland. Medical Microbiol 2012;61:261–5.

28. Kimpe A, Decostere A, Martel A, et al. Prevalence of antimicrobial resistance among pigeon isolates of Streptococcus gallolyticus, Escherichia coli and Salmonella enterica serotype Typhimurium. Avian Pathol 2002;31:393–7.

29. Ji F, Zhang D, Shao Y, et al. Changes in the diversity and composition of gut microbiota in pigeon squabs infected with Trichomonas gallinae. Sci Rep 2020;10: 19978.

30. Franssen FF, Lumeij JT. In vitro nitroimidazole resistance of Trichomonas gallinae and successful therapy with an increased dosage of ronidazole in racing pigeons (Columba livia domestica). Vet Pharmacol Ther 1992;15:409–15.

31. Seddiek Sh A, El-Shorbagy MM, Khater HF, et al. The antitrichomonal efficacy of garlic and metronidazole against Trichomonas gallinae infecting domestic pigeons. Parasitol Res 2014;113:1319–29.

32. Krautwald-Junghanns ME, Zebisch R, Schmidt V. Relevance and treatment of coccidiosis in domestic pigeons (Columba livia forma domestica) with particular emphasis on toltrazuril. J Avian Med Surg 2009;23:1–5.

33. Gozalo AS, Schwiebert RS, Lawson GW. Mortality associated with fenbendazole administration in pigeons (Columba livia). J Am Assoc Lab Anim Sci 2006; 45:63–6.

34. Howard LL, Papendick R, Stalis IH, et al. Fenbendazole and albendazole toxicity in pigeons and doves. J Avian Med Surg 2002;16(3):203–10.

Raptor Pediatrics

Abigail Duvall, DVM, DABVP-Avian Practice

KEYWORDS

- Raptor • Pediatric • Rehabilitation • Neonatal • Falcon

KEY POINTS

- Juvenile raptors are altricial and initially require heat support, though many species mature rapidly.
- Chicks are prone to imprinting and unless desired, steps must be taken to prevent this as they mature.
- Disease outbreaks can occur in captive breeding facilities, especially in those with large numbers of birds, making biosecurity of food sources and breeding birds crucial.
- Release of captive-reared raptors, even if originally born in the wild, must be done carefully to ensure survival post-release.

INTRODUCTION

Veterinarians may interact with neonatal and juvenile raptors in a variety of settings. Young raptors are frequently presented to wildlife rehabilitation centers after separation from their parents, often after falling from a nest. Healthy juveniles which are in the process of fledgling are also sometimes brought to rehabilitation centers by well-intentioned but misinformed members of the public. Captive breeding of raptors is also increasingly common, with some breeders producing only a few raptors per year and some large falcon breeding farms producing hundreds of falcons each year. Captive breeding of raptors was uncommon before the pioneering efforts of the Peregrine Fund which began in the 1970s in an effort to captive breed peregrine falcons (*Falco peregrinus*) for conservation.[1]

Within the context of this article, "raptor" will be used to refer to both diurnal members of the Accipitriformes, Cathartiformes, Falconiformes, and the nocturnal Strigiformes.[2] Although in the ornithological community there is a push to include the seriemas of the Cariamiformes, they will not be included here due to differences in life history and husbandry and a lack of traditional inclusion.[2]

HUSBANDRY AND MANAGEMENT OF JUVENILE RAPTORS

Raptor chicks, which are generally called eyasses by falconers, are altricial, and all species initially require external heat support when reared artificially. This is generally

Exotic Vet Care, 814 Johnnie Dodds Boulevard, Mt Pleasant, SC 29464, USA
E-mail address: add32@cornell.edu

Vet Clin Exot Anim 27 (2024) 359–378
https://doi.org/10.1016/j.cvex.2023.11.012
1094-9194/24/© 2023 Elsevier Inc. All rights reserved.

achieved through the use of an incubator or brooder, of which there are many styles available (**Fig. 1**). Initially, chicks may be brooded at 95°F (35°C) for most species, with a gradual decrease in temperature over time as chicks mature.[3] For many raptors native to North America, temperatures can be decreased by 5°F (2.8°C) every 3 days, with monitoring of the chicks to ensure comfort. Peregrine falcon chicks generally do not require heat after 10 days as long as temperatures do not fall below 70°F (21°C).[1] Cold chicks may huddle together, emit stress calls, and have slow emptying of the crop. Hot chicks may attempt to move away from heat, open mouth breathe, and splay out wings and legs. Creation of a temperature gradient within the brooding area can help to prevent overheating. Temperature can impact the digestion of food and the overall health of the chick. It is important that the flooring within the brooder be both easy to clean and disinfect and not too slick, to prevent splaying of the legs.[3]

If presented with a juvenile raptor of undetermined age, it is best to assume that if no contour or flight feathers are present and the chick is entirely downy that external heat support is essential. Older chicks with some contour feathers and the beginning of tail and wing feather growth will require less heat support. It can be helpful to seek out resources for aging nestling raptors in advance if expecting to work with them in rehabilitation. These are available for a variety of native species of raptor in North America, often due to field biologists needing to accurately age nestlings in field surveys. These may easily be found online and include guides for the American goshawk (*Accipiter atricapillus*), Swainson's hawk (*Buteo swainsoni*), red-tailed hawk (*Buteo jamaicensis*), ferruginous hawk (*Buteo regalis*), American kestrel (*Falco sparverius*), and turkey vulture (*Cathartes aura*).[4–9]

Most species will not immediately need to be fed after hatching. For falcons, initial feedings are generally within 8 to 12 hours of hatch.[1] Initial feedings are small and only

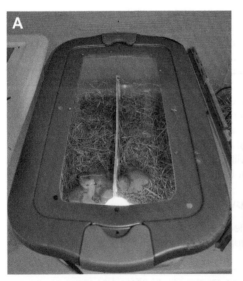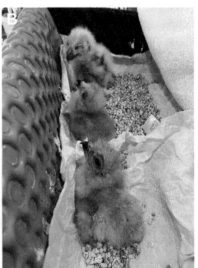

Fig. 1. Two different brooder setups. (*A*) Simple setup made from plastic tote with side-mounted 100 W incandescent bulb with hay substrate. (*B*) Setup similar to Peregrine Fund "K-pad" with water circulating pad on the side and under the pellet substrate such that the chicks can move toward the warm side with the pad or toward the cool side away from the pad.[1] (*Courtesy of* Jennifer Coulson, Pearl River, LA and David Kanellis, Las Vegas NV.)

partially fill the crop to avoid overwhelming the intestinal tract. It is often recommended that the meat initially offered to hatchlings be dipped in sterile saline to improve
hydration during feeding.[1] The size of feedings is gradually increased over the first
few days until enough food to fill the crop is safely given. The inclusion of bone within
the meat used for feeding is critical to avoid nutritional secondary hyperparathyroidism. Generally, this is achieved through the inclusion of bone finely ground into the
meat offered to young chicks and by offering whole prey with bone to older chicks
or parents rearing their own chicks.

The umbilicus should always be checked on newly hatched chicks and ideally
swabbed with iodine.[3] Unretracted yolk sacs or blood vessels may require urgent
and immediate attention.

In breeding operations using artificial incubation, it is common to hand-rear chicks
for around a week before placement with parents or foster parents so the chicks are
larger, stronger, and have better feeding responses.[3] Such chicks will not be imprinted
as they are returned for parent rearing early enough in their development, though
handling should still be minimized. If rearing raptors with the intention for later release
to the wild, care must be taken to avoid imprinting on humans. Ideally, this is done
through the use of non-releasable foster parents of the same species if possible. If
not, puppets designed to mimic the parent species and clothing which masks the
face and hands can be used with minimization of talking around chicks.

Regular weighing is recommended to track weight gain in chicks. Healthy chicks
should have a strong, vigorous response to feeding and should continuously gain
weight. Chicks that are unwell may be difficult to rouse for feeding, demonstrate
poor feeding responses, slow weight gain or failure to gain weight, and abnormal
vocalization. Dehydration may be noted by sinking of the eyes and changes to the
skin on the feet.[3] Any sign of regurgitation or true diarrhea should cause immediate
concern. Chicks which are intended to be parent-reared may be pulled temporarily
for treatment if needed.

The length of time which it takes for chicks to grow and fledge from the nest varies
greatly between species. Generally, chicks of smaller species fledge earlier than
larger species. Kestrels and screech owls (Megascops asio) may be flying by 4 weeks
of age. Red-tailed hawks fledge around 6 weeks of age and bald eagles (*Haliaeetus
leucocephalus*) around 12 weeks. This variation in rate of maturation is important as
mentally and physically, the chicks of larger species will have a longer period of time
in which they are considered to be nestlings. They have a longer period during which
imprinting needs to be avoided, and their musculoskeletal system is slower in
growth.

When handling juvenile raptors, the feet of downy juveniles without development of
contour feathers or those too young to stand are usually not strong enough to cause
injury. In fact, catching young raptors by the legs can lead to injury of the chick.[10]
Chicks should be caught from behind in a soft towel or blanket, with hands around
the outside of the body.[10] The older the juvenile, the more caution should be taken
in handling. The use of hoods or other visual barriers should always be considered
to reduce the stress of the juvenile raptors and to help avoid habituation and imprinting
of younger patients.[11]

Sick chicks benefit from general supportive care while attempting to find the underlying cause of illness. Hypothermia, dehydration, and hypoglycemia are all common in
ill neonatal raptors. All nestling raptors still in down benefit from external heat support
on initial presentation. The younger the chick, the more critical heat support becomes.
Fluids may be administered subcutaneously in the inguinal region, just as in adults. It is
more important in juveniles that these fluids be warmed before administration to

prevent hypothermia. Very young raptors may have increased fluid requirements when compared with adults, with a need for up to 50% more reported.[12] If needed, intraosseous or intravenous catheters can be placed for more urgent rehydration. The addition of up to 2.5% dextrose to administered subcutaneous, oral, intravenous, or intraosseous fluids is strongly recommended as often the last time in which the juvenile was fed is unknown.

Once stabilized, the underlying cause of illness can be determined. If large enough, blood may be collected from the jugular vein. Veins in the wings and legs are not well developed in very young chicks.

PROBLEMS DURING HATCHING

The hatching of healthy neonatal raptors is heavily dependent on incubation conditions. Eggs may be either hatched by parents or artificially incubated. In the case of artificial incubation, an attempt is made to replicate conditions under the parent bird. Temperature, humidity, turning, and ventilation must all be controlled. Tracking of egg weight loss during incubation can allow for modification of incubation conditions to improve the chances of a successful hatch. Ideally, falcon eggs should lose about 15% of their initial weight by the time of internal pipping and 18% by the time of hatch.[1] Similar rates of weights loss are reported for Harris' hawks (*Parabuteo unicinctus*).[13] Eggs which are noted to be losing too much weight in incubation can have the humidity in the incubator increased or can be moved to a separate incubator with higher humidity. In cases of continued severe weight loss, such as in abnormal porosity of the shell, a thin layer of nail polish or wax can be painted in vertical stripes along the length of the egg. Excessive application of any substance to the shell could cause embryonic death due to obstruction of pores in the shell through which gas exchange occurs, so this must be done with caution. Eggs losing insufficient weight may need to have a decrease in humidity.[1] If weight loss is predicted to be severely inadequate (< 11%), a small hole may be made over the air cell to aid in weight loss of the egg (**Fig. 2**).[13]

Complications during hatch are similar to those encountered in other species. Malpositions in the egg can occur, and some may result in fatal consequences. The malpositions described in poultry have been used to describe malpositions in psittacines and are useful in raptors as well (**Fig. 3**).[14] Chicks that are malpositioned within the shell are more likely to need assistance in hatching. Radiographs have been used to detect malposition before hatch in near-term California condor (*Gymnogyps californianus*) embryos, and this may be useful in other species.[15]

The time between initial internal pip and external pip, and from external pip to hatch, may vary between raptors. This information can be useful in deciding whether a chick may require assistance in hatching. The later in the process of hatching that assistance is needed, the safer it is to intervene. This is because it becomes increasingly likely that complete absorption of the yolk sac has occurred and that blood vessels have withdrawn. Too early an intervention can lead to fatal hemorrhage. Occasionally, a chick itself may damage a vessel in the process of hatching and can lose a significant amount of blood or even perish (**Fig. 4**).

If it is determined that a chick requires assistance, it is important to proceed slowly. In the case of a chick which has externally pipped and made at least some progress in its counterclockwise breaking of the shell, it is generally safe to remove small pieces of shell at a time, using sterile water to wet the shell membranes just ahead of where the chick's beak is located. If the membranes show prominent blood vessels, or bleeding is seen, no further shell should be removed. A small bleed can be stopped with a

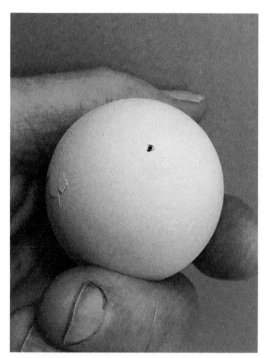

Fig. 2. Small hole made over the air sac in a Harris' hawk (*Parabuteo unicinctus*) egg to help increase weight loss. Note egg has subsequently pipped externally in a normal location at the time of photo. (*Courtesy of* Jennifer Coulson, Pearl River, LA.)

styptic pen or electrocautery pen and the egg returned to the incubator for a bit longer before attempting to aid the chick again.

To aid in determining whether a chick may need assistance in hatching, it is ideal to identify and describe normal times for various stages in hatching for the species being worked with (**Table 1**). If it is not possible to find this information in advance, it may be collected from within a breeding program for use in the future. For example,

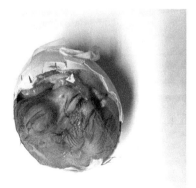

Fig. 3. Harris' hawk (*Parabuteo unicinctus*) chick with head over the right wing. Chick pipped internally but failed to hatch. (*Courtesy of* Jennifer Coulson.)

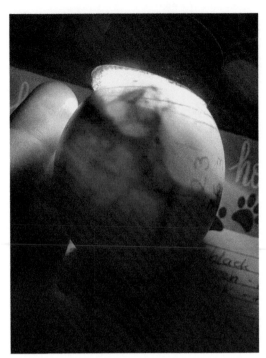

Fig. 4. Eurasian eagle owl (*Bubo bubo*) chick pipped internally but died of fatal hemorrhage. (*Courtesy of* David Kanellis.)

Table 1
Example of collection of useful normal hatching parameters for some species of raptors. Note that not all information may be available for all species

Species	Total Incubation Period (days)	Internal Pip (days)	Time from Internal to External Pip (hours)	Time from Start of Incubation to External Pip	Time from External Pip to Hatch (hours)
Harris' Hawk (*Parabuteo unicinctus*)[13]	30–33		Simultaneous or within 6 h		40
California Condor (*Gymnogyps californianus*)[15]	55–58	52–55	24–60		72
Peregrine falcon (*Falco peregrinus*)[1]	33–35	30–31	24–48		50
Bald eagle (*Haliaeetus leucocephalus*)[16,17]	34–37		12		24–48
Barn Owl (*Tyto alba*)[18]	27–35 (30)			25–33 (28)	36–48
American kestrel (*Falco sparverius*)[19]	28–30				55

determination of the normal time for external pip to complete hatch can allow for safe intervention if a chick takes substantially longer than normal.

CONGENITAL ABNORMALITIES

An incomplete absorption of the yolk sac is one of the most commonly encountered abnormalities in neonatal raptors following hatching. Usually, the entire yolk sac retracts within the umbilicus just before hatch.[1] An unretracted yolk can range from a small partial failure of retraction to a yolk sac which completely lays outside the body with a small portion of intestine. For a small, partial failure of retraction, coating the first two fingers and thumb of the dominant hand with sterile iodine while cradling the chick in the other hand, allows for the gentle massaging of the yolk sac through the umbilicus with gentle pressure. A sterile lubricated cotton tip applicator may also aid in this process. Once reduced, a single absorbable suture may be placed across the umbilicus if needed. Often, the natural contraction of the umbilicus renders this unnecessary.

In cases where a larger portion of the yolk sac or all of the yolk sac is unabsorbed, either complete amputation or partial amputation is possible. A sterile ligature may be placed across the yolk sac at the level at which amputation is desired and sterile scissors or radiosurgery used to remove the remainder of the tissue. In cases where intestine is exposed or where a partial unretracted umbilicius cannot be reduced manually, a small incision extending from the umbilicus cranially can be used to aid in reduction, with subsequent closure of the defect. Although manual reduction of a partially unretracted umbilicus can be performed in an awake chick, reduction of the yolk sac surgically should involve appropriate analgesia and anesthesia. Chicks seem to tolerate doses similar to those acceptable for adults; however, the lower end of dosing ranges may be selected as a precaution, especially in younger patients. There is a lack of data available for differences in drug metabolism between juvenile and adult raptors.

Congenital ocular abnormalities have been reported in a variety of raptor species. Microphthalmia was reported in 8 of 16 cases of suspected congenital ocular malformations in Accipitriformes, Falconiformes, and Strigiformes evaluated by Buyukmichi and colleagues.[20] They also found microphakia, congenital cataracts, retinal dysplasia, malformation of the ciliary body, choroid and pecten, and lentoid formation.[20] Colobomas have also been encountered in free-ranging hawks.[21] Abnormalities affecting vision in both eyes can raise concern for flying abilities later in life (**Fig. 5**).

In gyrfalcons (*Falco rusticolus*), and rarely in some hawks, feathering sometimes extends onto the feet. Individuals with one leg a different color than the other or "split" color patterns of dark and light can sometimes also arise. Gyrfalcons are increasingly bred for extreme coloration—very dark or very light patterns. There are no reported abnormalities associated with breeding used to achieve these colors at this time. Polydactyly has been reported in a saker falcon (*Falco cherrug*) and was recently observed in a red-tailed hawk (**Fig. 6**).[22] Occasionally, more severe musculoskeletal abnormalities may arise that are incompatible with long-term survival.[23] These may not always be reported or recorded, and many may only be mentioned anecdotally in literature.[24]

Infectious Etiologies

Omphalitis is a serious concern in raptor chicks. Affected chicks quickly lose vigor and develop discoloration around the umbilicus (**Fig. 7**).[1,25] Signs of sepsis are frequently seen at postmortem examination. Both vertically and horizontally transmitted infections have been reported. Gram-negative bacteria from the environment or food sources may cause mixed infections. The treatment of chicks with omphalitis can be

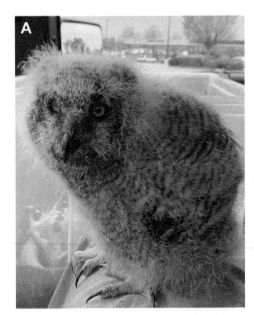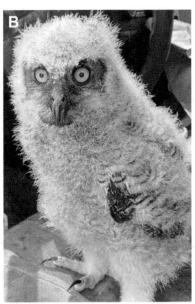

Fig. 5. (*A*) Bilateral congenital microphthalmia in a 17-day-old great-horned owl (*Bubo virginianus*) presented for rehabilitation as a nestling. The owl was found to be blind in both eyes as it developed was euthanized. (*B*) Normal chick of the same age and species for comparison. (*Courtesy of* Tyler Wright, Florence, SC.)

challenging due to poor vascular supply to the yolk sac. Although surgical removal of the yolk sac is recommended in such cases, chicks are generally unstable and frequently succumb to infection.[25] If there are repeated issues with omphalitis and sepsis in young chicks, an attempt must be made to screen parents and food sources to determine the origin of the infection.

Various bacterial infections can arise in young raptors, though there have been outbreaks of disease reported in large breeding facilities (**Table 2**). A common feature in most outbreaks is a suspicion of contaminated food as a source of infection, reinforcing a need for strict hygiene of food sourced to feed captive raptors. Other bacteria can and do cause infections, with Gram-negative bacteria frequently isolated in gastrointestinal and respiratory cases, and bacterial culture and sensitivity are always recommended when possible.[30]

Parasites can cause mortality and morbidity in nestling raptors. Simuliid flies have been reported to cause death of juvenile raptors and nestlings both in the wild and in captivity.[13,31,32] These biting flies can cause direct trauma and anemia in the process of feeding, secondary infections to wounds, and are so irritating that nestlings may fatally jump from the nest before ready to fledge in an attempt to escape. As there can be very large numbers of flies present during an outbreak, it is difficult to reduce fly numbers with treatment of the environment. Temporary movement of affected birds to enclosed barns may help to prevent injury.[13]

Protocalliphora larvae can be present in the ear canals of wild raptor chicks. In small numbers, they likely do not cause any harm and are self-limiting. When larger numbers of larvae are present, anemia, weight loss, and death have been reported in some raptors.[33] They can be treated with manual removal, though nitenpyram applied topically to the ear or administered orally is also effective.

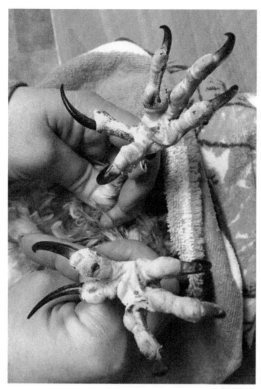

Fig. 6. Wild juvenile red-tailed hawk (*Buteo jamaicensis*) with polydactyly. (*Courtesy of* Dr. Claire Peterson, DVM.)

Coccidia of the genus *Caryospora* may cause significant outbreaks of clinical disease in young raptors in captivity. As they can be transmitted either directly via ingestion of contaminated food and water, or indirectly through consumption of infected prey serving as a paratenic host, it can easily spread.[34] Young raptors are most susceptible, especially during periods of stress. Clinical signs may include weight loss, loss of appetite, regurgitation, depression, diarrhea, hemorrhagic stool, and acute death.[35] Merlins seem to be particularly susceptible to infection.[35] Affected birds generally respond well to treatment with anticoccidial medications such as toltrazuril, clazuril, or amprolium, if treated early enough.

Cryptosporidium, especially *Cryptosporidium baileyi*, has been reported to cause small-scale outbreaks of upper respiratory disease on several falcon farms.[36] Affected birds may display conjunctivitis, tracheitis, and respiratory distress. *Cryptosporidium* may also cause loss of appetite, sneezing, and death in young chicks, presumably due to their relatively underdeveloped immune system.[36] Diagnosis can be challenging, though pale-staining ovoid structures may be seen with modified Wright-Giemsa (Diff-Quick) stains and follow-up biopsy or PCR testing can confirm suspected diagnosis.[36,37] Treatments found to be effective include paromomycin (100 mg/kg PO q12 for 7–12 days) and ponazuril (20 mg/kg PO q24 for 7 days).[36,38] As with many such outbreaks, quail or other birds used to feed the falcons are the presumed source of infection.[36–38]

Trichomoniasis caused by *Trichomonas gallinae* can be encountered in both captive bred and wild juvenile raptors. Called frounce by falconers, it usually presents as

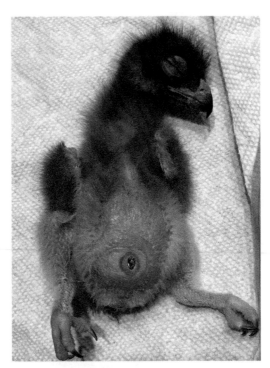

Fig. 7. African hawk eagle (*Aquila spilogaster*) chick displaying typical greenish discoloration around the umbilicus seen with omphalitis. Cultures revealed *E coli* within the yolk sac. (*Courtesy of* Dr Laura Jaworski, Port Jervis, NY).

caseous yellow-white plaques within the oropharynx. Affected birds may experience reduced growth, weight loss, and eventually, respiratory distress because the lesions grow.[26] It is most commonly encountered in raptors consuming pigeons, and shifts in diet in wild raptors to include more feral pigeon may increase frequency in wild nestlings.[39] Diagnosis is easily obtained with a warm saline wet mount, where motile organisms are seen.[3] Carnidazole is preferred for treatment as only a single dose of 100 mg/kg is generally needed, though metronidazole may also be used.[3] Candidiasis caused by the opportunistic yeast *Candida albicans* may also produce nearly identical lesions and clinical signs.[3,26] It is most common in very young raptors, especially following the prolonged use of antibiotics, or issues with food or feeding.[26] Gram staining of swabs from the mouth, esophagus, crop, or stool reveals small ovoid dark budding yeast, which may be treated with nystatin in most cases.[3] It is important to note that rarely *Capillaria* spp may cause oral lesions similar to those seen with trichomoniasis and candidiasis, and on wet mount of an oral swab, eggs of this parasite are seen.[3]

Aspergillus spp may cause respiratory disease in some species of juvenile raptors, especially gyrfalcons and their hybrids, goshawks, red-tailed hawks, rough-legged hawks (*Buteo lagopus*), snowy owls (*Bubo scandiacus*), ospreys (*Pandion haliaetus*), and golden eagles (*Aquila chrysaetos*).[40] In more predisposed species undergoing stress of initial handling or training, prophylactic treatment with itraconazole or terbinafine has been described.[40]

Viral disease outbreaks in captive breeding programs have been reported. Adenoviruses have caused perhaps the greatest mortality among captive Northern aplomado

Table 2
Reports of bacterial outbreaks in captive raptor breeding programs

Species	Bacteria	Clinical Signs	Pathology	Source	Treatment	Outcome
Falco spp.[26]	Ornithobacterium rhinotracheale	Inappetance, respiratory distress in 20%, death in 2/40 affected chicks	Severe acute serofibrinous airsacculitis, visceral pleuritis, hepatic/ splenic necrosis and hepatomegaly	4-week old cockerels	100 mg/kg intramuscularly (IM) long-acting doxycycline (Doxycyclin-SF; Ratiopharm, Ulm, Germany) followed by a second injection 3 d later	Only 1 further chick death; some adults still PCR + 1 year later
Aquila chrysaetos[27]	Pseudomonas aeruginosa	Sudden death, omphalitis in three chicks	Necrosuppurative omphalitis and pneumonia	Contamination of feeding utensils detected, quail presumed origin	Changes in hygiene/ husbandry	
European eagle owl (Bubo bubo), peregrine falcon (Falco peregrinus), buzzard (Buteo buteo), and lanner falcon (Falco biarmicus).[28]	Salmonella havana, S virchow, S livingstone	Late term embryonic and neonatal deaths; lethargy and food refusal; S livingstone acute respiratory signs, torticollis and death	S Havana systemic vasculitis; S virchow fibrinous polyserositis, duodenal abcessation; S livingstone fibrinous polyserositis liver and pericardium and valvular thromboendocarditis	Frozen day old chicks	Two peregrines and one eagle owl treated for S havana with enrofloxacin successfully, initiation of screening food sources	Decline in neonatal death rates in subsequent years, and no Salmonella detected in chicks

(continued on next page)

Table 2
(continued)

Species	Bacteria	Clinical Signs	Pathology	Source	Treatment	Outcome
Lanner falcon (*Falco biarmicus*), Lesser kestrel (*Falco naumanni*), Bonelli's Eagle (*Hieratus fasciatus*), Lappet-faced vulture (*Torgos tracheliotus*)[29]	*Mycoplasma spp* was thought to be primary cause for Lanners; *Salmonella*, *E coli*, *Pseudomonas*, *Staphylococci*, *Chlamydophila psittaci*, and one case of *Aspergillus fumigatus* also detected in other species.	Embryonic and neonatal sudden death	Not included in conference proceedings	Presumed vertical transmission of mycoplasma	Lanner pairs fed mice with 20 m/kg dose enrofloxacin for 7–10 d before breeding	Hatch rate increase from 47% to 70% for lanners

falcons (*Falco femoralis septentrionalis*), Taita falcons (*Falco fasciinucha*), and Mauritius kestrels (*Falco punctatus*).[41–43] Although many affected birds die without any signs, diarrhea and anorexia can be seen in some cases.[41] The mortality rates can be very high—in the aplomado outbreak 72/110 nestlings were affected and 62 died—a mortality rate of 86%.[43] As necrotizing hepatitis and splenitis with intranuclear viral inclusions has been described, collection of these tissues should be performed in suspected cases.[41]

Herpesviruses may cause acute decline and death in raptors and are generally diagnosed on postmortem examination due to challenges in obtaining antemortem samples. In birds who do demonstrate clinical signs, depression, regurgitation, lethargy, and biliverdinuria are seen up to 72 hours before death.[44] In the Middle East, outbreaks in large falcons have occurred and seem to be due to the feeding of pigeons contaminated with Columbid HV-1.[44] The same virus also causes fatal disease in owls.[44,45] Eosinophilic intranuclear inclusion bodies are seen within hepatocytes on histopathology, in contrast to basophilic inclusions generally encountered with adenovirus.[44] There seems to be no effective treatment, and infection is considered 100% fatal.[3,43]

Both West Nile virus and avian influenza may produce acute onset of neurologic signs in raptors. West Nile Virus is primarily transmitted by infected mosquitos and may cause a wide variety of clinical signs ranging from apparently asymptomatic infection to acute death. Torticollis, ataxia, seizures, loss of coordination, blindness, and pinching off of developing feathers may be seen.[46] Bald eagles, Cooper's hawks (*Accipiter cooperii*), and great horned owls (*Bubo virginianus*) seem to be prone to blindness, visual impairment, nystagmus, and abnormal pupillary light responses.[46] Northern goshawks (*Accipiter gentilis*) are prone to developing significant neurologic signs.[46] Juvenile raptors may be more susceptible to infection than adults.[47] Diagnosis can be confirmed via reverse transcriptase polymerase chain reaction (RT-PCR) of oral and/or choanal swabs or blood, or with paired antibody titers.[46] Affected birds may possibly recover with supportive care. Recent and historical outbreaks of avian influenza have caused significant mortality in adult, nestling, and juvenile raptors.[48,49] An acute onset of neurologic signs may be seen, with rapid progression in many cases, though some may recover with supportive care. State regulations may affect disposition of infected birds.[10] Virus isolation or PCR testing can usually be performed at state diagnostic laboratories from choanal or cloacal swabs.[10] In privately owned collections, falconers should be urged to avoid hunting waterfowl during outbreaks, practice strict biosecurity, and sanitize gear regularly.

DEVELOPMENTAL ABNORMALITIES

Neonatal raptors fed diets deficient in calcium or vitamin D3 may develop nutritional hyperparathyroidism, also called metabolic bone disease. Generally, such chicks present with angular limb deformities or folding fractures of the pelvic limbs. However, abnormalities in other bones are possible as well. In severe cases, seizures may also be seen. Early on, chicks may simply seem unable to stand and develop soiling of the feathers around the vent.[50] Although breeders generally take great care to avoid this, inexperienced parent birds may occasionally not feed chicks enough bone. In the United Kingdom, wild common buzzard (*Buteo buteo*) and golden eagle (*A chrysaetos*) chicks have been encountered with rickets due to a presumed shift toward readily available larger prey items which the parent birds found harder to break apart to feed to young chicks.[50] When feeding solely muscle meats, calcium: phosphorus ratios may be 1:17 to 1:44 versus the 1:1 to 2:1 range expected for whole prey diets.[3,50] In mild cases which are caught early, bandaging and calcium supplementation may be sufficient to correct deformities as bones may be quite malleable.[51] In more mature chicks, if limb abnormalities are not severe enough to warrant euthanasia, a de-rotational osteotomy may be performed. In such cases, an external tie-in fixator is generally used.[52]

Chicks housed on slick materials may develop outward splaying of the legs. As in psittacines, this can be corrected with the placement of soft "hobbles" made of tape or bandaging material that prevents the legs from slipping out from under the chick.[25]

Rarely, eyasses may develop a condition similar to "angel wing" in Anseriformes, which is a valgus deformity of the distal wing.[32] The cause of this deformity is not known; however, rapid growth rate may be a cause, as is seen in waterfowl. A low calcium:phosphorus ratio has also been proposed to play a role.[53] The rapid development of the primary feathers may cause hyperextension of the joint with subsequent outward rotation.[25] If not addressed promptly, this can become permanent and require de-rotational osteotomy to correct. Simple taping or bandaging of the wing with a figure-of-eight pattern to hold it in normal anatomic alignment can lead to rapid resolution in less than a week younger raptors, if performed soon after it is noted.[53] Bandages should not be left in place for more than a couple days in a row due to rapid growth rates, and physical therapy is recommended at least once every few days to avoid contracture of the propatagialis longus muscle and subsequent shortening of the propatagium.[53]

It is also possible for the alula to become medially displaced, most commonly in captive-reared falcons (**Fig. 8**).[54] There has not yet been any genetic, nutritional, or husbandry-related cause identified.[54] There are a couple of different surgical methods reported to attempt to reduce the alula into normal anatomic position, though this has mixed success.[53,54] Generally, suture is either passed through the calamus of feathers

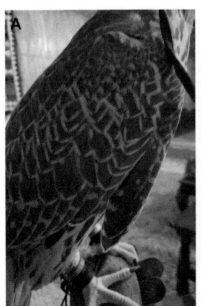 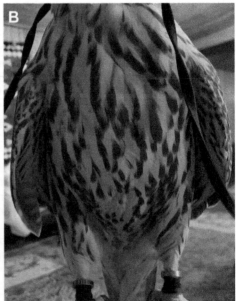

Fig. 8. (A) Medially displaced alula on the right wing in a juvenile captive bred saker falcon (*Falco cherrug*), lateral view. (B) Right wing (at left) demonstrating medially displaced alula. Left wing is normal.

of the alula and the calamus of an adjacent primary feather or suture is passed through the skin of the alula and the skin of the carpus.

Traumatic Injuries

Traumatic injuries in juvenile raptors are most commonly encountered in wildlife rehabilitation, where juveniles frequently fall from the nest and sustain injuries in the process. It is important to consider the incomplete ossification and rapid growth rates of juvenile raptors. Radiographically, very young raptors will seem to have incomplete joints due to a lack of secondary centers of ossification, and cartilaginous epiphyses, especially in the radius, ulna, and humerus (**Fig. 9**A).[55] The distal tibiotarsus and proximal tarsometatarsus have ossification of the tarsal bones, which mimic the appearance of epiphyseal growth plates in mammals.[55]

For surgical fixation of fractures of the long bones, sometimes modified versions of repairs used in adults may be attempted. The soft bones of a very young juvenile may not lend themselves to placement of a full IM pin with tie-in external skeletal fixator (see **Fig. 9**B). Care must be taken to consider that ends of long bones may be cartilaginous only and that pins may not hold in these areas. The placement of only an IM pin and the use of bandaging may be considered in very young chicks. In older chicks, techniques as used for adults are suitable and hatch year birds likely heal better than adults.[56]

In juvenile raptors being trained for falconry, fractures of the proximal one-third of the tibiotarsus are reported to be the most common fracture encountered.[57] It is possible that these fractures are more common in younger raptors due to their being tethered on too long a leash and more frequent and harder bating (jumping and flapping) in newly trained or untrained birds.[57]

Preventative Care

Generally, most captive bred raptors do not require extensive preventative care if breeders are careful in selection of food sources and maintenance of proper hygiene.

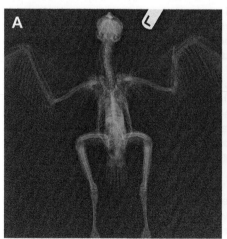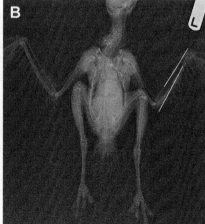

Fig. 9. (*A*) Ventrodorsal (VD) view of juvenile red-shouldered hawk (*Buteo lineatus*) with transverse mid-diaphyseal fractures of the left radius and ulna. The distal portions of many long bones are not yet ossified and therefore are not visible on radiographs. (*B*) Two weeks later, the same hawk has significant ossification of long bones. A single IM pin is present in both the radius and ulna. Pin in the radius is larger than ideal, but was the smallest available at the time of surgery.

A fecal examination consisting of both a direct wet mount and a fecal float is recommended to determine what, if any, parasitic treatment may be needed. A choanal swab collected for Gram stain and direct wet mount helps to evaluate for trichomonas, capillaria, and candida. For wild juveniles, treatment of the feathers with a pyrethrin or permethrin-based spray or powder is strongly recommended for hippoboscid flies, feather lice, and mites.[10] For raptors intended for long-term captivity, vaccination for West Nile Virus may be considered, as though vaccination may only be considered partially protective, in clinical trials in falcons it seems to reduce the severity of signs and shedding.[58] When available, recombinant vaccines may be preferable.[58] Sexing is not generally requested by breeders, as they will either have this testing performed on eggshells just after hatch, or will wait until the juveniles are large enough to determine gender by the markedly smaller size and weight of males of most raptor species. Rarely, in some individuals who are "in between" in weight, that is, large for a male but small for a female, DNA sexing on blood may be requested.

SPECIAL CONSIDERATIONS FOR RELEASE

For raptors raised with the intent to release into the wild, there must be a plan in place to condition them for eventual release. Adult raptors presented for rehabilitation have previously learned to fly, hunt, evade predation, and other health risks presented by humans (eg, electrocution, cars, and windows). Other than conditioning such birds physically, little is needed for successful release. A raptor reared in captivity from a young age is at a significant disadvantage for release, as they have never developed strong flight muscles, are vulnerable to predators, have not been taught hunting techniques by their parents, and lack a "safety net" of a parent to feed them when unsuccessful in initial hunting attempts. Imprinting can also be a serious impediment to release if a plan is not made to prevent it in young eyasses brought in for rehabilitation. Simply fixing medical issues and then rearing a juvenile raptor to fledging and releasing it is not sufficient to ensure its survival post-release. Ideally, wild foster parents would be used for chicks intended for release, however, placement into a wild nest is rarely practical unless a juvenile raptor has fallen from a nest and has been found to be healthy and can immediately be returned to the nest. A technique originally developed for building muscle condition in falconry raptors called "hacking" has been widely used in release of captive-reared aplomado and peregrine falcons in North America with great success, with reports for 10 week survival post-release in peregrines being over 90%.[59,60] This method has also been used by wildlife rehabilitation centers for other species, such as bald eagles.[61] Hacked juveniles are initially fed in a raised box before they are able to fly and are then offered food daily at the "hack site" after they have fledged and until they disperse, leaving the area. They stop coming to the site for food once they are successfully hunting on their own, much as how they would leave their wild parents.

Raptors which are not hacked need to exercise and have their ability to hunt assessed. In some programs, this may mean placement in a large flight cage with live prey offered for them to pursue. During a week or so in this flight cage, they are monitored to ensure that they are eating and are weighed periodically. Before release, they must meet predetermined criteria for weight, muscle mass and hunting success.[10] Some juvenile raptors may also be released following partial training with falconry techniques such as operant conditioning for free flight, which may improve fitness over traditional methods of conditioning for release as raptors can be flown over greater distances than is possible within aviaries.[62] Some juveniles may even be placed with falconers for conditioning and assessment of hunting skills before release.

Ultimately, more research into post-rehabilitation survival of juvenile raptors following methods other than hacking is needed to help guide best practices.

SUMMARY

Neonatal and pediatric raptor patients require special consideration in their medical care in comparison to adults. Long-term success in the management of the young raptor patient requires consideration of both the medical needs of the patient and long-term desired behavioral outcome.

CLINICS CARE POINTS

- Neonatal and young juvenile raptors are altricial and require external heat support and special care in feeding and handling to avoid imprinting.
- Outbreaks of disease in young raptors in a breeding program are often tied to infected food sources, and stringent biosecurity of food sources should be strongly encouraged.
- Fracture management in younger juveniles often requires modification of techniques used in adults due to the presence of growth plates and softer bone.
- Physical conditioning before release is of especial importance in the rehabilitation of very young birds of prey.

ACKNOWLEDGMENTS

The author would like to thank Jennifer and Tom Coulson and David Kanellis for sharing pictures for inclusion within the article. The author would like to thank Dr Laura Jaworski for sharing many pediatric raptor cases with her over the years, from which some of the photos also originate and Dr Claire Peterson also sharing a photo of a unique case of polydactylism. The author would also like to thank the Center for Birds of Prey and Avian Conservation Center for entrusting her to assist with the care of their raptors.

DISCLOSURE

The author has no commercial or financial conflicts of interest and no funding sources to disclose.

REFERENCES

1. Weaver JD, Cade TJ. Falcon propagation: a manual on captive breeding. Boise: The Peregrine Fund; 1983.
2. McClure CJW, Schulwitz SE, Anderson DL. Commentary: Defining raptors and birds of prey. J Rapt Res 2019;53(4):419.
3. Heidenreich M. Birds of prey: medicine and management. Oxford (United Kingdom): Blackwell Science; 1997.
4. Boal CW. A photographic and behavioral guide to aging nestling northern goshawks. Studies Av Biol 1994;16:32–40.
5. Moritsch MQ. Photographic guide for aging nestling ferruginous hawks. Boise, ID: United States Department of the Interior Bureau of Land Management; 1985.
6. Gossett DN, Makela PD. Photographic guide for aging nestling Swainson's hawks. Boise, ID: United States Department of the Interior Bureau of Land Management; 2005.

7. Moritsch MQ. Photographic guide for aging nestling red-tailed hawks. Boise, ID: United States Department of the Interior Bureau of Land Management; 1983.

8. Griggs GR. Guide for aging nestling American kestrels. Boise,ID: United States Department of the Interior Bureau of Land Management; 1993.

9. Nelson RW, Moore D, Kunnas F, et al. Turkey vultures: a photographic guide for aging nestlings. Edmonton (Canada): Alberta Sustainable Resource Development; 2009.

10. Scott DE. Raptor medicine, surgery and rehabilitation. 3rd edition. Boston: CABI; 2021.

11. Doss GA, Mans C. Changes in physiologic parameters and effects of hooding in red-tailed hawks (Buteo jamaicensis) during manual restraint. J Avian Med Surg 2016;30(2):12–132.

12. Huckabee JR. Raptor therapeutics. Vet Clin Exot Anim Pract 2000;3(1):91–116.

13. Coulson J, Coulson T. The Harris' Hawk Revolution. Pearl River (LA); 2012.

14. Schubot RM, Clubb KJ, Clubb SL. Psittacine aviculture: Perspectives, techniques and research. Loxahatchee (FL); 1992.

15. Ensley PK, Rideout BA, Sterner DJ. Radiographic imaging to evaluate chick position in California condor (Gymnogyps californianus) eggs, . Conference of the. Pittsburgh, PA: American Association of Zoo Veterinarians; 1994.

16. Maestrelli JR, Wiemeyer SN. Breeding Bald eagles in captivity. Wilson Bull 1975; 87(1):45–53.

17. Wiemeyer SN. Captive Propagation of bald eagles at Patuxent wildlife research center and introductions into the wild, 1976-80. J Raptor Res 1981;15(3):68–82.

18. Marshall JD, Hager CH, McKee G. The barn owl egg: Weight loss characters, fresh weight prediction and incubation period. J Raptor Res 1986;20(3):108–12.

19. Snelling JC. Artificial incubation of sparrow hawk eggs. J Wild Man 1972;36(4): 1299–304.

20. Buyukmihci NC, Murphy CJ, Schulz T. Developmental Ocular Disease of Raptors. J Wildl Dis 1988;24(2):207–13.

21. Lord FD. An anomalous condition in the eye of some hawks. Auk 1956;73:451–3.

22. Samour J. Observations from the field: five-toed falcon. Exot Dvm 2000;2(1):5.

23. Barreiro A, Fdez De Troconiz P, Vila M, et al. Congenital skeletal abnormalities in a Tawny owl chick. Avian Dis 2003;47(3):774–6.

24. Cooper JE. Veterinary aspects of captive birds of prey. (United Kingdom): Cherington; 1985.

25. Bailey T, Magno MN. Neonatology. In: Samour J, editor. Avian medicine. 3rd Edition. St. Louis (MO): Elsevier; 2016.

26. Hafez HM, Lierz M. Ornithobacterium rhinotracheale in nestling falcons. Avian Dis 2010;54(1):161–3.

27. Rosas AG, Perez JG, Paras A, et al. Diagnostic Investigation of Pseudomonas aeruginosa infection in chicks of Golden Eagle (Aquila chrysaetos), Scarlet Macaw (Ara macao), and Horned Guan (Oreophasis derbianus) in captivity. Proceedings of the Am Assoc of Zoo Veterinarians Conference 2009.

28. Battisti A, Di Guardo G, Umberto A, et al. Embryonic and neonatal mortality from salmonellosis in captive bred raptors. J Wildl Dis 1998;34(1):64–72.

29. Lublin A, Gerchman I, Mechani S, et al. Etiology of pre-hatching mortality of raptors. Proceedings of the Association of Avian Veterinarians 2008.

30. Jones MP. Raptors: pediatrics and behavioral development and disorders. In: Chitty J, Lierz M, editors. Manual of raptors, pigeons and passerine birds. Gloucester (UK): British Small Animal Veterinary Association; 2008. p. 157–75.

31. Smith RN, Cain SL, Anderson SH, et al. Blackfly-induced mortality of nestling red-tailed hawks. The Auk 1998;115(2):368–75.
32. Franke A, Lamarre V, Hedlin E. Rapid nestling mortality in arctic peregrine falcons due to the biting effects of black flies. Arctic 2016;69(3):281–5.
33. Dykstra CR, Hays JL, Simon MM. Protocalliphora (Diptera: Calliphoridae) infestations of nestling red-shouldered hawks in southern Ohio. Wilson J Ornith 2012; 124(4):783–7.
34. Juarez A, Garcia YM, Sauza RP, et al. Prevalence of Caryospora (Apicomplexa: Eimeriidae) oocysts in the environment of a gyrfalcon (Falco rusticolus) breeding center in the United Arab Emirates. J Avian Med Surg 2020;34(2):152–7.
35. Forbes NA, Simpson GN. Caryospora neofalconis: an emerging threat to captive raptors in the United Kingdom. J Avian Med Surg 1997;11(2):110–4.
36. Van Zeeland YRJ, Schoemaker NJ, Kik MJL. Upper respiratory tract Infection caused by Cryptosporidium baileyi in three mixed-bred falcons (Falco rusticolus ×Falco cherrug). Avian Dis 2008;52(2):357–63.
37. Barbon AR, Forbes N. Use of paromomycin in the treatment of a cryptosporidium infection in a gyr falcon (Falco rusticolus) and a hybrid gyr/saker falcon (Falco rusticolus X Falco cherrug). Zurich, Switzerland: Proc. 9th European Association of Avian Veterinarians Conference; 2007. p. 191–7.
38. Van Sant F, Stewart GR. Ponazuril used as a treatment for suspected cryptosporidium infection in 2 hybrid falcons. Milwaukee, Wisconsin: Proc. 30th Association of Avian Veterinarians Conference; 2009.
39. Dudek BM, Kochert MN, Barnes JG, et al. Prevalence and risk factors of trichomonas gallinae and trichomonosis in Golden Eagle (Aquila chrysaetos) nestlings in western North America. J Wildl Dis 2018;54(4):755–64.
40. Arne P, Risco-Castillo V, Jouvion G, et al. Aspergillosis in wild birds. J Fungi 2021; 77(3):241.
41. Van Wettere AJ, Wunschmann A, Latimer KS, et al. Adenovirus infection in Taita falcons (Falco fasciinucha) and hybrid falcons (Falco rusticolus x Falco peregrinus). J Avian Med Surg 2005;19(4):280–5.
42. Schrenzel M, Oaks JL, Rotstein D, et al. Characterization of a new adenovirus species in falcons. J Clin Microbiol 2005;43(7):3402–13.
43. Forbes NA, Simpson GN, Higgins RJ, et al. Adenovirus infection in Mauritius kestrels (Falco punctatus). J Avian Med Surg 1997;11(1):31–3.
44. Raghav R, Samour J. Inclusion body herpesvirus hepatitis in captive falcons in the Middle East: A review of clinical and pathological findings. J Avian Med Surg 2019;33(1):1–6.
45. Rose N, Warren AL, Whiteside D. Columbid Herpesvirus-1 mortality in great horned owls (Bubo virginianus) from Calgary, Alberta. Can Vet J 2012;53(3): 265–8.
46. Vidana B, Busquets N, Napp S, et al. The role of birds of prey in West Nile Virus epidemiology. Vaccines 2020;8(3):550.
47. Smith KA, Campbell GD, Pearl DL. A retrospective summary of raptor mortality in Ontario, Canada (1991-2014), including the effects of West Nile Virus. J Wildl Dis 2018;54(2):261–71.
48. Nemeth NM, Ruder MG, Poulson RL, et al. Bald eagle mortality and nest failure due to clade 2.3.4.4 highly pathogenic H5N1 influenza a virus. Sci Rep 2023; 13:191.
49. Shearn-Boschler V, Knowles S, Ip H. Lethal infection of wild raptors with highly pathogenic avian influenza H5N8 and H5N2 viruses in the USA, 2014-2015. J Wildl Dis 2019;55(1):164–8.

50. Forbes NA, Flint CG. *Raptor nutrition*, . Honeybrook Animal Foods. UK: Evesham; 2000.
51. Kim HJ, Kim KT. A case of rickets in an artificially raised white-tailed eagle (Haliaeetus albicilla) chick at a zoo. J Vet Med Sci 2023;85(5):584-6.
52. Kuzma AB, Hunter B. Osteotomy and derotation of the humerus in a turkey vulture using intramedullary polymethymethacrylate and bone plate fixation. Can Vet J 1989;30.
53. Zsivanovits P, Monks DJ, Forbes NA. Bilateral valgus deformity of the distal wings (angel wing) in a northern goshawk (accipiter gentilis). J Avian Med Surg 2006; 20(1):21-6.
54. Barbon AR, de la Fuente JG, Fischer D. Surgical technique to correct alula malposition in falcons. 11th European Association of Avian Veterinarians Conference and 1st European College of Zoological Medicine Meeting. Madrid (Spain), April 26-30, 2011. p. 105-107.
55. Naldo JL, Samour JH, Bailey TA. Radiographic monitoring of the ossification of long bones in houbara (*Chlamydotis undulata macqueenii*) and Rufous-Crested (*Eupodotis ruficrista*) bustards. J Avian Med Surg 1997;11(1):25-30.
56. Bueno I, Redig PT, Rendahl AK. External skeletal fixator intramedullary pin tie-in for the repair of tibiotarsal fractures in raptors: 37 cases (1995-2011). J Am Vet Med Assoc 2015;247(10):1154-60.
57. Hatt J-M. Hard Tissue Surgery. In: Chitty J, Lierz M, editors. Manual of raptors, pigeons and passerine birds. Gloucester (UK): British Small Animal Veterinary Association; 2008. p. 157-75.
58. Angenvoort J, Fischer D, Fast C, et al. Limited Efficacy of West Nile virus vaccines in large falcons (Falco spp.). Vet Res 2014;45(1):41.
59. Powell LA, Calvert DJ, Barry IM, et al. Post-fledging survival and dispersal of peregrine falcons during a restoration project. J Raptor Res 2002;36(3):176-82.
60. Perez CJ, Zwank PJ, Smith DW. Survival, movements and habitat use of Aplomado falcons released in Southern Texas. J Raptor Res 1996;30(4):175-82.
61. Meyers JM, Miller DL. Post-release activity of captive- and wild-reared bald eagles. J Wild Manag 1992;56(4):44-749.
62. Holz PH, Naisbitt R, Mansell P. Fitness level as a determining factor in the survival of rehabilitated peregrine falcons (Falco peregrinus) and brown goshawks (Accipiter fasciatus) released back into the wild. J Avian Med Surg 2006;20(1): 15-20.

Updates for Reptile Pediatric Medicine

La'Toya V. Latney, DVM, DECZM (Zoo Health Management), DABVP (Reptile/Amphibian), CertAqV

KEYWORDS

- Congenital disorders • Hypovitaminosis A • Hypovitaminosis D • *Salmonella*
- Spider ball python • Reptile pediatric medicine

KEY POINTS

- A 10 hr low UVB irradiance exposure, and a diet of Vitamin A dusted, Vitamin D dusted gut loaded insects, prevented nutritional hyperparathyroidism and fibrous osteodystrophy documented in hatchling veiled chameleons.
- Hatchling bearded dragons provided minimum 2-hour UVB exposure daily are able to maintain serum vitamin D levels that ensure healthy growth. Oral Vitamin D3 supplementation alone, at 3 month or 6 months or age, is ineffective in raising plasma concentrations to the levels seen with UVB-exposed animals.
- Adult female bearded dragons lose the ability to maintain serum calcidiol levels in the absence of UVB exposure at 11 weeks.
- Silkback and Leatherback bearded dragons experience higher evaporative water loss than normal scale phenotypes and lack parietal-eye UVB detection. They also do not display basking behaviors that link elevated UVB exposure to thermoregulatory basking. They bask under high UVB exposure at cold temperatures which is rarely a paired thermoregulatory phenomenon in the wild.
- Spider ball python phenotypes have proven congenital developmental malformations of the stato-acoustic organs, which results in vestibular clinical signs and a lack of spatial orientation.

INTRODUCTION

Pediatrics is the branch of medicine that provides health care to infants, children, adolescent, and young adults. In reptile medicine, this encompasses the health of hatchlings, juveniles, and those that have just reached the biologic hallmark to reproduce. This requires that a practitioner develop knowledge of developmental disorders, common estimations of sexual maturity for several species, seasonal egg laying timelines, clutch size estimations, and knowledge of diseases most likely to affect the life of

Avian and Exotic Medicine & Surgery, The Animal Medical Center, 510 East 62nd Street, New York, NY 10065, USA
E-mail address: latoya.latney@amcny.org

Vet Clin Exot Anim 27 (2024) 379–409
https://doi.org/10.1016/j.cvex.2023.11.013
1094-9194/24/© 2023 Elsevier Inc. All rights reserved.

a hatchling during its continued development into adulthood. "Adulthood" in this case, may not be unequivocally compared to sexual maturity, as several species are bred in captivity before reaching the known age of reproduction commonly noted for their wild counterparts.[1] Perinatology and reproductive disease, while closely connected to pediatric medicine, is beyond the scope of this article; however, robust overviews are available elsewhere.[2,3] This article serves to provide an overview of the most common conditions of neonate, juveniles, and young adults, which include congenital and developmental disorders, trauma and husbandry-related disease, nutritional disorders, and infectious disease.

Congenital Diseases & Developmental Disorders

With the United States and Europe serving as the world's largest consumer markets for reptiles, the demand for hard-to-obtain species and species with unique variations has been a strong driver of captive breeding practices among herptile enthusiasts.[4] Gross congenital aberrations largely arise from environmental causes (**Fig. 1**), whereas discrete aberrations appear to result from recessive autosomal gene manifestations.[5] In the herptile pet industry, intensive breeding practices, environmental variability, and the breeding of genetically aberrant offspring for distinctive color morph and scale patterns, have resulted in "common" congenital and developmental disorders. The consequences of these practices include, but are not limited to, stunted growth, failure to thrive, calvaria malformations, neurologic disease, and integument-alterations that can result in high rates of evaporative water loss[6] and neoplasia.[7] A brief overview of common periods for developmental hallmarks for commonly kept pet species is available in **Table 1**.[8–17]

While reviews of other taxa highlight a low incidence of congenital abnormalities, in herpetofauna, reports of the most commonly affected systems include skeletal, muscular, and central nervous systems.[5] A robust review of the anomalies that arise from rare aberrations during gametogenesis, fertilization, blastogenesis, embryogenesis, or fetogenesis is well described elsewhere.[5] These result in rare cephalic malformations, bicephaly, ocular malformations, and spinal deformities. In clinical practice, practitioners are often faced with developmental disease that (1) arose from deficits in hatchling health, (2) disease that arose due to selective breeding for phenotype

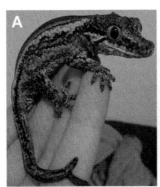 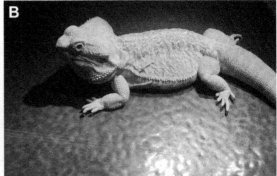

Fig. 1. (*A*) A juvenile female gargoyle gecko (*Rhacodacytulus auriculatus*) with a functional congenital tail abnormality. The pet was named "Lernaea" after the common anchorworm fish parasite which has a similar shape as the pet's tail. (*B*) Congenital brachygnathia in a central bearded dragon (*Pogona vitticeps*). ([A] Photograph courtesy of Colin McDermott, VMD, DABVP (Reptile/Amphibian), CertAqV.)

Table 1
Overview of clutch size, gestation, sexual maturity, size, and longevity for common captive species

Species	Clutch Size, Gestation	Sexual Maturity	Adult Size	Longevity in Captivity (years)	Source
Chelonians					
Red Eared Slider (*Trachemys scripta elegans*)	6–20 (13) eggs, 60–95 ds. Usually 1 clutch per year, can be up to 4. April–October	Male: 2–5 years Female: 5–8 years	10–29 cm SVL Males: 9–11 cm, 0.5–1.5 kg Females: 15–20 cm, 2.5–3.2 kg	30–50	8
West African Mud (*Pelusios castaneus*)	11–18 eggs, 53–59 ds. Nesting occurs during dry season, egg laying occurs Feb–March (northern hemisphere), and July to September (Southern hemisphere) Females clutch twice yearly	Morphologic changes noted for adults: • Loss of narrow median keel • Flattening of carapace • Curved sides on the first vertebral scute • A deep acute angle is noted in the notch between plastron anal scutes	7–11 inches SVL Males: 12.7 ± 2.6 cm Females: 13.5 ± 3.7 cm	30–50	9
Eastern Painted (*Chrysemys picta*)	4–15 eggs, 72–80 ds. Mate once yearly late spring, egg laying early summer	Male: 3–5 years Females: 6–10 years	Males: 7.0–9.5 cm juvenile, 300 g Females: 10.0–13.0 cm plastron length juvenile, 500 g Adults: up to 25.0 cm after reaching sexual maturity	30–40	8
Eastern Box Turtle (*Terrapene carolina Carolina*)	3–8 eggs, 90 ds. Nesting occurs from May through July. A female may lay fertile eggs for up to 4 years after one successful mating	5 years of age, both male and female	11–18 cm	60–100	8

(continued on next page)

Table 1
(continued)

Species	Clutch Size, Gestation	Sexual Maturity	Adult Size	Longevity in Captivity (years)	Source
Chinese Box Turtle (*Cuora flavomarginata*)	2–9 eggs, 68–101 ds. Breeding can occur throughout the year but is most common from November to March, Nesting May through September	Male: 13 years Female: 14 years	12.0–19.0 cm	Unknown, author has treated several 20–30 years old	8
Red-footed tortoise (*Chelonoidis carbonaria*)	2–15 eggs, 117–158 ds. Mating occurs throughout the year but nesting occurs June to September.	5 years, both male and female	Males up to 35 cm in length Females up to 29 cm Weight: up to 9 kg	Up to 50 years	8,10
Russian Tortoise (*Testudo horsfieldii*)	1–4 eggs, 84–126 ds. Breeding occurs from April–May.	8–10 years	Female: 20–25 cm Male: 17–20 cm 400–600g	50–80	11,13
African Spurred-Thighed Tortoise (*Centrochelys sulcata*)	15–30 eggs, up to 8 months Mating September through November, nesting in autumn	5 years	36–50 kg	Up to 54 years	8,13
Leopard Tortoise (*Stigmochelys pardalis*)	5–30 eggs, 9–14 months. Breeding occurs once yearly, May to October.	Males: 5–6 years Females: 5 years	30–70 cm, with an average carapace length of 45 cm 18–54 kg	50–100 years	8,13
Greek Tortoise (*Testudo graeca*)	1–3 clutches of 2–19 eggs annually between May and July	8–10 years	Females: 0.7–2.25 kg, 14.5–21.9 cm Males: 0.420–2.70 kg, 13.5–24.1 cm	50–100 in captivity	12,13

Species	Reproduction	Sexual maturity	Size	Lifespan	References
Hermann's Tortoise (Testudo hermanni)	3 eggs, 80–100 ds Breeding occurs once yearly, at the end of hibernation (late February), with nesting beginning in May and ending in July.	Based on carapacial length Males: > 12 cm Females: > 14 cm	12–23 cm Weight: 2–2.5 kg	40–60 years	8,13
Lacertilia					
Central Bearded Dragon (Pogona vitticeps)	Up to 24 eggs, 55–75 ds. Mating: Sept to March in Australia. Up to 9 clutches per year in captivity, seasonal breeding in the wild	1–2 years, author has seen follicular development in dragons 4–6 months old	33–61 cm	5–15	8
Leopard Gecko (Eublepharis macularius)	2 eggs, 55 ds Up to 6 clutches per year	16–24 months	20—25 cm, 50–80 g	5–20	8
Green Iguana (Iguana iguana)	10–30 eggs, 59–84 (69) d	Male: 3–4 years Female: 3–5 years	1.6–2 m, 4–8 kg	10–20	8
Savannah Monitor (Varanus exanthematicus)	20–50 eggs, 5–6 months	1.5–2 years	2 m, 1–70 kg	10–12	8
Crested Gecko (Rhacodactylus ciliatus)	2 eggs, 90–190 ds	Male:9–12 months Female: 12 months	20 cm, 30–35 g	10–20	8
Common Blue Tongue Skink (Tiliqua scincoides)	10–15 live young, 3–5 month before birth in Dec to April. Clutch: once yearly, some skip a year	18–36 months	30–38 cm, 450–500 g	9–20	13.–15
Serpentes					
Corn snake (Pantherophis guttatus)	10–30 eggs, 60–65 ds	600 ds (19 months)	61–182 cm, 900 g	23–32	8

(continued on next page)

Table 1
(continued)

Species	Clutch Size, Gestation	Sexual Maturity	Adult Size	Longevity in Captivity (years)	Source
California Kingsnake (Lampropeltis zonata)	2–8 eggs, 62 ds Breeding from April through early June, Oviposition occurs in late May to July	2–3 years	Up to 122.5 cm	26 years	8,13
Western Hognose (Heterodon nasicus)	4–20 eggs, 50–65 ds	Male: 12 months, Females: 21 months	Males: 45–60 cm Females: up to 91 cm Weight: 80–350 g	15–20	8
Ball Python (Python regius)	7–11 eggs, 44–54 ds	Male: 16–18 months Female: 27–31 months	0.9–1.3 m	20–30	8
Green Tree Pythons (Morelia viridis)	6–32 eggs, 39–65 ds	Male: 2.4 years Female: 3.6 years	1.5–2.2 m	15–20	8
Boa constrictors (Boa constrictor)	Viviaparous: 10–64 (24) live young, 152–243 ds. Breed every other year, April-August	2–3 years	1–4 m	25–35	8
Burmese pythons (Python molurus)	Oviparous: 100 (4) eggs, 60–90 ds	2–3 years	7.6 m	10–15	8
Blood Pythons (Python brongersmai)	Oviparous: 12–30 eggs, 60–70 ds	2–4 years	Male: 91–152 cm Female: 122–183 inches	20	16,17
Reticulated Pythons (Python reticulatus)	Oviparous: 8–150 (25–50), 60–90 ds	Males: 3–5 years Female: 4 years	1.3–9 m (150 kg average)	15–22	8

variation in color,[6,7,18–20] body size,[21,22] and scale morphology,[23,24] (3) deficits in maternal health, and/or (4) the direct consequences of malnutrition or infectious diseases.

Omphaloceles
During the last stages of post-ovopositional development, embryonic growth and neonate survival are largely dependent on yolk sac resorption. In some cases, failed resorption of the yolk sac from the umbilicus can occur (**Fig. 2**). In rare cases, schistosomus reflexus syndrome can occur when there is a fissure and failure of the coelomic wall to close during development, resulting in the expulsion of abdominal viscera from the defect.[5] This is most commonly reported in chelonians[25] and rarely in snakes.[26]

Failure to thrive
This term is used often to describe neonates that are not growing or those that maintain a negative energy balance due to congenital factors, concurrent disease, and improper environmental conditions during development. It is important to note that not all hatchlings are expected to survive in the wild and each neonate may not have the resources to develop to adulthood.[27] Failure to thrive often results in loss of life prior to the animal reaching 1 year of age (**Fig. 3A**), the causes of which may escape antemortem diagnosis, but that result in an inability to grow due to aberrant metabolism or malnutrition. The term "stunting" often refers to animals that fail to grow to expected adult size, which may also be due to congenital factors, improper environmental conditions during development, nutritional deficiencies, and/or infectious disease co-morbidities. Some can reach developmental milestones, surviving to adulthood with excellent husbandry and supportive care (**Fig. 3B and C**).

DISORDERS ASSOCIATED WITH COLOR AND SCALE PHENOTYPES

Congenital neurologic conditions have been reported in spider color morph scale color pattern in ball pythons (*Python regius*). A survey to breeders and a call for ethical

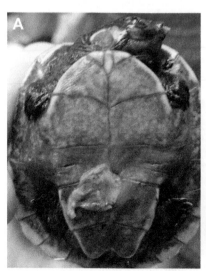
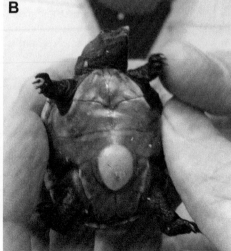

Fig. 2. (*A*) Hatchling Arrau turtle (*Podocnemis expansa*) with delayed yolk sac absorption. (*B*) Hatchling *Podocnemis expansa*, omphalocele. (Photograph courtesy of Colin McDermott, VMD, DABVP (Reptile/Amphibian), CertAqV.)

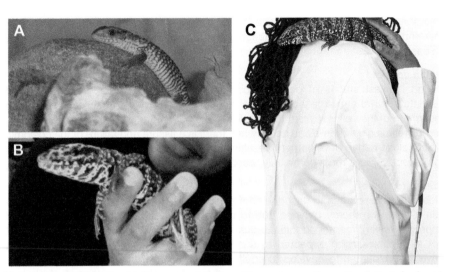

Fig. 3. (*A*) A 6-month-old Savannah monitor (*Varanus exanthematicus*) that had not increased in size for over a year despite normal prey intake and experienced an acute cardiac arrest. Histopathology confirmed the absence of adipose reserves necessary for normal metabolism and growth, noting failure to thrive as the cause of death. (*B*) An unknown age, presumed hatchling Colombian tegu (*Tupinambis teguixin*), photographed here after 1 year of ownership by the author. (*C*) The same Colombian tegu experienced a growth surge after 6 years in captivity and is pictured here after 15.5 years in captivity with the author. Note the tegu is smaller than reported normal sizes by hobbyists and in wild specimens.

breeding sanctions for captive ball pythons was first reported in 2014.[7] Clinicians and breeders alike noted a described "wobbler" syndrome in the spider phenotype of ball pythons, resulting in clinical signs described as side-to-side head tremors, incoordination, erratic corkscrewing of the head and neck, inhibited righting reflex, torticollis, poor muscle tone, and loose grip with the tail (**Fig. 4**).[7] A genetic mutation linked to the color pattern appeared to be the cause, as breeders reported spider ball python offspring that lack the pattern, even those born from severely affected females, do not express wobbler symptoms. A recent magnetic resonance (MR) and computed

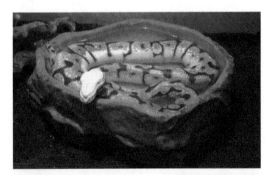

Fig. 4. A reported 6-month-old spider ball python that suffers from vestibular disease. Although the patient thrives with help during feeding to improve strike accuracy, the pet often displays clinical assigns associated with a lack of spatial orientation, as seen here while soaking and resting in a water bowl. (Photograph courtesy of Susan Tyson, MS, VMD.)

tomography (CT) study confirmed that there are no spinal or vertebral canal abnormalities in spider morphs, as compared to wild type phenotypes; however, there are abnormalities in osseous and neural parts of the inner ear.[18] In 5 clinically-affected spider balls, MR and CT imaging revealed that the semicircular canals of the inner ear were asymmetrical and widened, and the diameter of the inner ear compared to width of the telencephalon and medulla and the dimension of the vitreous bodies, were also significantly different when compared to wild type anatomy.[18] In a subsequent study, comparative μ-CT scans revealed that clinically-affected spider ball pythons have neural-crest associated developmental malformations of the stato-acoustic organs, specifically the saccular and the semicircular canals.[19] These confirmed inner ear abnormalities likely result in the manifestation of a loss of spatial orientation caused by vestibular system malfunction.[18]

Another congenital aberration that has led to concerns for welfare is the coveted scale variation phenotype in central bearded dragons (*Pogona vitticeps*). It has been determined that 1 copy of a mutant allele (genotype Sca/sca) results in the leatherback phenotype, that is a bearded dragon that exhibits scales of reduced prominence compared with the wild-type phenotype.[23,28] Two copies of the mutant allele (genotype Sca/Sca) result in a completely scaleless animal, known as a silkie or silkback phenotype.[23,28] To date, there are 2 studies that reveal physiologic consequences of gene patterns that reduce the scale coverage and size in bearded dragons. Sakich and colleagues experimentally demonstrated that on average silkbacks lost water evaporatively at about twice the rate that wild-types dragons and that leatherbacks were closer in their rates of evaporative water loss to silkbacks than they were compared to wild-types.[23] They also report that despite the significant differences in evaporative water loss, there was no significant change in thermal preference suggesting a lack of plasticity in thermal preference in response to an increase in the rate of evaporative water loss.

An additional study by the same team reviewed self-exposure to ultraviolet (UV) irradiation, noting 3 clinically relevant concerns.[24] First, they noted that silkies on average spent less time under high levels of UV irradiation, which may be adaptive due to the reduced scale thickness. Second, bearded dragons housed at cooler temperatures chose higher UV irradiances. The reason for this is unclear, but they postulate that dragons use UV irradiance as a proximate cue for thermoregulation. There is a chance that the photostatic behavior is programmed, as high UV irradiance and high temperatures would be naturally experienced together in the wild. In captivity, this could result in reduced thermoregulatory behaviors that affect overall health, independent of the photoisomerization of pre-vitamin D_3 to cholecalciferol. Lastly, they noted a significant difference in the chosen irradiation for UVA and for combined UVA + UVB, but not for UVB when considered alone without UVA. They suggest whatever mechanism these bearded dragons use to detect their UV light exposure level appears to be sensitive to UVA but not to UVB. These findings all suggest that the reduced scaling of the leatherbacks and silkbacks may alter their photoregulatory behavior due to how much light is detected by their parietal eye and its lens-like structure, the pineal gland, or may result from alterations of the pineal gland-associated genes.[24]

TRAUMA AND HUSBANDRY-RELATED DISEASES
Iatrogenic Trauma

In the last 30 years, several recommendations for improved husbandry and feeding practices have been made available to the public through veterinary resources as textbooks, care guides, and pamphlets provided by major pet store chains. Prey-induced injury remains a common presentation in the author's practice, including insect-induced injury (**Fig. 5**) and often rodent bite-induced injury. In a cross-sectional study that surveyed ball python vendors at the North American Reptile Breeder's Conference in 2018, information regarding breeding practices, pet demographics, finances, husbandry, diet, temperature, humidity, housing, income, and veterinary care practices of hobbyists and breeders was ascertained.[29] The 50-item survey returned 50 responders. When asked if live prey was fed to adults, 42% reported feeding live prey and 2% reported feeding a mix of frozen-thawed and live prey. The size of the aquariums/breeding racks was also noted in this survey of breeders, and despite welfare-guided recommendations for tank sizes that allow adult animals to stretch out at least two-third the length of the body (at least 48 inches), the median length reported in the survey was 40 inches.[29] It becomes very apparent how a live prey item could injure a snake that has little room to escape or retreat. Bites to the face are common and can cause severe osteomyelitis to the jaw bones,[30] However, with prolonged exposure, prey injuries can be more extensive and even fatal (**Fig. 6A**).

In addition to prey-induced trauma in hatchlings and juveniles, it is not uncommon to see conspecific trauma as well. Most reptiles are solitary by nature and may tolerate the presence of other reptiles of the same species for a short period. Neonatal bearded dragons are known to aggregate for thermoregulation when heat and light sources are limited.[31] However, it is not uncommon to see hatchlings participate in cannibalism or sustain digit and partial limb amputations (**Fig. 6B and C**).

NUTRITIONAL DEFICIENCIES
Hypovitaminosis D

Hypovitaminosis D has been historically one of the most reported conditions in captive reptiles and yet we lack studies that outline species-specific requirements for cholecalciferol, tolerance to dietary supplementation of vitamin D_3, dependency on and/or use of photodynamic conversion of 7-dehydrocholesterol, and how these requirements vary for each species based on life stage (ie, growth, reproduction). While excellent overviews of calcium homeostasis in reptiles are detailed in several articles,[32–34] reviews of studies that discover species-specific requirements and examine patient-driven behavioral and dietary choices in response to deficiencies are limited.[35] Much of the work published in reptile nutrition outline minimal dietary requirements for common captive species,[36,37] how to optimize the nutritive profile of insect prey,[38–42] and determine optimal UVB exposure parameters to improve calcium absorption and vitamin D_3 synthesis[43] to thwart the occurrence of nutritional hyperparathyroidism and subsequent conditions, including severe osteopenia, fibrous osteodystrophy,

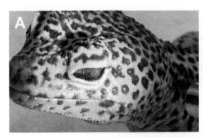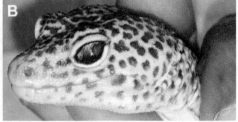

Fig. 5. (*A*) A 7- month-old male leopard gecko that sustained OS corneal injury caused by a superworm (*Zoophobas morio*) during mastication. (*B*) The same patient 3 weeks later with conservative treatment course of saline ophthalmic drops, systemic anti-inflammatory (oral meloxicam), and antibiotic (oral enrofloxacin) therapy.

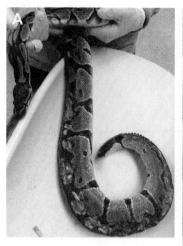
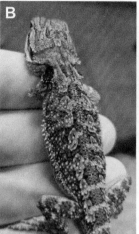
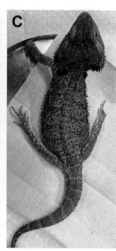

Fig. 6. (*A*) An 8-month-old ball python (*Python regius)* traumatized by a live small rat left unattended in the cage during a feeding attempt. (*B*) Traumatic amputation of the left forelimb sustained by being caged with another subadult bearded dragon. (*C*) A subadult bearded dragon that underwent traumatic digit and limb amputations as a hatchling when housed with several dragons in a single tank. Note the proprioceptive deficit of the left forelimb.

mandibular jaw shortening, pathologic fractures, tetany, gastrointestinal stasis, and cloacal prolapses (**Figs. 7–9**).

Variations in Response to Ultraviolet Irradiance

It has been shown that diurnal reptiles produce cholecalciferol at different exposure times when compared to crepuscular and nocturnal reptiles. Each species' mechanism for cholecalciferol production differs based on their ecology. When comparing 2 species of Jamaican anoles, the shade-dwelling species (*Anolis lineatopus merope*) had a higher rate of photoconversion than the basking species (*A. sagrei*), while simultaneously consuming less dietary vitamin D.[44] UVB-exposed crepuscular house geckos (*Hemidactylus turcicus*) convert UVB radiation to increased serum vitamin D$_3$ levels more effectively as compared to the diurnal spiny tailed lizard (*Sceloporus olivaceus*).[45] While there is evidence that diurnal snakes, such as cornsnakes (*Pantherophis guttatus*),[46] ball pythons,[47] and Burmese pythons (*Python bivittatus*), can produce cholecalciferol after UVB exposure,[48] its clinical importance for captive species remains debated as cross-sectional studies that concurrently evaluate bone density assessment, all Vitamin D metabolites (25-hydroxycholecalciferol or calcidiol, dihydroxycholecalciferol or calcitriol) and parathyroid hormone (PTH) concentrations are unavailable. In 1 study evaluating the biochemical and electrolyte differences in captive indoor-housed and outdoor-housed indigo snakes (*Drymarchon couperi*) within their native range in Florida, all male and female snakes housed outdoors predictably produced higher calcidiol levels than their indoor counterparts and decreases were also noted in ionized calcium, phosphorus, and total calcium in the indoor groups for both males and females.[49] Indigo snakes, wild and captive, have historically been reported to have higher serum calcium and phosphorus levels relative to other squamates and chelonians.[49,50] As North America's largest diurnal and partially fossorial snake, it is interesting to note this biochemistry variation when evaluating their natural

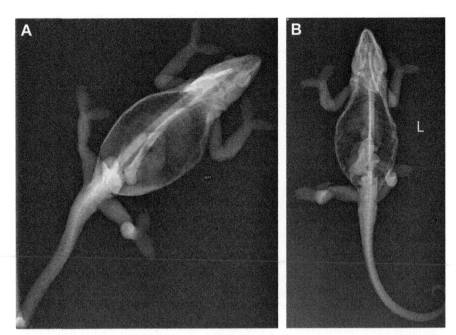

Fig. 7. (*A*) Radiograph of a 6-month-old, veiled chameleon (*Chamaeleo calyptratus*) with severe gastric distension, osteopenia, and a malunion folding fracture of the right femur. This pet suffered from severe hyovitaminosis D and nutritional hyperparathyroidism. (*B*) Radiograph of the same chameleon 2 years later with persistent osteopenia despite normal serum calcium levels and UVB therapy, as fibrous tissue has replaced the osteoid matrix, preventing cortical calcium replacement after being subjected to see hypovitaminosis D and subsequent hypocalcemia as a juvenile. Slight improvements in cortical bone density can be appreciated in the coccygeal vertebrae and skull; however, osteopenia of the long bones persists.

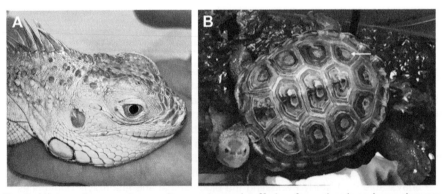

Fig. 8. (*A*) Juvenile green iguana (*Iguana iguana*) suffering from class long bone changes associated with nutritional hyperparathyroidism. Note the shortened mandible length which occurs due to demineralization and fibrous replacement of the osteoid, resulting in a pliable mandible or "rubber jaw." (*B*) A hatchling diamond back terrapin (*Malaclemys terrapin*), confiscated from the wild and retained in a captive environment without UVB supplementation or dietary calcium supplementation for 6 months. The carapace and plastron were compressible on palpation due to prolonged hypocalcemia and secondary fibrous osteodystrophy. Note the concavity of the embryonic scutes on the carapace (*white arrow*). (Photograph courtesy of John Mastrobuono, VMD.)

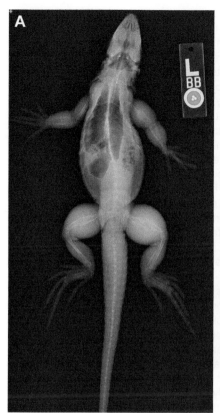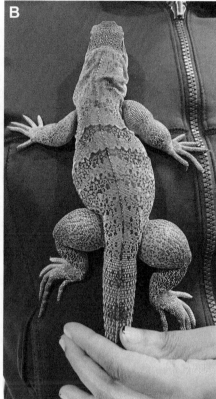

Fig. 9. (*A*) Radiograph of a 2-year-old *Ctenosaura similis*, revealing signs of fibrous osteodystrophy. In this chronic case, note the polyostotic lesions seen as periosteal reactions of the left humerus, right, and left femurs. Exuberant fibrocartilaginous deposition along the periosteal surfaces can lead to progressive pressure atrophy of the surrounding muscles and the (*B*) pseudo hypertrophy appearance of the limbs observed grossly. This is the result of chronic hypocalcemia as a hatchling and juvenile.

diet, which often includes hatchling and juvenile terrapins, tortoises, even small alligators, all vertebrates with modified skin that contains dermal bone.

While diet likely plays a significant role in reported variations in serum calcidiol levels of captive snakes, current evidence suggests that snakes have biologically retained the ability to produce cholecalciferol and to modulate calcidiol and other vitamin D metabolites. This reserved photodynamic function appears to be true for those of the closely related Varanidae family. As carnivorous hunters that consume large vertebrate prey, they also produce cholecalciferol when exposed to artificial UVB light.[51,52] Lack of oral supplementation and UVB exposure can result in chondroid metaplasia and fibrous osteodystrophy if nutritional needs are unmet.[53]

Vitamin D_3 supplementation has remained somewhat controversial given that iatrogenic vitamin D_3 toxicity has been reported.[54,55] The decision to provide oral supplementation is governed by several factors, including health status (eg, growth, reproductive status, clinical presumption of deprivation, etc.), UVB exposure and intensity, normal dietary exposure to vitamin D_3, and vitamin D_3 dose recommendations.

In veiled chameleons, the enteric vitamin D_3 steroid receptor (VDR) and cytosolic calcium-binding protein, calbindin D28k (Cb-D28k), have been found to have increased immunohistochemical expression in the duodenum of hatchlings supplemented with oral calcium, vitamin A, and oral vitamin D_3 as compared to those provided UVB exposure alone.[56] This suggests a genetically inducible mechanism to improve oral absorption of vitamin D_3 may be present in some omnivorous, insectivorous, or carnivorous squamates, especially during the early life phase of growth.

Studies in panther chameleons reveal that increases in self-basking behavior were associated with appropriate levels of serum vitamin D_3 levels to compensate for decreased oral vitamin D_3 supplementation.[57] Alternatively, in another study in the same species, the same author found that reproductively active female panther chameleons had an increased mortality when fed a diet high in vitamin D (9.1 IU/g cholecalciferol).[58] A deprivation study performed in juvenile black-throated monitor lizards (*Varanus albigularis*) revealed that, after 87 days of not having oral or UVB-induced vitamin D_3 sources, UVB exposure for 20 minutes daily failed to restore normal serum vitamin D_3 levels. Oral administration of vitamin D_3 (10,000 IU/kg) once weekly for 92 days did stop the decline of and caused a 600% increase in serum vitamin D_3 levels as compared to pre-deprivation levels. However, this dose is too high for maintenance and could cause toxicity.[55]

In those black-throat monitor lizards, it is of note that the duration and source of UVB exposure only allowed for a 14.2% conversion of provitamin D_3 to pre-vitamin D_3. In another study evaluating serum calcidiol levels and behavior changes when comparing a female and a male captive Komodo dragons (*V. komodoensis*) shifted from indoor to outdoor exhibits, a 98% increase in serum vitamin D_3 levels was noted in the female when moved outdoors and an increase in locomotion behavior was noted in the male when moved outdoors.[59] Interestingly, when the UVB bulbs were tested, the authors found that the bulbs only produced the desired UV irradiance for 3.5 months. While these studies conclude that UVB-exposure timelines and source are important, they also conclude that UVB irradiance should be monitored routinely, as even current hobbyist-based recommendations of replacing UVB-producing bulbs every 6 months may be inaccurate.

Although UVB-associated hypervitaminosis D_3 has not been documented, UV lamps that produced too high of an output have been shown to cause basal cell generation, epidermal necrosis, and keratoconjunctivitis in a captive ball python and a blue-tongue skink.[60] It has been found that nocturnal leopard geckos (*Eublepharis macularius*) use UVB light for vitamin D_3 synthesis[61] and that short duration of 2 hours daily (1 hour in the morning, 1 hour in the evening) may be best for captive pets using a UVB irradiance of 12 to 2L watts/cm^2 with hides provided.[62] Behavioral enrichment studies have shown that this species specifically prefers warm shaded areas to prolonged open-space exposure, which mirrors its wild behavioral ecology as a desert gecko exposed to severe heat extremes and predation risk in their native regions.[63] The use of the hide becomes incredibly important, as the aforementioned UVB study revealed no significant difference in "time under the hide" between the UVB exposure and control groups, suggesting selective dermal absorption of UVB in short time frames. A prior study in captive geckos that did not provide hides yet tested UVB exposure, resulted in increased ecdysis and presumed skin damage.[64]

Given the variations in biologic need, vitamin D source among many reptiles, and the real clinical concern for oral dose toxicity, the inherent need to develop UVB exposure guidelines for captive species becomes imperative, as no report of hypervitaminosis D_3 secondary to UVB exposure has been published. Of the reports available, variable responses to artificial light supplementation and natural light supplementation and patient-selective oral vitamin D_3 supplementation have been documented for several captive species, highlighting the need for species-specific studies that consider confounders such as native versus non-native geographic location for natural light exposure, life stage, calcium and vitamin D_3 requirements, and evaluation of adaptive or inducible enteric mechanisms of vitamin D_3 oral absorption.

Studies in captive veiled chameleons,[56,65] captive panther chameleons,[57] and captive bearded dragons[66–68] have demonstrated behavioral UVB basking preferences to increase serum levels of vitamin D_3. **Table 2** summarizes studies aimed at providing supplementation recommendations for neonates, hatchlings, and reproductive females.

UVB supplementation in chelonian species has been well studied, yet comparative studies that evaluate natural versus artificial UVB light in hatchlings and young adults are scarce, with reports for Hermann's tortoises (*Testudo hermanni*),[69,70] Blanding's turtles (*Emydoidea blandingii*),[71] and red-eared sliders (*Trachemys scripta elegans*)[72] available and summarized in **Table 2**. In Hermann's tortoises, 3 to 8-year-old young adults exposed to mercury-vapor and fluorescent lamps had significantly lower cholecalciferol levels by Day 35 when compared to a group that experienced natural light exposure in their native geographic range. In the same species, a bone density study was explored comparing normal native diet with UVB exposure versus commercial vegetable diet with native UVB exposure.[69] In 10-month-old hatchling Hermann's tortoises fed a native diet of dandelions (*Taraxacum officinale*), clover (*Trifolium* spp.), mallow (*Malva* spp.), ribwort plantain (*Plantago lanceolata*), wood sorrels (*Oxalis* spp.), and creeping cinquefoil (*Potentilla reptans*), under natural UVB exposure, normal bone density was reported. In a cohort fed natural diet but housed indoors with artificial UVB exposure, the highest incidence of pyramiding was noted in this group with increased bone density. The cohort housed indoors with artificial UVB and fed commercial produce, including 50% chicory (*Cichorium intybus*), 35% red radish (*Cichorium intybus* var *foliosum*), 7.5% endive (*Cichorium endivia* var *crispum*), and 7.5% escarole (*Cichorium endivia* var *latifolium*), had the greatest body weights, yet decreased occurrence of pyramiding (20%) as compared to the indoor, normal diet group. The cohort fed a natural diet and housed outdoors for natural UVB exposure in their native range had no increases in bone density assessment and pyramiding was absent. While this study may suggest a produce-based diet may improve oral calcium levels when a non-native diet is unavailable, calcium utilization in hatchlings appears heavily influenced by appropriate levels of UVB irradiation and pyramiding can result even when intaking a native diet.[69]

Insect Prey Feeding Practices and Supplementation

Invertebrate nutrient composition has been formally studied for more than 60 years and excellent reviews are available that provide baseline nutrient content and offer ways to supplement insects to improve critical nutrient consumption for captive insectivores.[40–42,73] Resources that examine evidence-based feeding practices for juvenile and young adult insectivorous reptiles are scarce. In a recent study evaluating the feeding practices of bearded dragons amongst pet owners, approximately one-half (55.3%) of the respondents reported feeding too many larval and adult insects and approximately one-half (47.4%) of the respondents reported not feeding enough leafy greens.[74] Of 327 respondents, 92.4% reported providing UVB for the bearded dragons, 70.6% gut-loaded their insect prey, 20% calcium-dusted their insect prey, and 68% dusted with calcium plus vitamin D_3 powder. Interestingly, this aticle cites vitamin D_3 disparities in captive insects and notes that wild insects have higher vitamin D_3 content. UVB exposure has been shown to increase vitamin D_3 levels in

Table 2
UVB irradiance, natural UVB light exposure, and oral vitamin D studies in hatchling, juvenile, and young adult reptiles

Species (Study Design)	UVB Exposure (Artificial, Natural, Absence of UVB)	Comparisons of Artificial UV Source to Oral Supplementation	Reference
Bearded Dragon (*Pogona vitticeps*)			
n = 25 captive juvenile dragons studied for 11 weeks, different artificial UVB sources and natural light	• Highest serum levels were noted in dragons exposed to compact fluorescent lighting, when compared to mercury vapor, hard quartz fluorescent, and incandescent and natural light (geographic location was the state of Virginia in the United States). • All dragons had osteodystrophic changes on bone histopathology		67
n = 22 captive female dragons previously afforded artificial UVB		• After 11 weeks of not receiving UVB exposure, females were able to maintain serum vitamin D metabolites for 83 ds; however, total calcium, ionized calcium, and phosphorus declined over time within reference range	68
n = 84 hatchlings, studied with UVB and oral vitamin D supplementation, serum levels measured at 3 months and 6 months of age		• At 3 months old, oral vitamin D supplementation (35 IU/M) did not increase serum levels. Animals not exposed to UVB light selected feed items richer in vitamin D. • At 6 months old, 2 hours of UVB exposure enabled adequate physiologic concentrations of plasma vitamin D metabolites to be maintained in growing bearded dragons. • Oral supplementation is ineffective in raising plasma concentrations of vitamin D3 to the levels seen with UVB -exposed animals	69

n = 15 captive-bred, subadult, male bearded dragons, feed crickets, salad and pinkies. Provided 2-hour daily exposure to LED-UVB producing bulb, fluorescent-UVB producing bulb, or incandescent-no UVB activity bulb for 11 months.	• Plasma concentration for 25-OHD3 in the LED group was greater than for the UVB group • Decreases in serum iCa was noted for LED and UVB groups over time • Decreases in serum Total Ca was noted in the UVB group over time • Decreases in serum Vitamin D3 was noted in LED and non UVB groups over time	43

Veiled Chameleon (Chamaeleo calyptratus)

n = 56 hatchlings, divided into 6 groups, stratified by calcium, UVB, cholecalciferol, and Vitamin A supplementation for 6 months	• Best prevention for nutritional hyperparathyroidism = 12% calcium gut-loaded locusts (48 h), Vitamin A dusted (75 mg/kg), Vitamin D dusted (0.625 mg/kg) with 10 hour/day low irradiation UVB exposure (3–120 μW/cm2)	65
n = 56 hatchlings, divided into 6 groups, stratified by calcium, UVB, cholecalciferol, and Vitamin A supplementation for 6 months	• Vitamin D steroid hormone receptor (VDr) and cytosolic calcium-binding protein (C-albindin D28k (Cb-D28k) immunohistochemical reactions were found in the duodenum. • Cb-D28k IHC immunoreactions were higher in hatchlings that received Ca, vitamin A, and oral vitamin D supplemented hatchlings as compared to UVB treated only group. • There was a tendency to increased VDR immunoreactions when animals were not supplemented (groups UV and None); however, VDR induction was not able to cover the deficiency in these 2 groups where most of the individuals developed nutritional hyperparathyroidism and associated osteopathic disease	56

(continued on next page)

Table 2
(continued)

Species (Study Design)	UVB Exposure (Artificial, Natural, Absence of UVB)	Comparisons of Artificial UV Source to Oral Supplementation	Reference
Panther Chameleon (*Furcifer pardalis*)			
n = 26 juvenile females		• When dietary intake of cholecalciferol was low (1–3 IU/g), they exposed themselves to significantly more UV-producing light. • When intake was high (9–129 IU/g), they exposed themselves to less UV- producing light.	57
Hermann's Tortoise (*Testudo hermanni*)			
n = 18, age 3–8, previously hibernated outdoors. Stratified groups by mercury vapor, UVB exposure, compact fluorescent UVB exposure, and natural lighting outdoors (geographic range: native European country)	Cholecalciferol levels were significantly lower by Day 35 for mercury-vapor and fluorescent lamps exposed turtles when compared to natural light exposure in their native geographic range		69
n = 26, 1 month old hatchlings	Higher bone mineral density of captive-raised tortoises was morphologically associated with a higher incidence of pyramidal growth in captive-raised groups.		70
Blanding's Turtles (*Emydoidea blandingii*)			
n = 16 hatchling Blanding's turtles. Eighthatchlings were afforded UVB 23-W fluorescent bulbs 12 h/day for 6 months	25-OHD3 concentrations being 5.5 times higher in the UVB group than in the controls		71
Red Readed Sliders (*Trachemys scripta elegans*)			
n = 12 yearling red eared sliders, stratified in groups of UVB versus no UVB supplementation under captive conditions for 30 ds. All turtles were previously housed outdoors for and removed during aestivation, allowed 7 ds to acclimate to captive conditions prior to study onset.	25-OHD3 concentrations differed significantly between turtles provided supplemental UV radiation (71.7 ± 46.9 nmol/L) as compared to those not provided UV radiation (31.4 ± 13.2 nmol/L)		72

invertebrate prey.[75] In addition to using critically-evaluated gut-loading diets,[40–42,73] this may be a simple, employable practice recommendation for pet owners to improve vitamin D_3 concentrations in invertebrate prey.

While several insect prey items have become more readily available at retail pet stores, helpful food labels that overview their nutrient content are not available. In general, the author reminds consumers of the following to guide their choices. First, all larvae that are designed to pupate into beetles and/or moths are usually high in fat and protein content. The larval and nymph forms of beetles and roaches contain more fat than their adult counterparts. Second, insects such as migratory locusts (*Locusta migratoria*), silkworms (*Bombyx mori*), flies, and earthworms (*Lumbricus terrestris*) appear to have a leaner protein content and can be more vitamin dense based on natural retinol levels or natural calcium levels (eg, solider fly larvae). Third, digestion of "healthy" bugs can be variable among species. Black soldier fly larvae (*Hermetia illucens*), naturally high in calcium content, have been shown to be expelled undigested in the feces of mountain chicken frogs (*Leptodactylus fallux*)[37] and calcium absorption from the dense exoskeleton or cuticle was limited in leopard geckos[76] after consumption. Mastication or maceration of this larval species still did not improve calcium bioavailability during digestion; however, gut-loading the insect did significantly improve calcium absorption. Lastly, the practice of feeding a valid nutrient-dense diet to prey at least 24 hours prior to consumption, can radically alter the nutrient profile of the prey to improve the overall nutrition of the insectivore.[40–42,73,76]

Hypovitaminosis A

Hypovitaminosis A has been historically reported in captive reptiles.[37] In a retrospective study of leopard geckos that examined diagnosis and treatment of ophthalmic disease, 46% of 112 geckos had ophthalmic disease and hypovitaminosis A was identified as an important risk factor.[77] Subsequently, reports of oral vitamin A supplementation have been explored in this species. In a black soldier fly larvae fed a Vitamin A-loaded diet (20,000 ug/kg dry matter basis to result in a larval concentration of 1000 ug/kg), leopard geckos that ingested these supplemented larvae had improved hepatic vitamin A levels based on biopsy.[41] In a comparison study evaluating beta-carotene assimilation, leopard geckos that received 0.1 mL of carrot juice per 50 g of body weight administered orally once weekly, developed higher hepatic vitamin A concentrations, than those geckos supplemented with 0.1 mL of cod liver oil per 50 g of body weight orally once weekly after 10 weeks. This study not only offers a practical supplementation reference, it also demonstrates that this species, as an obligate insectivore, can convert dietary beta-carotene into vitamin A.[78]

INFECTIOUS DISEASES

There are a number of infectious diseases that threaten the health of neonates, juvenile, and young adult reptiles. In herpetofauna, a large number of emerging infectious diseases have been reported in the last 10 years, requiring revisions of previous references due to host-shifts and novel disease presentations that have jarred microbiologists, parasitologists, mycologists, and virologists alike. Detailed overviews of emerging diseases are available in 2 Veterinary Clinics of North America, Exotic Animal Practice (VCNA) reviews.[79,80] Due to the reptile pet trade and near dissolution of geographic barriers for native and international diseases, the author recommends that clinicians pay attention to reports of foreign disease phenomena in *captive* and *wild* reptiles. Global has become local, and pathologists in our field identify new threats to captive and local wildlife species, daily. **Table 3** highlights diseases of

Table 3
Critical infectious diseases in juvenile and young adult reptiles[80–84]

		Species Affected	Disease Hallmarks, Diagnosis	Treatment	Biosecurity
Viruses	Adenovirus	*Chelonian variants:* Siadenovirus (Sulawesia Adv1), BxAdv1 (Box Turtle) *Lizard Variants:* Agamid Adenoviruses (AgAdv1, AgAdv2), Gecko, Chameleon and Skink adenoviruses (EuAdV1, GeAdV-1, ScAdV-1, ChAdv-1) Helodermatid strains (HeAdV1, HeAdV2) Varanid AdV1 Anolis Adv1 *Snake Variants:* SnAdv 1, SnAdv 2, SnAdv3	*All Species:* Weight loss, anorexia and diarrhea secondary to hepatic necrosis. CNS signs include circling, abrupt paresis, and opisthotonos Vasculitis, Coelomitis *Diagnostics:* PCR of feces, TEM	Supportive Care, including fluid therapy, warm water soaks, systemic and topical antibiotics, and nutritional support	Environmentally stable. Remove organic debris with soap and water followed by use of a 10% bleach solution on cages and hard surfaces, allowing for a 10-min contact time. Quarantine new dragons, snakes, and tortoises upon entry into new collections and submit feces for PCR and/or TEM.
	Iridovirus	*Chelonians:* Frog Virus 3 (FV3) – Ranavirus *Lizards:* FV3, Invertebrate Iridovirus *Snakes:* Erythrocytic virus	*Chelonians:* severe conjunctivitis, palpebral edema, ocular and nasal discharge, oral plaques and abscessation, and severe subcutaneous edema of the neck *Diagnostics:* qPCR can be performed on oral swab, blood, and even on bone for autolyzed samples postmortem	Supportive, including fluid therapy, warm water soaks, systemic and topical antibiotics, nutritional support, Vitamin A and D3 supplementation, and potential anti-viral therapy	Quarantine sick testudines from other turtles and from amphibian collections. Chlorhexidine (0.75%), sodium hypochlorite (3.0%), and Virkon S (1.0%) inactivate ranaviruses after 1 min of exposure

		Species/Strains	Clinical Signs	Treatment	Prevention
	Arenavirus	*Snakes:* Inclusion Body Virus (UGV1–3) (ICTV) common in US, GoGV, (ROUTV and UHV), (CASV), (TSMV-2)	*Clinical Signs:* Pythons-opisthotonus, loss of righting reflex, head tilt, disequilibrium, incoordination, and sudden death. Boas can be asymptomatic and survive for years. *Diagnostics:* RT-PCR can be performed on esophageal swabs, liver biopsy, ELISA peripheral blood sample	Pythons: none Boas: quarantine, supportive care	Do not breed positive animals Control positive arthropod vectors
	Serpentovirus (Nidovirus)	*Chelonians:* Bellinger River snapping turtle (Myuchelys georgesi) *Lizards:* Veiled Chameleons, shingle back lizards (Tiliqua rugosa) *Snakes:* Captive boids, colubrids	*Clinical Signs:* increased oral mucous secretion, oral mucosal reddening, dyspnea, anorexia, and weight loss Lesions: Severe proliferative pneumonia, stomatitis, tracheitis, esophagitis Dx: RT-PCR oral/choanal swabs	Supportive care	Quarantine, complete with separate caretakers, equipment, food, and bedding. Accelerated hydrogen peroxide, Simple Green, or F10
Parasites	*Cryptosporidium*	*Chelonians:* C. ducismarci, & a separate novel Genus-partially characterized *Lizards & Snakes:* C. serpentis, C. varanii, C. baileyi, several unidentified strains	*Clinical Signs* *Chelonians:* chronic diarrhea, decreased appetite, pica, decreased growth rate, weight loss, lethargy, and passing undigested feed *Squamates:* strains are organ specific. C.serpentis causes a hypertrophic gastritis, gastric mucosa, causing a mid-body swelling, regurgitation and chronic wasting. C.varanii causes	*Hermann's Tortoises:* Paromomycin, 100 mg/kg PO q24 h for 7 ds, eliminated clinical signs and led to negative test results for 9 months *Bearded dragons:* Treatments of 100 mg/kg PO q24 h for 7 ds then 360 mg/kg PO q48 h for 10 ds revealed an absence of intestinal cryptosporidium on histopathology	Cryptosporidium are resistant to most disinfectants and survive well in the environment for many months Disinfection can be achieved with steam-treatment, formalin (10%), glutaraldehyde (2.65%), and possibly 5% to 10% ammonia solution may be effective on clean, smooth, impermeable surfaces

(continued on next page)

Table 3
(continued)

	Species Affected	Disease Hallmarks, Diagnosis	Treatment	Biosecurity
		intestinal inflammation and chronic wasting. *Diagnostics:* PCR of gastric washes or feces. Coccidia stain acid-fast	*King Cobra (Ophiophagus Hannah):* 360 mg/kg PO twice weekly for 6 weeks	13 min with 6% hydrogen peroxide for good reduction of infectivity, with excellent decontamination expected for 10% hydrogen peroxide after 2 hours
Intranuclear Coccidiosis	*Chelonians:* Reported in several tortoise species, box turtles in Germany, the United States.	*Clinical Signs:* mild chronic conjunctival or nasal erythema or discharge, severe gasping, subcutaneous edema, ulceration of the cloacal mucosa. Additional signs can include anorexia, lethargy, lack of normal diurnal behavior patterns, increased respiratory effort, mouth breathing, rapid weight gain or loss. *Diagnostics:* qPCR swabs from the conjunctiva, oral and choanal mucosa, and cloaca. Wright Giemsa stains of nasal discharge	Attempts with Ponazuril and Tonazuril are anecdotally reported. Chronic infection, even after treatment response in lowering qPCR, recrudescence is common months later	in general, coccidian oocysts are highly stable in the environment. I would preferentially remove soil, or do a prolonged high-temperature burn. Studies in other unsporulated Eimeria species recommend ammonium hydroxide, 5% and 10%, and phenol 10%

Fungal Disease	Onygenales	*Chelonians: Emydomyces testavorans* *Lizards: Nannizziopsis guarroi, N. chlamydospora, N. draconii, N. barbata, N. dermatitidis, Nannizziopsis crocodili P. australasiensis* *Snakes: Ophidiomyces ophiodiicola, P. tardicrescens, Paranannizziopsis crustacea, P. californiensis, P. longispora, P. californiensi*	*Lesions:* Epithelial inclusion cysts, defined as cystic structures within the dermis lined by keratinized stratified squamous epithelium and containing necrotic bone and keratin debris. Ulcerative shell and skin lesions of freshwater aquatic chelonians *Diagnostics:* Fungal PCR, avoid temperature extremes, heat may degrade DNA	Voriconazole at 10 mg/kg PO q24 h has been shown to be better tolerated in bearded dragons. Terbinafine 5 mg/kg terbinafine PO every 24 h has been shown to help in refractory cases. Itraconazole can cause high mortality in dragons. Terbinafine nebulizations have been shown to achieve effective serum levels in cottonmouth snakes. Intraconazole (Oral: 10 mg/kg q24 every 7 ds for 3 weeks) and eniconazole (Topical: 2 mg/mL every 4 ds for 1 month) have been used with success in treating Bocourt's water snakes and a Pueblan Milk Snake	3% and 10% Bleach, Benzalkonium chloride 0.16%, 70 & ethanol (Contact time 2, 5, 10 mins) Lysol power bathroom cleaner, Lysol all-purpose cleaner, CLR, 409, NPD quaternary ammonium 0.4%, 70% Ethanol (Contact 10 mins) Nolvasan 2%, Simple Green, Spectracide Immunox (propiconazole) in High and Low formulations – does NOT inactive spores
Bacteria Disease	*Devriesea Agamarum*	*Lizards:* agamid, iguanid, and euphlebarid species	*Lesions:* Severe hyperkeratotic dermatitis, cellulitis, and potential septicemia *Diagnosis:* Culture	Cetiofur at 5 mg/kg q24 h for 18 ds in bearded dragons and 12 ds in *Uromastyx* sp. resulted in clinical resolution. Enrofloxacin was not effective Ceftazidime 10 mg/kg IM q72 for 15 ds, effective in *Uromastyx* species	Can exist in humid sand and distilled water for over 5 months, and remains in dermal crusts for up to 57 ds. *Disinfection:* 5-min contact time minimum: sodium hypochlorite (0.05%–0.5%), chlorhexidine (0.05%–0.5%), boric acid (0.01%), and ethanol (70%)

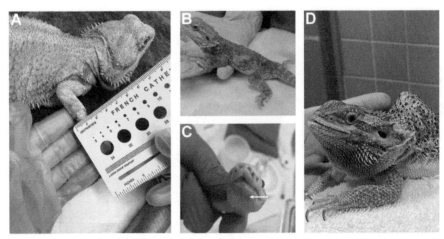

Fig. 10. (*A*) A 5-month-old female intact central bearded dragon (*Pogona vitticeps*) present-ing for recurrence of *Nannizziopsis guarroi* infection of the right antebrachium, despite treatment with extensive surgical debridement and voriconazole. Terbinafine was adminis-tered for 3 weeks to help assist control of this infection. (*B*) A 4-month-old male intact bearded dragon presenting with severe dermatitis, confirmed *Nannizziopsis guarroi* via po-lymerase chain reaction (PCR). (*C*) A 4-month-old captive ball python (*Python regius*) pre-sented with retained shed and cheilitis (*white arrow*), direct microscopy confirmed the presence of fungal hyphae and fungal PCR confirmed *Ophidiomyces ophidioocola*. (*D*) juve-nile bearded dragon that has survived "stepped on" trauma to the spine as a hatchling, also presenting with prognathism and cheilitis. Direct microscopy and culture confirmed *Devrie-sea agamarum*.

interest that have become more prominent in the literature in the last decade. Among all families, fungal disease (**Fig. 10**), viral disease, and gram-positive bacterial infec-tions (see **Fig. 10**) have increased in prevalence in captive and wild reptile species; however, parasite infections[81] are still commonly reported (**Figs. 11** and **12**).

Unfortunately, a large zoonotic outbreak of reptile-associated *Salmonella* has been reported in pet bearded dragons.[85] In a recent zoonotic disease compendium review for non-traditional pets, the Center for Disease Control conducted a review of

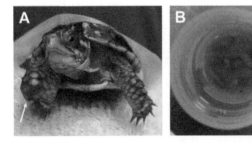
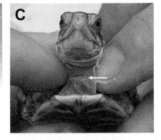

Fig. 11. (*A*) Juvenile ornate boxturtle (*Terrapene ornata ornata*) with a right branchial swelling and associated superficial lesion suffering from cutaneous myiasis (*Cistudinomyia cistudinis* bot fly larvae) (*yellow arrow*). Housed outdoors prior, the patient had been in an endemic area where bot flies were reported. (*B*) Photograph of larval species removed from several forelimb and hindlimb swellings. (*C*) Bot extraction site (*white arrow*) long the ventral cervical area, healed by second intention 7 days after extraction.

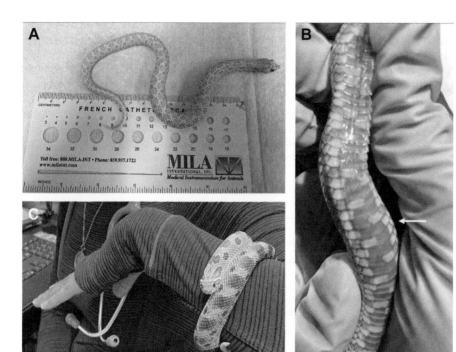

Fig. 12. (A) A 6-month-old Western Hognose snake (*Heterodon nasicus*) that presented with neurologic signs and generalized osteopenia lack of growth despite having a robust appetite. Fecal culture confirmed *Salmonella sp.* and *Cryptosporidium serpentis* on PCR. (B) The same western hognose developed a large midbody swelling, commonly seen with hypertrophic gastritits caused by *Cryptosporidium serpentis (yellow arrow).* (C) Photograph of an adult 2-year-old young adult male western hognose normal SVL length and size. SVL, snout to vent length.

outbreaks between 1996 and 2017 and noted that *Salmonella* bacteria caused 81% of 243 non-traditional pet-associated outbreaks and case reports.[86] There were 64 outbreaks associated with pet reptile species, 17 outbreaks associated with small mammal and rodent pets, 8 outbreaks caused by captive fish, and 105 outbreaks associated with backyard chickens. These current studies confirm that *Salmonella* is still the most common reported zoonotic disease among pet reptiles in the United States and remains a continued concern despite advances in client education and in the overall care of pet reptiles.

SUMMARY

Reports of phenotype-based breeding practices have been shown to negatively impact the captive welfare of ball pythons and bearded dragons which may result in modified husbandry recommendations in affected pets. While access to veterinary-driven care guides and recommendations for captive reptiles have improved, nutritional and husbandry imbalances continue to plague the pet industry. Prey-induced trauma continues to occur due to owner feeding practices and is largely preventable with improved client-education. Hypovitaminosis D continues to be a common condition seen in juvenile reptiles, and current studies report that both oral and UVB supplementation may be necessary in captive hatchling reptiles to prevent osteopathic changes associated with nutritional hyperparathyroidism. While species-specific studies that evaluate species-specific vitamin D metabolism and utilization are scarce, there is mounting evidence that suggests the photodynamic production of vitamin D via UVB exposure (natural and artificial) is a retained mechanism in snakes, and that genetic induction of vitamin D receptors in the duodenum of veiled chameleons is directly affected by oral vitamin D_3 supplementation *and* UVB exposure. Oral beta-carotene assimilation and conversion to retinol have been demonstrated in leopard geckos and warrants exploration in other insectivorous and carnivorous species. Classic and emerging infectious diseases continue to afflict young reptiles, and practitioners should continue to review the literature to inform best diagnostic practices.

CLINICS CARE POINTS

- A 10-h, low UVB irradiance exposure and a diet of gut-loaded insects dusted with vitamins A and D prevented nutritional hyperparathyroidism and fibrous osteodystrophy in hatchling veiled chameleons.

- Hatchling bearded dragons provided at least 2 hours of UVB exposure daily can maintain serum vitamin D levels that ensure healthy growth. Oral vitamin D3 supplementation alone, at 3 month or 6 months or age, is ineffective at raising plasma concentrations to the levels seen with UVB-exposed animals.

- Adult female bearded dragons lose the ability to maintain serum calcidiol levels in the absence of UVB exposure at 11 weeks without UVB exposure.

- Silkback and leatherback bearded dragons experience higher evaporative water loss than normal scale phenotypes and lack parietal-eye UVB detection. They also do not display basking behaviors that link elevated UVB exposure to thermoregulatory basking. They bask under high UVB exposure at cold temperatures which is a rarely paired thermoregulatory phenomenon in the wild.

- Spider ball python phenotypes have proven congenital developmental malformations of the stato-acoustic organs, which result in vestibular clinical signs and a lack of spatial orientation.

- Carrot juice supplementation once weekly resulted in increased hepatic retinol concentrations in leopard geckos, which may help reduce ophthalmic disease caused by hypovitaminosis A.

DISCLOSURE

The author has nothing to disclose and is unaware of any conflicts of interest.

REFERENCES

1. Raiti P. Husbandry, diseases, and veterinary care of the bearded dragon (*Pogona vitticeps*). J. Herp Med. Surg 2012;22(3–4):117–31.
2. Keller KA. Reptile perinatology. Vet Clin North Am Exot Anim Pract 2017;20(2): 439–54.
3. Knotek Z, Cermakova E, Oliveri M. Reproductive medicine in lizards. Vet Clin North Am Exot Anim Pract 2017;20(2):411–38.
4. Valdez JW. Using Google trends to determine current, past, and future trends in the reptile pet trade. Animals 2021;11(3):676. Available at: https://www.mdpi.com/2076-2615/11/3/676. Accessed March 7, 2023.
5. de Carvalho MP, Lewbart GA, Stewart JR, et al. Normal and Abnormal Reptile Development. In: Garner MM, Jacobson ER, editors. Noninfectious diseases

and pathology of reptiles2, 2nd edition. Boca Raton: CRC Press; 2020. p. p157–204.

6. Guo L, Bloom J, Sykes S, et al. Genetics of white color and iridophoroma in "Lemon Frost" leopard geckos. PLoS Genet 2021;17(6):e1009580.

7. Rose MP, Williams DL. Neurological dysfunction in a ball python (*Python regius*) colour morph and implications for welfare. J Exot Pet Med 2014;23(3):234–9.

8. Animal Diversity Web hosted by the at the University of Michigan Museum of Zoology. Available from: https://animaldiversity.org/. Accessed 27 May 2023.

9. Bour R, Luiselli L, Petrozzi F, et al. *Pelusios castaneus* (Schweigger 1812) – West African Mud Turtle, Swamp Terrapin. In: Rhodin AGJ, Pritchard PCH, van Dijk P, et al, editors. Conservation biology of freshwater turtles and tortoises: a compilation project of the IUCN/SSC tortoise and freshwater turtle specialist group. Chelonian Research Monographs; 2016. p. 1–11. https://doi.org/10.3854/crm.5.095.castaneus.v1. http://www.iucn-tftsg.org/cbftt/.

10. Red Footed Tortoise, Smithsonian's National Zoo & Conservation Biology Institute. Available at: https://nationalzoo.si.edu/animals/red-footed-tortoise Accessed 27 May 2023.

11. Bauer T, Reese S, Koelle P. Nutrition and husbandry conditions of Palearctic tortoises (*Testudo* spp.) in captivity. J. Appl. Anim. Welf 2019;22(2):159–70.

12. Türkozan O, Javanbakht H, Mazanaevz L, et al. *Testudo graeca* Linnaeus 1758 (Eastern Subspecies Clades: *Testudo g. armeniaca, Testudo g. buxtoni, Testudo g. ibera, Testudo g. terrestris, Testudo g. zarudnyi*) – Armenian Tortoise, Zagros Tortoise, Anatolian Tortoise, Levantine Tortoise, Kerman Tortoise. In: Rhodin AGJ, Iverson JB, van Dijk PP, et al, editors. Conservation biology of freshwater turtles and tortoises: a compilation project of the IUCN/SSC tortoise and freshwater turtle specialist group. Chelonian Research Monographs; 2023. p. 121–33. https://doi.org/10.3854/crm.5.120.eastern.graeca.v1.2023. Available at: www.iucn-tftsg.org/cbftt/.

13. Paré JA, Lentini AM. Reptile geriatrics. Vet Clin North Am Exot Anim Pract 2010; 13(1):15–25.

14. Eastern Blue Tongue Skink Natural History, SeaWorld. Available at: https://seaworld.org/animals/facts/reptiles/eastern-blue-tongued-skink/Accessed 27 May 2023.

15. Eastern Blue Tongue Skink Natural History. Available at: https://australian.museum/learn/animals/reptiles/eastern-blue-tongue-lizard/Accessed 27 May 2023.

16. Malaysian Blood Python Natural History, iNaturalist.org Available at: https://www.inaturalist.org/taxa/32162-Python-brongersmai. Accessed on July 24, 202.

17. Blood Python Natural History, Lehigh High Valley Zoo. Available from: https://www.lvzoo.org/animals/blood-python/Accessed 24 July 2023.

18. Schrenk F, Starck JM, Flegel T, et al. Comparative Assessment of Computed Tomography and Magnetic Resonance Imaging of Spider Morph and Wild Type Ball Pythons (*Python regius*) for Evaluation of the Morphological Correlate of Wobble Syndrome. J Comp Pathol 2022;196:26–40.

19. Starck JM, Schrenk F, Schröder S, et al. Malformations of the sacculus and the semicircular canals in spider morph pythons. PLoS One 2022;17(8):e0262788.

20. Brown AR, Comai K, Mannino D, et al. A community-science approach identifies genetic variants associated with three color morphs in ball pythons (*Python regius*). PLoS One 2022;17(10):e0276376.

21. Scagnelli AM, Biswell E. Diagnosis and treatment of unilateral renal dysplasia in a super dwarf reticulated python (*Python reticulatus*). J Exot Pet Med 2022; 40:52–7.

22. De Vosjoli P, Klingenberg R. Burmese pythons: plus reticulated pythons and related species. Mount Joy: Fox Chapel Publishing; 2012.
23. Sakich NB, Tattersall GJ. Bearded dragons (*Pogona vitticeps*) with reduced scalation lose water faster but do not have substantially different thermal preferences. J Exp Biol 2021;224(12):jeb234427.
24. Sakich NB, Tattersall GJ. Regulation of exposure to ultraviolet light in bearded dragons (*Pogona vitticeps*) in relation to temperature and scalation phenotype. Ichthyol Herpetol 2022;110(3):477–88.
25. Bárcenas-Ibarra A, Rojas-Lleonart I, Lozano-Guzmán RI, et al. Schistosomus reflexus syndrome in olive ridley sea turtles (*Lepidochelys olivacea*). Vet Path 2017; 54(1):171–7.
26. de Carvalho MP, Sant'Anna SS, Grego KF, et al. Microcomputed tomographic, morphometric, and histopathologic assessment of congenital bone malformations in two neotropical viperids. J Wildl Dis 2017;53(4):804–15.
27. Monks D, Doneley B. Reptile Paediatrics. In: Reptile medicine and surgery in clinical practice. Oxford: John Wiley & Sons Ltd; 2017. p. p105–13.
28. Sommella TM, Mailloux R, de Vosjoli P, et al. The bearded dragon manual: expert advice for keeping and caring for a healthy bearded dragon. 2nd edition. Mount Joy: Companion House Books; 2016.
29. Cacioppo JA, Perry SM, Rockwell K, et al. A Survey of Husbandry and Breeding Techniques in the Ball Python (*Python regius*) Pet Trade. J Herp Med Surg 2020; 31(1):25–35.
30. Latney LV, McDermott C, Scott G, et al. Surgical management of maxillary and premaxillary osteomyelitis in a reticulated python (*Python reticulatus*). J Am Vet Med Assoc 2016;248(9):1027–33.
31. Khan JJ, Richardson JM, Tattersall GJ. Thermoregulation and aggregation in neonatal bearded dragons (*Pogona vitticeps*). Physiol Behav 2010;100(2):180–6.
32. Rivera S, Lock B. The reptilian thyroid and parathyroid glands. Vet Clin North Am Exot Anim Pract 2008;11(1):163–75.
33. Klaphake E. A fresh look at metabolic bone diseases in reptiles and amphibians. Vet. Clin. North Am.: Exot. Anim. Pract 2010;(13):375–92.
34. Vergneau-Grosset C, Péron F. Effect of ultraviolet radiation on vertebrate animals: update from ethological and medical perspectives. Photochem Photobiol Sci 2020;19(6):752–62.
35. Oonincx D, van Leeuwen J. Evidence-based reptile housing and nutrition. Vet Clin North Am Exot Anim Pract 2017;20(3):885–98.
36. Maslanka MT, Frye FL, Henry BA, et al. Nutritional considerations. In: Warwick C, Arena PC, Burghardt GM, editors. Health and welfare of captive reptiles. Cham: Springer International; 2023. p. p447–85.
37. Boyer TH, Scott PW. Nutrition. In: Mader DR, Divers SJ, Stahl SJ, editors. Reptile and Amphibian medicine and surgery. 3rd edition. St. Louis: WB Saunders; 2019. p. 201–23.
38. Dierenfeld ES, King J. Digestibility and mineral availability of phoenix worms, *Hermetia illucens*, ingested by mountain chicken frogs, *Leptodactylus fallax*. J. Herp Med. Surg 2008;18(3):100–5.
39. Attard L. The development and evaluation of a gut loading diet for feeder crickets formulated to provide a balanced nutrient source for insectivorous amphibians and reptiles. Guelph, Ontario, Canada: University of Guelph; 2013. Available at:.
40. Latney LV, Toddes BD, Wyre NR, et al. Effects of various diets on the calcium and phosphorus composition of mealworms (*Tenebrio molitor* larvae) and superworms (*Zophobas morio* larvae). Am J Vet Res 2017;78(2):178–85.

41. Boykin KL, Mitchell MA. Evaluation of vitamin A gut loading in black soldier fly larvae (*Hermetia illucens*). Zoo Biol 2021;40(2):142–9.

42. Boykin K, Bitter A, Mitchell MA. Using a Commercial Gut Loading Diet to Create a Positive Calcium to Phosphorus Ratio in Mealworms (*Tenebrio molitor*). J Herpetol Med Surg 2021;31(4):302–6.

43. Cusack L, Rivera S, Lock B, et al. Effects of a light-emitting diode on the production of cholecalciferol and associated blood parameters in the bearded dragon (*Pogona vitticeps*). J Zoo Wildl Med 2017;48(4):1120–6.

44. Ferguson GW, Gehrmann WH, Karsten KB, et al. Ultraviolet exposure and vitamin D synthesis in a sun-dwelling and a shade-dwelling species of *Anolis*: are there adaptations for lower ultraviolet B and dietary vitamin D3 availability in the shade? Physiol Biochem Zool 2005;78(2):193–200.

45. Carman EN, Ferguson GW, Gehrmann WH, et al. Photobiosynthetic opportunity and ability or UVB generated vitamin synthesis in free living house geckos (*Hemidactylus turcicus*) and Texas spiny lizards (*Sceloporus olivaceus*). Copeia 2000;(1):245–50.

46. Acierno MJ, Mitchell MA, Zachariah TT, et al. Effects of ultraviolet radiation on plasma 25-hydroxyvitamin D3 concentrations in corn snakes (*Elaphe guttata*). Am J Vet Res 2008;69(2):294–7.

47. Hedley J, Eatwell K. The effects of UV light on calcium metabolism in ball pythons (*Python regius*). Vet Rec 2013;173(14):345.

48. Bos JH, Klip FC, Oonincx DG. Artificial ultraviolet B radiation raises plasma 25-hydroxyvitamin D3 concentrations in Burmese pythons (*Python bivittatus*). J Zoo Wildl Med 2018;49(3):810–2.

49. Bogan JE Jr, Cray C, Rick M, et al. Comparison of selected blood parameters of captive eastern indigo snakes (*Drymarchon couperi*) housed indoors vs. outdoors in Central Florida, USA. J Herpetol Med Surg 2020;30(3):165–72.

50. Knafo SE, Norton TM, Mitchell M, et al. Health and nutritional assessment of free-ranging eastern indigo snakes (*Drymarchon couperi*) in Georgia, United States. J Zoo Wildl Med 2016;47(4):1000–12.

51. Gyimesi ZS, Bums RB III. Monitoring of plasma 25-hydroxyvitamin D concentrations in two Komodo dragons, *Varanus komodoensis*: a case study. J Herpetol Med Surg 2002;12(2):4–9.

52. Gillespie D, Frye FL, Stockham SL, et al. Blood values in wild and captive Komodo dragons (*Varanus komodoensis*). Zoo Biol 2000;19(6):495–509.

53. Scott GN, Cullen J, Bakal RS, et al. Nutritional fibrous osteodystrophy with chondroid metaplasia in a Nile monitor, *Varanus niloticus*. Vet Rec Case Rep 2018; 6(4):e000590.

54. Vergneau-Grosset C, Carmel ÉN, Raulic J, et al. Vitamin D toxicosis in a blue-tongued skink (*Tiliqua scincoides*) presented with epistaxis and tongue discoloration. J Herpetol Med Surg 2020;30(4):224–31.

55. Ferguson GW, Gehrmann WH, Peavy B, et al. Restoring vitamin D in monitor lizards: exploring the efficacy of dietary and UVB sources. J Herpetol Med Surg 2009;19(3):81–8.

56. Haxhiu D, Hoby S, Wenker C, et al. Influence of feeding and UVB exposition on the absorption mechanisms of calcium in the gastrointestinal tract of veiled chameleons (*Chamaeleo calyptratus*). J Anim Physiol Anim Nutr 2014;98(6):1021–30.

57. Ferguson GW, Gehrmann WH, Karsten KB, et al. Do panther chameleons bask to regulate endogenous vitamin D3 production? Physiol Biochem Zool 2003; 76(1):52–9.

58. Ferguson GW, JonesJ R, Gehrmann WH, et al. Indoor husbandry of the panther chameleon *Furcifer pardalis*: effects of dietary vitamins A and D and ultraviolet irradiation on pathology and life-history traits. Zoo Biol 1996;15(3):279–99.

59. Wood MN, Soltis J, Sullivan KE, et al. UV irradiance effects on komodo dragon (*Varanus komodoensis*) vitamin D3, egg production, and behavior: A case study. Zoo Biol 2023. https://doi.org/10.1002/zoo.21801.

60. Gardiner DW, Baines FM, Pandher K. Photodermatitis and photokeratoconjuncti-vitis in a ball python (*Python regius*) and a blue-tongue skink (*Tiliqua* spp.). J Zoo Wildl Med 2009;40(4):757–66.

61. Ooninex DG, Diehl JJ, Kik M, et al. The nocturnal leopard gecko (*Eublepharis macularius*) uses UVb radiation for vitamin D3 synthesis. Comp Biochem Physiol B Biochem Mol Biol 2020;250:110506.

62. Gould A, Molitor L, Rockwell K, et al. Evaluating the physiologic effects of short duration ultraviolet B radiation exposure in leopard geckos (*Eublepharis macular-ius*). J Herpetol Med Surg 2018;28(1–2):34–9.

63. Bashaw MJ, Gibson MD, Schowe DM, et al. Does enrichment improve reptile wel-fare? Leopard geckos (*Eublepharis macularius*) respond to five types of environ-mental enrichment. Appl Anim Behav Sci 2016;1(184):150–60.

64. Watson MK, Mitchell MA. Vitamin D and ultraviolet B radiation considerations for exotic pets. J Exot Pet Med 2014;23(4):369–79.

65. Hoby S, Wenker C, Robert N, et al. Nutritional metabolic bone disease in juvenile veiled chameleons (*Chamaeleo calyptratus*) and its prevention. J Nutr 2010;140: 1923–31.

66. Kroenlein KR, Zimmerman KL, Saunders G, et al. Serum vitamin D levels and skeletal and general development of young bearded dragon lizards (*Pogona vit-ticeps*), under different conditions of UV-B radiation exposure. J Anim Vet Adv 2011;10(2):229–34.

67. Ooninex DG, Van De Wal MD, Bosch G, et al. Blood vitamin D3 metabolite con-centrations of adult female bearded dragons (*Pogona vitticeps*) remain stable af-ter ceasing UVb exposure. Comp Biochem Physiol B Biochem Mol Biol 2013; 165(3):196–200.

68. Ooninex DG, Stevens Y, Van den Borne JJ, et al. Effects of vitamin D3 supple-mentation and UVb exposure on the growth and plasma concentration of vitamin D3 metabolites in juvenile bearded dragons (*Pogona vitticeps*). Comp Biochem Physiol B Biochem Mol Biol 2010;156(2):122–8.

69. Selleri P, Di Girolamo N. Plasma 25-hydroxyvitamin D3 concentrations in Her-mann's tortoises (*Testudo hermanni*) exposed to natural sunlight and two artificial ultraviolet radiation sources. Am J Vet Res 2012;73(11):1781–6.

70. Gramanzini M, Di Girolamo N, Gargiulo, et al. Assessment of dual-energy X-ray absorptiometry for use in evaluating the effects of dietary and environmental management on Hermann's tortoises (*Testudo hermanni*). Am J Vet Res 2013; 74(6):18–924.

71. Hoskins A, Thompson D, Mitchell MA. Effects of artificial ultraviolet B radiation on plasma 25-hydroxyvitamin D3 concentrations in juvenile Blanding's turtles (*Emy-doidea blandingii*). J Herpetol Med Surg 2022;32(3):225–9.

72. Acierno MJ, Mitchell MA, Roundtree MK, et al. Effects of ultraviolet radiation on 25-hydroxyvitamin D3 synthesis in red-eared slider turtles (*Trachemys scripta el-egans*). Am J Vet Res 2006;67(12):2046–9.

73. Finke MD, Dunham SU, Kwabi CA. Evaluation of four dry commercial gut loading products for improving the calcium content of crickets, *Acheta domesticus*. J Herpetol Med Surg 2005;15(1):7–12.

74. Barboza TK, Abood SK, Beaufrère H. Survey of Feeding Practices and Supplement Use in Pet Inland Bearded Dragons (*Pogona vitticeps*) of the United States and Canada. J Herpetol Med Surg 2022;32(3):187–97.

75. Oonincx DG, Van Keulen P, Finke MD, et al. Evidence of vitamin D synthesis in insects exposed to UVB light. Sci Rep 2018;8(1):10807.

76. Boykin KL, Carter RT, Butler-Perez K, et al. Digestibility of black soldier fly larvae (*Hermetia illucens*) fed to leopard geckos (*Eublepharis macularius*). PLoS One 2020;15(5):e0232496.

77. Wiggans KT, Guzman DS, Reilly CM, et al. Diagnosis, treatment, and outcome of and risk factors for ophthalmic disease in leopard geckos (*Eublepharis macularius*) at a veterinary teaching hospital: 52 cases (1985–2013). J Am Vet Med Assoc 2018;252(3):316–23.

78. Cojean O, Lair S, Vergneau-Grosset C. Evaluation of β-carotene assimilation in leopard geckos (*Eublepharis macularius*). J Anim Physiol Anim Nutr 2018; 102(5):1411–8.

79. Latney LV, Wellehan JF. Selected emerging infectious diseases of Squamata: an update. Vet Clin North Am Exot Anim Pract 2020;23(2):353–71.

80. Adamovicz L, Allender MC, Gibbons PM. Emerging infectious diseases of chelonians: An update. Vet Clin North Am Exot Anim Pract 2020;23(2):263–83.

81. O'Toole CJ, Quesenberry K, Latney LV, et al. Computed tomography of cutaneous myiasis in an ornate box turtle (terrapene ornata ornata). J Zoo Wildl Med 2021; 52(3):1090–4.

82. Wellehan JF, Jacobson E, Stilwell J, et al. Testudine Intranuclear Coccidiosis (TINC). J Herpetol Med Surg 2022;32(2):144–54.

83. Bogan JE Jr. Gastric cryptosporidiosis in snakes, a review. J Herpetol Med Surg 2019;29(3–4):71–86.

84. Bogan JE Jr, Hoffman M, Dickerson F, et al. Evaluation of paromomycin treatment for *Cryptosporidium serpentis* infection in eastern indigo snakes (*Drymarchon couperi*). J Herpetol Med Surg 2021;31(4):307–14.

85. Kiebler CA, Bottichio L, Simmons L, et al. Outbreak of human infections with uncommon Salmonella serotypes linked to pet bearded dragons, 2012–2014. Zoonoses and Public Health 2020;67(4):425–34.

86. Varela K, Brown JA, Lipton B, et al. A review of zoonotic disease threats to pet owners: A compendium of measures to prevent zoonotic diseases associated with non-traditional pets such as rodents and other small mammals, reptiles, amphibians, backyard poultry, and other selected animals. Vector Borne Zoonotic Dis 2022;22(6):303–60.

Wildlife Pediatrics

Ernesto Dominguez-Villegas, DVM, DACVPM, CWR

KEYWORDS

- Pediatrics ● Wildlife ● Orphan ● Rehabilitation ● Hand-rearing ● Nutrition ● Release

KEY POINTS

- Neonate wildlife medicine follows the same principles for all other species.
- Hydration, heat support, and adequate nutrition are critical during the initial care of neonate wildlife.
- Some specific knowledge of the ecology, biology, and specific problems encountered by the various species is necessary, to provide adequate care to wildlife.
- Drug use in wild animals is considered extra-label and as such drug residues are a potential public health risk.
- The goal of wildlife neonate medicine is to provide temporary care, husbandry, and nutrition, to restore the health of the individuals to be released back into the wild.

INTRODUCTION

It has been estimated that tens of thousands of wild animals are injured attributable to human causes daily on the United States.[1] In spring and summer months, wildlife rescuers will experience an increase in calls, most of which will involve young animals. A young wild animal stands a greater chance of surviving as an adult and leading a normal life if raised by a wild parent. From wild parents, young learn where to forage and hunt, what to eat, what to be afraid of, and where to find shelter. By growing up in the wild, they will also acquire valuable and necessary social skills.[1]

Several misconceptions about wildlife often lead to unnecessary human intervention or disturbance. For example, handling wildlife expands on the myth that infant animals will be immediately abandoned by their parents once touched by humans. Although it is true that wild infants should not be handled more than is necessary, casual handling of a baby will not result in parental abandonment. Wildlife displays a high degree of fidelity to their offspring, sometimes to the extreme of aggressive defense. Certain species, such as Eastern cottontail rabbits (*Sylvilagus floridanus*) and white-tailed deer (*Odocoileus virginianus*), have a distinct strategy of distant parental attention. This method keeps adults distant so as not to attract attention to the concealed rabbit nest or the cryptic coloration of a young fawn during daylight hours. Often the public views infrequent nest visitation of Eastern cottontails as nest abandonment or neglect when the nest,

Southwest Virginia Wildlife Center, 5985 Coleman Road, Roanoke, VA 24018, USA
E-mail address: e.dominguezv22@gmail.com

Vet Clin Exot Anim 27 (2024) 411–430
https://doi.org/10.1016/j.cvex.2023.11.014
1094-9194/24/© 2023 Elsevier Inc. All rights reserved.

vetexotic.theclinics.com

in fact, is being properly attended by the mother. If nests in groomed yards are uncovered by mowing or other activities, most infants can be successfully renested by placement in the same area, covering the nest with natural vegetation and keeping domestic pets restrained. Second, there is the misconception that human rearing of wild infants is an acceptable alternative to parent animals raising its own offspring. Humans make very inadequate surrogate parents for wild infants despite their ability to properly nourish them. There is far more parental investment in young than merely feeding. Species recognition, sibling interaction and rivalry, and learning wild food sources are only a few of the critical skills necessary for successful survival. Artificial hand-rearing should only be attempted when every possible attempt to return the wild infant to its proper parents has been exhausted. In the process of hand-rearing, wild infants often become habituated to the presence of humans and domestic pets. These young lose their natural protective survival skills, one of which is aversive fear of humans. Birds are known to experience a process termed imprinting, where during a specific critical time period they fix their species recognition and future social and courtship behaviors on the largest object in their immediate area. In addition, male white-tailed deer raised in the presence of humans have been known to seek human sparring partners during the fall rutting season, leading to human fatalities.[2]

Human–wildlife conflict are difficult to measure, but the analysis of records from wildlife rehabilitation facilities has shown potential as a technique for characterizing human impacts on wildlife.[3]

Juvenile animals feature heavily in admissions to wildlife centers.[4] The International Wildlife Rehabilitation Council defines wildlife rehabilitation as the "treatment and temporary care of injured, diseased, orphan, and displaced indigenous animals, and the subsequent release of healthy animals to appropriate habitats in the wild."[5]

In wildlife rehabilitation, it is necessary to be able to determine what kind of care is needed to restore a wild patient to good health and for return to the wild, not just to save its life. It is also critical to realistically assess and understand who has the training and resources to provide what level of care. An awareness of both the kind of care that is required and the capacity of available care providers is essential in the realistic triage of patients and development of a treatment plan that is workable in a wildlife rehabilitation setting. A good working relationship between the veterinarian and the cooperating wildlife rehabilitators will greatly improve decision-making and increase the potential for successful outcome for wild patients.[6]

The process of rehabilitation is inherently stressful for wildlife, and maintaining the individual animal's welfare at the center of the rehabilitation process requires deliberate, timely, and humane decision-making. The welfare of wild animals can be improved by preventing human-related causes of admission, providing much-needed resources and support for those animals in rehabilitation, further developing evidence-based wildlife rehabilitation methods and welfare measures, increasing engagement of the veterinary profession, harmonizing regulatory oversight with standards of care, training, and accountability, and raising public awareness regarding the steps that can be taken to mitigate the number of wild animals in need of rehabilitation.[6,7]

Some veterinarians will allow clients, members of the public, local animal control officers, animal welfare organizations, or the wildlife rehabilitators themselves to drop off wild animal patients needing care so they can be seen when time permits throughout the day.

Veterinary first aid provision during triage follows the same basic principles as domestic species. Where treatment is carried out, it is essential that the long-term future of the casualty animal is continually considered where release remains the only goal. Some specific knowledge of the ecology, biology, and specific problems encountered by the various species is necessary.[4]

In most states and provinces, there are wildlife-specific guidelines, requirements, and prohibitions related to the captive care of wild species, including housing requirements for specific animal groups, prohibition of exposure of wild patients to domestic animals or the public, and certain occupational health and safety requirements, especially related to zoonotic diseases, such as rabies. Veterinarians should be aware of the local, state, and/or national/federal laws that are required to provide care for wildlife animals, including juvenile animals.

LEGAL ASPECTS OF TREATING WILDLIFE

In virtually all instances, licensed veterinarians can lawfully admit and treat a wild animal that requires medical attention.[5,6,8–10] However, once an animal has been medically treated and stabilized, further steps should be taken to transfer the animal to a licensed or permitted wildlife rehabilitation facility. Regulations may vary around the world, but in the United States, every state has its own set of regulations that govern the wildlife native to that state, but all contain a general provision that prohibits the temporary or permanent possession of almost all species of native wild animals. As mentioned earlier, most state wildlife rehabilitation regulations are silent on any prohibition of a veterinarian rendering immediate, emergency medical assistance to a wild animal in need. Some public health or wildlife agencies have reporting and surveillance requirements for cases of various diseases observed or suspected. Those of public health importance may include rabies, plague, tularemia, or hantavirus, and state wildlife agencies may request information on cases of parvovirus, white-nose syndrome, West Nile virus, highly pathogenic influenza virus, and Newcastle's disease virus. Those agencies should be contacted in advance for their reporting, and surveillance requirements and the information should be maintained in a readily accessible location.[8–13] Veterinary practitioners should report injuries caused by illegal activities such as gunshot wounds to nongame species to local, state, or federal wildlife authorities.[12]

Drug use in wild animals is considered extra-label and as such is regulated by the Food and Drug Administration (FDA) through the Animal Medicinal Drug Use Clarification Act. This act is divided into food-producing animals and non-food-producing animals. Drug residues in game animals are a potential public health risk to those who consume the meat. Game animals are defined by the FDA as "an animal, the products of which are food that is not classified as livestock, sheep, swine, goat, horse, mule or other equine, or as poultry or fish." Game animals include mammals such as deer, antelope, rabbit, squirrel, opossum, raccoon, nutria, or muskrat and nonaquatic reptiles such as land snakes. The FDA classifies wild game birds as "poultry" and includes "migratory waterfowl or game birds, pheasant, partridge, quail, grouse, or pigeon." Practitioners need to be aware of potential meat withdrawal times (ie, the time between drug administration and when the meat can safely be consumed by a human) when administering drugs to game species during or just before established hunting and trapping seasons. There are very few established withdrawal times for wildlife, and practitioners should check the Food Animal Residue Avoidance Database for guidance on drug administration in game species that could be consumed.[12]

GENERAL CARE OF ORPHANED WILDLIFE

Orphaned neonatal wildlife accounts for one of the largest causes of admissions to wildlife rehabilitation centers and highlights an opportunity for conservation education regarding when wildlife is truly orphaned and requires professional intervention.[3]

All presentations of orphaned wildlife should be considered emergencies. Juvenile animals have limited fluid and energy stores, and after a short period of time (ie, hours), they may develop negative energy balance and dehydration.[10] Veterinary care during the admission and triage of orphaned wildlife follows the same basic principles as that of domestic species. Where treatment is carried out, it is essential that the long-term future of the casualty animal is continually considered where release remains the ultimate goal. Specific knowledge of the ecology, biology, and specific problems encountered by the various species is necessary.[4,14,15]

A good working relationship between the veterinarian and the cooperating wildlife rehabilitators will greatly improve decision-making and increase the potential for a successful outcome for wild patients.[6] Veterinary practices are usually unsuitable places to hand raise young wild animals. Many species require frequent feeding over much of each 24-hour period, as often as every 20 minutes in some species, which may be a strain on clinic staffing.[16]

The most important assessment is to determine if the young animal is truly orphaned. Well-intentioned individuals may assume an animal is orphaned when it is not. If uninjured, chicks may be returned to nests and young mammals reunited with their parents. To reduce the number of unnecessary admissions into human care, veterinarians and wildlife rehabilitators should actively attempt to reunite wild healthy offspring with their parents.[10,16]

Restraint and handling procedures are stressful for wildlife. Before handling any wildlife, one should set out a clear checklist of procedures that need to be performed on the animal, as well as all equipment or medications that are needed.[17]

Hydration, temperature and heat support, and adequate nutrition are critical during the initial care of neonate wildlife. Neonates are usually hypothermic and unable to thermoregulate on arrival. Generally, the younger the animal, the more supplemental heat must be provided, and as the animal matures, less supplemental heat is needed. Infants should be warmed to normal body temperature before completing the physical examination, administering fluids, or feeding.[1,10,12,13,16–20] Assume most wildlife patients are 10% dehydrated on admission. Once infants are at normal body temperature, weigh them, and administer warm fluids to correct hydration deficits. Routes of administration include oral (PO), subcutaneous (SC), intraosseous (IO), and intravenous (IV). Maintaining humidity at 50% to 70% in housing helps prevent ongoing dehydration.[10,12,16,17]

On admission, neonatal mammals and precocial birds are frequently hypoglycemic. Young animals have higher glucose requirements than do most adults of their species. This increased requirement is a result of the high level of energy needed for maintaining metabolic function, growth, and normal blood glucose levels. Once the infant is warmed and well-hydrated, appropriate species-specific diets may be fed. Neonates of most species have a stomach or crop capacity of ~50 mL/kg. Often the first few feedings of orphans are slow. Aspiration often occurs as a result of poor feeding techniques.[10,12,16,17] Aspiration pneumonia is a common reason for fatality in orphaned animals.[12]

Provide analgesia and anti-inflammatory medications if needed. Determine appropriate housing. The main goals are safety and to reduce stress on the animal by preventing noise and visual stimulation. In general, minimize contact to people and domestic animals.[10,12,16,17,21]

ORPHANED WILD BIRDS

There are two types of neonatal birds: altricial or precocial (**Fig. 1**). Most species are altricial; that is, species hatched with few or no feathers, with their eyes closed and entirely dependent on their parents for food and warmth. Conversely, precocial

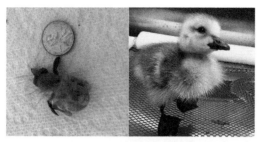

Fig. 1. Comparison between an altricial bird (*left*) and a precocial one (*right*).

species hatch with a good coat of down feathers and an ability to leave the nest immediately and follow its parents.[10,13,16,22]

Correct identification of neonate birds can be difficult and challenging, when the general practitioner does not work with wild bird species frequently (**Fig. 2**).[16,23–25] Several resources are available which can aid on the identification on neonatal birds such as https://sites.tufts.edu/babybirds/.[26] It is challenging to provide a comprehensive account of avian neonatology, because significant differences exist between the medical conditions that altricial and precocial species are susceptible to. In addition, great variations are found in the husbandry and rearing methods for the different avian groups.[22]

Newly arrived altricial chicks that are too young or too debilitated to stand must be supplied with a comfortable nest (**Fig. 3**). Precocial young can be housed in boxes or plastic containers like those for adults.[10,13,16,22,25] Generally, orphaned chicks should be kept in a temperature between 85° and 95° F (29° and 35° C). Ultimately, the temperature selected should be based on the age and plumage of the animal. In general, the highest temperatures are reserved for the hatchlings, moderate temperatures for the nestlings, and lowest for the fledglings.[10,13,15,22,25,27–29]

Neonate birds should be weighed daily.[10,13,16,22] Nutritional requirements of wild species are not well known and are usually extrapolated from domestic species.[10,13,16,22] Avoid physical contact during the feedings whenever possible. Hatchling birds are prone to imprint. Feeding the birds using a surrogate (eg, puppet look-a-like) or by hiding behind a blanket or towel will ensure the animal does not imprint onto humans. Placing a mirror in front of the animal so that its own reflection is the only animal it can see may also be done. Feeding intervals for birds should be consistent to promote regular gastrointestinal transit times. Comfortable, well-hydrated chicks will rest quietly in the nest between meals, eat enthusiastically when food is offered, feel warm and fleshy to the touch, and produce well-formed droppings approximately as often as fed.[10,13,15,22,25,27–29]

The most common medical conditions in orphaned birds are:[10,16]

- Hypothermia
- Dehydration
- Hypoglycemia
- Internal and external parasites
- Metabolic bone disease
- Other skeletal disorders
- Wounds and fractures
- Aspiration pneumonia
- Crop stasis
- Accidental crop burns

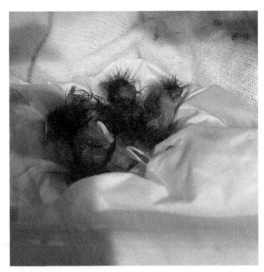

Fig. 2. Nestling Eastern bluebird (*Sialia sialis*), which is commonly mistaken for American robins (*Turdus migratorius*).

Physical Examination

Once warm and stable, each chick should receive a physical examination. Examinations should be performed in a systematic manner to avoid missing injuries or medical problems. Always be gentle.

A visual examination of the chick's attitude, posture, droppings, signs of bleeding, ectoparasites, and feeding response can be performed when the chick arrives in the container. Determine if the animal is altricial or precocial, try to identify the species, and evaluate if the eyes are opened or closed. Continue your examination in a systematic manner, to look for symmetry, wounds, evidence of hemorrhage or hematomas, musculoskeletal abnormalities, feather condition, if the crop and ventriculus are full or empty, and the conformation and integrity of the beak.[16,23,30]

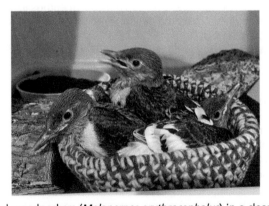

Fig. 3. Red-headed woodpeckers (*Melanerpes erythrocephalus*) in a clean nest.

Treatments

As mentioned before, the three most important aspects of the care and treatment of orphaned chicks are to provide heat, keep them hydrated, and provide of adequate nutrition.

Rehydration can be achieved orally or through SC routes. Human infant electrolyte formulas, lactated Ringer's solution, or Plasma-Lyte A are the author's preferred rehydrating solutions. The total amount of fluids should be divided and administered several times a day. Although the average chick needs 50 mL/kg/day, small passerines may need up to 300 mL/kg/day.[16,23–25,28,29,31–33] Altricial birds that are gaping can be orally hydrated until they defecate and urinate (**Fig. 4**). In larger birds, oral fluids can be administered by a gavage tube. If the oral route is not feasible or the bird is severely dehydrated, administer fluids two to three times a day.[16,23–25,28,29,31–33]

To treat for internal and external parasites, a herd or flock approach is preferred versus an individual approach. The development of flock treatment plans should be based on identification of the bird species and which parasites are commonly a problem for that species.[16] Fecal flotation and centrifugation techniques are quick and accurate to identify most gastrointestinal parasites. Empirical antiparasitic treatment is recommended if any clinical signs consistent with parasitic diseases (diarrhea, reduced average weight gain, and continuous dehydration).

Metabolic bone disease develops quickly in wild orphans fed inadequate diets, as fast as a few days in rapidly growing species, and it is usually due to inadequate dietary calcium and phosphorus. Growing chicks require a dietary ratio of elemental calcium to phosphorus of ~2:1 by weight. Fractured limbs must be considered life-threatening in wild chicks because they need to have fully functional limbs to qualify for release. Advanced metabolic bone disease may be fatal or require euthanasia.

Treatment involves feeding an appropriately nutritious diet in adequate amounts and frequency, providing supplemental calcium, exposing the animal to natural sunlight, and maintaining adequate hydration.[16,23,28,29] Owing to its low calcium concentration, using calcium glubionate to correct dietary calcium requires unrealistically large volumes to be fed. Calcium carbonate is a better alternative, as it provides ~400 mg elemental calcium per gram.[16]

Wounds should be cleaned, debrided, and closed primarily whenever possible. Analgesia is always warranted before treatment. Judicious use of antibiotics should be considered. The same principles of wound management in adult animals can be applied to wounded wild chicks.[1,10,16–18,20,23,25,27–29,31–41]

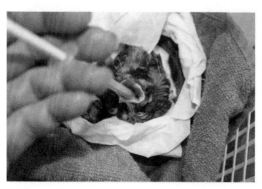

Fig. 4. Oral hydration of a nestling American robin (*Turdus migratorius*) with a 1 mL syringe.

Nutrition and Suggested Diets

High animal protein, moderate fat, and low-carbohydrate diets are adequate for most altricial birds, with some exceptions. Vitamins A, D, and E, calcium, and taurine are likely deficient in almost all insect diets. Several commercial products intended for raising parrots are inadequate for wild altricial chicks.[14,16,24]

Offer fledglings ample wild-type diet in a visually engaging presentation as soon as they are old enough to stand and move about their enclosure.

Songbirds, swifts, and woodpeckers have high growth rates. Chicks generally eat 50 mL/kg per meal and should be fed repeatedly over the course of 12 to 14 hours each day. Hatchlings should be fed every 15 to 30 minutes, nestlings every 20 to 45 minutes and older birds every hour until weaned. The latter species and corvids should show strong feeding reflex and stop gaping when full (**Fig. 5**).[16,23,24] Overfeeding may cause crop distension with poor motility, yeast or bacterial overgrowth, and diarrhea.

Feeding down the esophagus or crop is safer than just offering food cranial to the oropharynx. Chicks cannot breathe and are at risk of aspiration when the oral cavity is full of food.[14,16,23–25,28,34] Feed hatchlings a more dilute diet and fledglings a thicker diet. Always clean birds during and after feeding.[10]

Hummingbird hatchlings may weigh as little as 0.25 g and must be fed every 10 to 20 minutes. Feeding hummingbird chicks commercial hummingbird nectars or sugar water rapidly leads to malnutrition.[16] In the author's experience, a supportive diet for hummingbird chicks can be prepared by diluting 5 to 7 g of Nektar-Plus (Nekton USA, Arcata, CA) and 1 to 2 g of whey protein powder in 50 mL of distilled water. Administer food when the bird is accepting it, verifying the crop's size, and stop delivering food when the crop feels full.

Pelican and cormorant chicks imprint on humans easily. These species should always be fed with puppets simulating the parents and conversation should not be held around the chicks. Chicks may pick food up from the floor or may require feeding pieces of fish with hemostats or tongs. Train the chick to learn to eat from a dish as early as possible. Thiamine and vitamin E supplementation is critical in these species.[23,32]

For raptors, follow the same imprinting guidelines as for pelicans, using puppets for each feeding or methods to disguise the human face and body. Hatchlings and

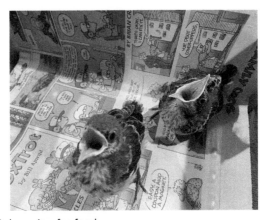

Fig. 5. Nestling birds gaping for food.

nestlings must be fed with long forceps or tongs. When very young, they may require a meal every 2 to 3 hours.[28,29]

Precocial species, if weak or stressed, might need to be stimulated to feed or to be force fed. Once warm, hydrated, and safe, most species will eat on their own. Correct species identification is needed as some species may require different foods (eg, live prey) and protein levels during growth.[16,25]

In general, waterfowl have nutrient requirements different from other poultry species, specifically an increased need for the B vitamins such as niacin, choline, and biotin.[16,25] One commercially available diet specifically designed for wild waterfowl is commercially available (Mazuri, St Louis, MO, USA).

Pigeons and doves receive crop milk from their parents, and it is the primary food for around 10 days. The composition of crop milk is like that found in mammals but lacks carbohydrates; it contains water, fat, protein, and ash. Some formulas to mimic crop milk have been reported, including mixing one hard-boiled egg yolk (mashed), 3 tablespoons of mixed baby multi-cereal, 3 tablespoons of powdered oatmeal, and 3 tablespoons of cornmeal.[10]

ORPHANED WILD MAMMALS

When found, injured, sick, or orphaned neonates are commonly dehydrated, hypothermic, and hypoglycemic. All infant mammals should be warmed to their normal temperature, before administering anything through the oral route. Orphaned mammals that are dehydrated or hypothermic will reduce their caloric intake.

All orphaned mammals should be provided an enclosure that is dry and warm and has appropriate nesting material. Excessive humidity often leads to the development of severe dermatitis.[1,2,4,10,12,16–20,30,33,35,38,42] Orphaned mammals do not need to be bathed or washed. All feeding utensils should be cleaned or disinfected before being used to limit the transfer of infectious diseases between patients. Orphans should be weighed daily, and their diet modified if necessary.

Each species of mammal produces its own specific milk. It is impossible to replicate these milks, but substitutes can be made up. Marsupial milk contains almost no lactose, whereas in Eutherian species, lactose is the predominant saccharide.[10,14,16,30,43–52]

Generally, once infant mammals are warm and hydrated, nutrition should start. Gradual introduction of milk replacement formulas causes fewer gastrointestinal problems. A common practice is to follow these steps.

- Oral electrolytes and hydration on the first two feeds
- The third feed should be 75% oral electrolytes and 25% milk substitute
- The following feed 50% electrolyte and 50% milk replacer;
- The fifth feed 25% electrolytes and 75% milk substitute
- Finally, 100% of the ideal milk replacer for the species.

Administering oral electrolytes and milk replacement formulas can be challenging and there is always a risk of aspiration pneumonia. The use of small syringes and nipples makes it easier to control the flow of fluid (**Fig. 6**). Some species benefit more from being gavage by orogastric tube, instead of syringe or bottle fed.

Newborns will have to be fed as often as every 3 to 4 hours to get the nutrition and calories they need.[30,44,48–50,52] Infants should be fed in the prone position, stomach down, with the chin raised so that the face is forward (**Fig. 7**). After each feeding, all mammals that still have closed eyes should be stimulated to urinate and defecate.

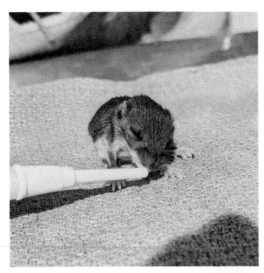

Fig. 6. Small syringe and small nipple or tip to feed small mammals.

Fecal and urinary output of each orphan should be monitored closely and at each feeding. A reduction in output may suggest dehydration or decreased gastrointestinal transit.

Common medical problems include:

- Hypothermia
- Dehydration
- Hypoglycemia
- Omphalitis, which should be treated locally and/or systemically as necessary
- Wounds and fractures

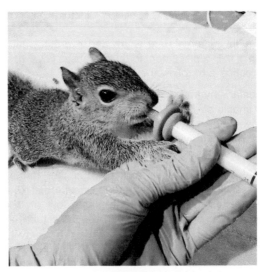

Fig. 7. Infant Eastern gray squirrel (*Sciurus carolinensis*) being fed in prone position, stomach down, with the chin raised so that the face is forward.

- External and internal parasites
- Septicemia, commonly caused by *Escherichia coli*, *Clostridium* spp, *Salmonella* spp, and *Pasteurella* spp
- Digestive disorders
- Aspiration pneumonia
- Metabolic bone disease.

Rodents and Lagomorphs

The mortality rate for young rodents is high, especially for smaller species such as mice, rats, and squirrels. Owing to their higher metabolism, rodents and lagomorphs require higher fluid and caloric rates compared with any other mammals. If dehydrated, the use of warm SC fluids at a rate of 60 to 100 mL/kg/day is indicated. If hydrated, start oral electrolytes at 4% of body weight.

Squirrels open their eyes between 4 and 5 weeks of age, and at that point, they can urinate and defecate without stimulation. Milk replacement formulas with 16% protein and 20% fat are optimal for individuals less than 50 g. Formulas with 10% protein and 25% fat are a reasonable option for squirrels more than 50 g. Feed 5% body weight per feed initially, gradually increasing the amount as the squirrel grows. At 100 g, feed about 7% body weight per feeding.[16,47,51,53,54] A suggested feeding schedule for three different species of squirrels is shown in **Tables 1–3**.

Eastern cottontail rabbits that are furred, with eyes open, ears erect and greater than 5 inches (12.7 cm) long are likely old enough to survive on their own.[16,55,56] Neonates range from 15 to 25 g have no fur and tightly closed eyes and ears. By days 4 to 7, fur starts to develop, and the young are about 3 to 4 inches (7.6–10.1 cm) in length and weight 25 to 35 g. By 7 to 10 days, the eyes and ears usually start to open, weights range from 35 to 40 g, and the young are fully furred.

Rabbit mothers feed their infants only two to three times in a 24-hour period. The infants hide in the nest and are left alone for the rest of the day. This feeding schedule should be replicated in wildlife rehabilitation settings.[13,16] The stomach capacity of an infant rabbit is greater than that of most mammals of comparable size. When calculating formula amounts, use 8% to 10% of their body weight. There is much debate about the best formula to feed orphaned juvenile cottontail rabbits. In general, formulas with 30% to 40% protein and more than 40% fat are recommended.[56] Infant cottontails require stimulation of the anogenital region to urinate and defecate. Young

Table 1
Feeding schedule for Eastern gray squirrels (*Sciurus carolinensis*) based on age and weight

Age	Estimated Weights	Amount per Feeding in mL	Feedings per day
0–1 wk	15–35 g	½–1	6+
2 wk	36–55 g	2–2 ½	5
3 wk	56–78 g	3–5	4
4 wk	79–106 g	6–7 *(begin mush bowl and soft snacks)*	3
5 wk	107–125 g	8–10	3
6 wk	126–144 g	10–12 *(introduce small dish of water)*	2
7 wk	145–175 g	10–12	1
8 wk	176–199 g	Mush bowl and post-wean diet	0

Adapted from Southwest Virginia Wildlife Center.

Table 2
Feeding schedule for fox squirrels (*Sciurus niger*) based on age and weight

Age	Estimated Weights	Amount per Feeding in mL	Feeding per day
0–1 wk	18–35 g	½–2	6
2 wk	40–60 g	2–4	5
3 wk	60–90 g	4–6	5
4 wk	105–140 g	8–10	4
5 wk	140–165 g	9–12	3
6 wk	170–200 g	12–15	3
7 wk	210–250 g	15–18 *(begin mush bowl and soft snacks)*	3
8 wk	220–290 g	18 *(add natural foods)*	2
9–10 wk release at 12–14 wk	300–500 g	18–20	1 wean by 10 wk

Adapted from Southwest Virginia Wildlife Center.

rabbits may start to eat vegetation as early as day 10 and are usually weaned by about day 15. A suggested feeding schedule for rabbits is shown in **Table 4**.

Marsupials

Infants weighing less than 30 g have a poor prognosis and should be euthanized, particularly if they are cold to the touch when presented or with a history of being attached to a dead jill. Virginia opossums (*Didelphis virginiana*) longer than 6 inches (15 cm) (not including the tail) are likely old enough to survive on their own.[16,57] Housing juvenile opossums must take into consideration the unique environment the mother's pouch would normally provide. Opossums are generally orphaned in groups and should be kept together for comfort and warmth.[57]

Opossum infants do not have the same suckling reflex that most mammals have, nor do they possess the oral or extremity musculature to hold a teat. They are normally attached to their mother's teat constantly during the nursing period of several months. The teat is long and thin and may reach the neonate's stomach.[13] Orogastric gavage is the most recommended technique to feed opossums (**Fig. 8**).

Table 3
Feeding schedule for flying squirrels (*Glaucomys* spp.) based on age and weight

Age	Estimated Weights	Amount per Feeding in mL	Feeding per day
0–1 wk	6–8 g	¼–½	6
2 wk	9–12 g	½–¾	5
3 wk	13–15 g	¾–1	4
4 wk	16–20 g	1–2 *(begin mush bowl and soft snacks)*	3
5 wk	21–26 g	2–2 ½ *(introduce small dish of water)*	2
6 wk	27–35 g	2 ½–3	1
7 wk	36–46g	Mush bowl and post-wean diet.	0
8 wk	47–51 g	FULLY WEANED	NONE

Adapted from Southwest Virginia Wildlife Center.

Table 4
Feeding schedule for Eastern cotton tails (*Sylvilagus floridanus*) based on age and weight

Age in d	Estimated Weights	Amount of Formula per Feeding	Feedings per day
0–8	25–59 g	10% body weight (BW)	2
9–10	60–65 g	10% BW	2
11–14	66–70 g	10% BW	2
15–18	71–85 g	10% BW *(offer fresh tender greens and hay)*	1
19–20	86–95 g	5% BW *(offer fresh tender greens and hay)*	1
21–23	96–100 g	Just offer fresh greens, hay, and rabbit pellet food	0
24	>105 g	Ready for release	0

Adapted from Southwest Virginia Wildlife Center.

Milk replacer formulas with 25% to 30% of protein and 30% to 40% fat are adequate for hand raising opossums. Weaning occurs around 95 days of age.[43,57] The proposed feeding schedule is shown in **Table 5**.

Opossums are nocturnal, so they are very efficient at producing endogenous vitamin D without exposure to sunlight and require little UVB light or vitamin D supplementation. However, they are susceptible to nutritional secondary hyperparathyroidism if fed a diet with an inappropriate calcium:phosporus (Ca:P) ratio. Internal and external parasites can often be a serious problem.

Pyrantel (10 mg/kg) is a safe empirical choice for a dewormer. Fleas are often a serious problem, causing life-threatening anemia in older haired babies. Selamectin (6–10 mg/kg) is safe for haired babies more than 50 g and is often used prophylactically on initial presentation. A common syndrome in young opossums is dermal septic necrosis, also known as "crispy-ear syndrome." Amoxicillin-clavulanic acid is a good empirical choice to treat this condition.[57]

Raccoons and Skunks

Always wear personal protective equipment when handling racoons and skunks. These species are common hosts for rabies virus and *Baylisascaris procyonis*. People

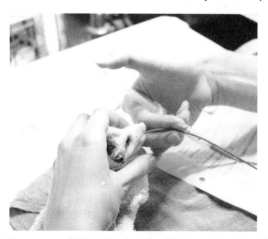

Fig. 8. Infant Virginia opossum (*Didelphis virginiana*) being tube fed with orogastric tube.

Table 5
Feeding schedule for Virginia opossums (*Didelphis virginiana*) based on weight

Estimated Weights	Amount per Feeding in mL	Feeding per day
21–30 g	1	5
31–40 g	1 $\frac{1}{4}$–1 $\frac{3}{4}$	4
41–54 g	1 $\frac{1}{4}$–2 *(begin to offer mush bowl)*	3
55–74 g	2 $\frac{1}{2}$–3 $\frac{1}{2}$ cc *(add soft foods and dish of water)*	2
75–100 g	4–5 *(introduce small mouse pieces)*	1
101–200 g	Juvenile meal (see menu) and a mouse.	NONE

Adapted from Southwest Virginia Wildlife Center.

working with raccoons should have rabies preexposure inoculations and biennial titer checks.

Newborns weigh 60 to 75 g with eyes and ears sealed. Young raccoons and skunks may be bottle-fed or fed via orogastric tube. Feed 5% by volume of body weight. Milk replacer formulas with 40% of protein and 25% fat are adequate for hand raising raccoons and skunks.[16,58] Neonates should start to defecate and urinate without stimulation at 4 to 6 weeks of age. To prevent future wildlife human conflicts, preventing imprinting in these species is of high importance.

Mustelids

Infant mustelids are born with eyes and ears closed, covered with a very fine hair coat, and are totally dependent on their mother for care. Several commercial formulas are available and have been used successfully. Fox Valley Animal Nutrition, Inc (Lake Zurich, IL, USA) and Zoologic Milk Matrix (PetAg, Hampshire, IL, USA) offer several milk replacer formulas that can be adapted to the specific needs of the species. The estimated gastric capacity is 5% to 7% of body weight.

The following feeding schedule can be used for North American river otters (*Lontra canadensis*):[59]

- 0 to 2 weeks: feed every 2 to 3 hours (including overnight)
- 3 to 4 weeks: feed 5 to 6 times per day, every 3 hours (no overnight feeds)
- 5 to 6 weeks: feed 5 times per day, every 3 to 4 hours
- 7 to 8 weeks: feed 4 to 5 times per day, every 4 hours (introduce fish)
- 9 to 10 weeks: feed 4 times per day (decreasing formula with weaning).

Carnivores

Young wild canids should never be raised alone; they are highly social and it is essential that they are raised with conspecifics. Red fox (*Vulpes vulpes*) kits weigh about 85 to 110 g at birth and measure 6 to 8 inches (15–20 cm) in length. Pups are weaned at about 5 weeks of age, and the food provided should replicate what is available in the wild.[60]

Gray fox (*Urocyon cinereoargenteus*) kits are altricial and average 85 g at birth with a body length of 3 to 5 inches (7–13 cm). At birth, the neonates do not seem foxlike. Gray fox pups are weaned at 7 to 8 weeks of age when they weigh on average 1 kg.

Newborn coyotes (*Canis latrans*) weigh approximately 300 to 350 g. By 4 weeks of age, after weaning has occurred, the social hierarchy has been established.

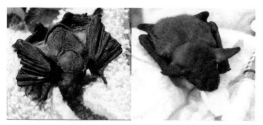

Fig. 9. Comparison between a dehydrated bat pup and one euhydrated.

The ability of pups and kits to swallow does not fully develop until about 3 weeks of age. Foxes and coyotes should be fed around 5% of their body weight every 4 hours.[60,61]

Before working with wild bears, veterinarians should ensure that state laws permit veterinary care and rehabilitation.[62–65] Black bears have one to six cubs (average 2–3) weighing approximately 200 to 450 g are born in January or early February. The eyes are initially closed and open around day 25. The cubs emerge from the den in April or May when the cubs weigh approximately 2 to 5 kg. Bear milk contains high concentrations of protein, fat, and minerals but low concentrations of carbohydrates. Milk from American black bears (*Ursus americanus*) consist of approximately 44.5% total solids, 24.5% fat, 0.4% lactose, 8.8% casein, 5.7% whey protein, 1.8% ash, 0.41% calcium, and 0.28% phosphorus.[63–67] Following rehydration, some bear care facilities choose to start feeding full-strength formula, whereas others gradually increase the percentage of formula to rehydrating solution in stepwise daily increments. The volume of food delivered at each meal is approximately 10% of the bear's body weight divided into 2 to 6 feedings per day.

Bats

Always wear personal protective equipment when handling bats. They are hosts for rabies virus. Bat pups are born during the summer and are quite large in relation to the adult (as much as 30%–40% of the mother's body weight). Most species are born naked with closed eyes. Eyes generally open within days after birth. Hypothermia and dehydration are quite common in orphaned pups and should be addressed immediately (**Fig. 9**).[68] Once the pup is warm to the touch, it may be hydrated with electrolytes using SC or oral routes, depending on the degree of dehydration. A small-tipped cannula or plastic catheter tip on a 1 mL feeding syringe can facilitate oral feedings for mildly dehydrated neonates. After rehydrating, food may be introduced via a commercial milk replacer such as Esbilac (Pet-Ag, Inc, Hampshire, IL 60140), KMR (Pet-Ag, Inc), or Fox Valley 32/40 (Fox Valley Animal Nutrition, Inc, Lakemoor, IL 60051). Neonates can succumb quickly to aspiration pneumonia. Care must be taken to prevent aspiration during feedings.

Cervids

Birth weight of white-tailed deer averages between 2.5 and 4.0 kg (5.5–17.6 lbs.). Fawns triple their weight in their first month of life and are weaned between 8 and 12 weeks of age. Their spotted hair coat remains until autumn when their first molt occurs.[69]

Fawns readily imprint on caregivers and inappropriate interactions may impact their chances for release. Fawns should be raised in groups with minimal human contact.[16]

Table 6
Feeding schedule for white-tailed deer (*Odocoileus virginianus*) based on weight

Age	Estimated Weights	Amount per Feeding in Oz	Feeding per day
0–1 wk	0.45–1.36 kg	12 oz AM 8 oz noon 12 oz PM	3
1–2 wk	1.36–4.54 kg	12 oz	2
3–5 wk	4.54–6.81 kg	16 oz	2
6–7 wk	6.81–9.09 kg	16 oz AM 12 oz PM	2

Adapted from Southwest Virginia Wildlife Center.

Mildly dehydrated fawns should get 30 to 50 mL/kg SC on admission. If moderately to severely dehydrated, place an IV catheter and give 90 mL/kg/day IV.[16,69]

Newborn to 2-day-old fawns require colostrum for the first 24 to 48 hours. Commercial goat colostrum formulas are a replacement option. Milk replacement formulas that have a content of 30% protein and 40% fat, or goat and lamb's milk, are adequate for most cervids. Fawns may be fed by hand initially but as soon as they are suckling consistently, the bottles should be offered in a rack feeder. A proposed feeding schedule is shown in **Table 6**. Fawns will require stimulation to urinate and defecate until at least 16 days of age.

Neonatal cervids are susceptible to hypoglycemia, which can be secondary to diarrhea, sepsis, or malnutrition. Treatment for hypoglycemia is recommended when blood glucose levels are less than 3.3 mmol/L (60 mg/dL) in white-tailed deer or black-tailed or mule deer (*Odocoileus hemionus*).[69]

SUMMARY

The principles of triage, evaluation, and care of neonate wildlife are universal and applicable as they are to other domestic, zoologic, or exotic species. Hydration, temperature and heat support, and adequate nutrition are critical during the initial care of neonate wildlife. A few modifications are needed to provide adequate care to wildlife, with the goal to be released back into the wild.

DISCLOSURE

The author has nothing to disclose.

REFERENCES

1. Dmytryk R. Wildlife search and rescue: a guide for first responders. Chischester West Sussex, UK: John Wiley & Sons; 2012.

2. Burton DL, Doblar KA. Morbidity and mortality of urban wildlife in the midwestern United States. presented at. Proc 4th International Urban Wildlife Symposium; 2004. https://ag.arizona.edu/pubs/adjunct/snr0704/snr07042m.pdf.

3. Long RB, Krumlauf K, Young AM. Characterizing trends in human-wildlife conflicts in the American Midwest using wildlife rehabilitation records. PLoS One 2020;15(9):e0238805.

4. Mullineaux E. Veterinary treatment and rehabilitation of indigenous wildlife. J Small Anim Pract 2014;55(6):293–300.
5. Miller EA. Minimum standards for wildlife rehabilitation. 4th edition. St. Cloud, MN: National Wildlife Rehabilitators Association; 2012.
6. Clark EE Jr. The veterinary practitioner and the wildlife rehabilitator: building the right relationship and touching all the bases. In: Hernandez SM, Barron HW, Miller EA, et al, editors. Medical management of wildlife species: a guide for practitioners. NJ, USA: Wiley Online Library; 2019. p. 97–104.
7. Willette M, Rosenhagen N, Buhl G, et al. Interrupted lives: welfare considerations in wildlife rehabilitation. Animals 2023;13(11):1836.
8. Mullineaux E. Legal responsibilities of veterinary professionals when working with wildlife centres. Companion Animal 2016;21(10):592–7.
9. McCallum H, Hocking BA. Reflecting on ethical and legal issues in wildlife disease. Bioethics 2005;19(4):336–47.
10. Bewig M, Mitchell MA. Wildlife. In: Mitchell MA, Tully TN, editors. Manual of exotic pet practice. St. Louis, MO: Elsevier; 2009. p. 493–529, chap 19.
11. Casey A, Miller EA. Regulatory and legal considerations in wildlife medicine. In: Hernandez SM, Barron HW, Miller EA, et al, editors. Medical management of wildlife species: a guide for practitioners. NJ, USA: Wiley Online Library; 2019. p. 1–9, chap 1.
12. McRuer DL, Barron H. Wildlife. In: Carpenter JW, editor. Exotic animal formulary. 5th eedition. MO, USA: Elsevier; 2018. p. 616–35.
13. Ruth I. Wildlife care basics for veterinary hospitals: before the rehabilitator arrives. Washington, DC: Humane Society of the United Sates; 2002.
14. Robbins C. Wildlife feeding and nutrition. New York, NY: Academic Press; 2012.
15. Stocker L. Practical wildlife care. Ames, IA: John Wiley & Sons; 2005.
16. Gage LJ, Duerr RS. Principles of initial orphan care. In: Hernandez SM, Barron HW, Miller EA, et al, editors. Medical management of wildlife species: a guide for practitioners. NJ, USA: Wiley Online Library; 2019. p. 145–57, chap 12.
17. Myers DA. Common procedures and concerns with wildlife. Vet Clin Exot Anim Pract 2006;9(2):437–60. https://doi.org/10.1016/j.cvex.2006.03.005.
18. Cox SL. Medical management of wildlife species: a guide for practitioners. J Wildl Dis 2020;56(4):971–2.
19. Meredith A. Wildlife triage and decision-making. In: Mullineaux E, Keeble E, editors. BSAVA manual of wildlife casualties. 2nd edition. Gloucester: British Small Animal Veterinary Association; 2016. p. 27–36.
20. Quattrucci DJ. Emergency wildlife care and management. Worcester: Worcester Polytechnic Institute; 1999.
21. Thompson P. Wildlife rehabilitation manual. Washington, USA: Washington State Department of Fish and Wildlife; 2015.
22. Bailey T, Magno MN. Reproduction. In: Samour J, editor. Avian medicine. 3rd edition. MO, USA: Elsevier Health Sciences; 2015. p. 557–66, chap 15.
23. Duerr RS, Gage LJ. Hand-rearing birds. 2nd edition. Hoboken, NJ: John Wiley & Sons; 2020.
24. Welte SC, Miller EA. Natural history and medical management of passerines, galliformes, and allies. In: Hernandez SM, Barron HW, Miller EA, et al, editors. Medical management of wildlife species: a guide for practitioners. NJ, USA: Wiley Online Library; 2020. p. 197–213.
25. Goodman M. Natural history and medical management of waterfowl. In: Hernandez SM, Barron HW, Miller EA, et al, editors. Medical management of

wildlife species: a guide for practitioners. NJ, USA: Wiley Online Library; 2020. p. 229–45.

26. Berkowitz A, Grogan D. Baby Birds. A site to help you with identification. Tufts University; 2023. https://sites.tufts.edu/babybirds/. Accessed September 17, 2023.

27. Fusté E, Obon E, Olid L. Hand-reared common swifts (Apus apus) in a wildlife rehabilitation centre: assessment of growth rates using different diets. Journal of zoo and aquarium research 2013;1(2):61–8.

28. Rayman B, Duerr R. Raising Orphaned Raptors. LafeberVet. 2023. Avaialble at: https://lafeber.com/vet/raising-orphaned-raptors/. Accessed June 06, 2023.

29. Scott D. Natural history and medical management of raptors. In: Hernandez SM, Barron HW, Miller EA, et al, editors. Medical management of wildlife species: a guide for practitioners. NJ, USA: Wiley Online Library; 2020. p. 215–28.

30. Cowen S. Care and hand-rearing of young wild animals. BSAVA Manual of wildlife casualties. 2nd edition. Gloucester: British Small Animal Veterinary Association; 2016. p. 73–80.

31. Anderson DL. Waterfowl rehabilitation: A primer for veterinarians. Semin avian exot pet med 2004;13(4):213–22.

32. Duerr RS. Medical and surgical management of seabirds and allies. In: Hernandez SM, Barron HW, Miller EA, et al, editors. Medical management of wildlife species: a guide for practitioners. NJ, USA: Wiley Online Library; 2019. p. 247–58.

33. Carlson D, Ruth I. Wildlife care for birds and mammals: 7 volume basic manual wildlife rehabilitation series. 3rd edition. Madison, CT: Bick Pub. House; 1997.

34. Samour J. Avian medicine. 3rd edition. St. Louis, MO: Elsevier; 2015.

35. Cope HR, McArthur C, Dickman CR, et al. A systematic review of factors affecting wildlife survival during rehabilitation and release. PLoS One 2022;17(3): e0265514.

36. Hall E. Release considerations for rehabilitated wildlife. presented at: Australian National Wildlife Rehabilitation Conference 2005; Surfers Paradise.

37. Hanson M, Hollingshead N, Schuler K, et al. Species, causes, and outcomes of wildlife rehabilitation in New York State. PLoS One 2021;16(9):e0257675.

38. Hernandez SM, Barron HW, Miller EA, et al. Medical management of wildlife species: a guide for practitioners. NJ, USA: Wiley Online Library; 2020.

39. Jacobs SK. Healers of the wild: rehabilitating injured and orphaned wildlife. 2nd edition. Boulder, CO: Johnson Books; 2003.

40. Jorquera CB, Moreno-Switt AI, Sallaberry-Pincheira N, et al. Antimicrobial resistance in wildlife and in the built environment in a wildlife rehabilitation center. One Health 2021;13:100298.

41. Latas PJ, Rescue. rehabilitation, and release of psittacines: an international survey of wildlife rehabilitators. J Wildl Rehabilitation 2019;39(3):15–22.

42. Grogan A, Kelly A. A review of RSPCA research into wildlife rehabilitation. Vet Rec 2013;172(8):211.

43. Green B, Krause WJ, Newgrain K. Milk composition in the North American opossum (Didelphis virginiana). Comp Biochem Physiol B Biochem Mol Biol 1996;113(3):619–23.

44. Iverson SJ. Milk composition and lactation strategies across mammalian taxa: implications for hand-rearing neonates. presented at: proceedings of the Seventh Conference on Zoo and Wildlife Nutrition. Knoxville: AZA Nutrition Advisory Group; 2007.

45. McDonald JE Jr, Fuller TK. Effects of spring acorn availability on black bear diet, milk composition, and cub survival. J Mammal 2005;86(5):1022–8.

46. Mueller C. Changes in the nutrient composition of milk of black-tailed deer during lactation. J Mammal 1977;58(3):421–3.

47. Nixon CM, Harper W. Composition of gray squirrel milk. Ohio J Sci 1972; 72(1):3–6.

48. Novak M, Szenci O. Artificial milk for wildlife orphaned neonates. Veterinarska stanica. 2024;55(1):111-123.

49. Paul G, Friend DG. Comparison of outcomes using two milk replacer formulas based on commercially available products in two species of infant cottontail rabbits. J Wildl Rehabil 2017;37(1):13–9.

50. Robbins CT, Moen AN. Milk consumption and weight gain of white-tailed deer. J Wildl Manag 1975;39:355–60.

51. Grant K. Nutrition of tree-dwelling squirrels. Vet Clin Exot Anim Pract 2009;12(2): 287–97.

52. Gage LJ. Hand-rearing wild and domestic mammals. Ames, IA: John Wiley & Sons; 2008.

53. Levy IH, Keller KA, Allender MC, et al. Prognostic indicators for survival of orphaned eastern gray squirrels (Sciurus carolinensis). J Zoo Wildl Med 2020; 51(2):275–9.

54. Miller EA. Natural history and medical management of squirrels and other rodents. In: Hernandez SM, Barron H, Miller EA, et al, editors. Medical management of wildlife species: a guide for practitioners. NJ, USA: Wiley Online Library; 2020. p. 167–84.

55. Principati SL, Keller KA, Allender MC, et al. Prognostic indicators for survival of orphaned neonatal and juvenile eastern cottontail rabbits (Sylvilagus floridanus): 1,256 Cases (2012–17). J Wildl Dis 2020;56(3):523–9.

56. Tseng FS. Natural history and medical management of lagomorphs. In: Hernandez SM, Barron H, Miller EA, et al, editors. Medical management of wildlife species: a guide for practitioners. NJ, USA: Wiley Online Library; 2020. p. 185–96.

57. Gardner A. Natural history and medical management of opossums. In: Hernandez SM, Barron H, Miller EA, et al, editors. Medical management of wildlife species: a guide for practitioners. NJ, USA: Wiley Online Library; 2020. p. 297–311.

58. Schott R. Natural history and medical management of procyonids: emphasis on raccoons. In: Hernandez SM, Barron HW, Miller EA, et al, editors. Medical management of wildlife species: a guide for practitioners. NJ, USA: Wiley Online Library; 2020. p. 271–82.

59. Abou-Madi N. Natural history and medical management of mustelids. In: Hernandez SM, Barron H, Miller EA, et al, editors. Medical management of wildlife species: a guide for practitioners. NJ, USA: Wiley Online Library; 2020. p. 283–96.

60. Lord J, Miller EA. Natural history and medical management of canids: emphasis on coyotes and foxes. In: Hernandez SM, Barron H, Miller EA, et al, editors. Medical management of wildlife species: a guide for practitioners. NJ, USA: Wiley Online Library; 2020. p. 313–25.

61. Kelly TR, Sleeman JM. Morbidity and mortality of red foxes (Vulpes vulpes) and gray foxes (Urocyon cinereoargenteus) admitted to the Wildlife Center of Virginia, 1993–2001. J Wildl Dis 2003;39(2):467–9.

62. Alt GL, Beecham JJ. Reintroduction of orphaned black bear cubs into the wild. Wildl Soc Bull (1973-2006) 1984;12(2):169–74.
63. Beecham J. Orphan bear cubs. London, UK: Rehabilitation and release guidelines WSPA; 2006.
64. Rogers LL. Aiding the wild survival of orphaned bear cubs. Wildl Rehabil 1985;4: 104–11.
65. McRuer D, Ingraham H. Natural history and medical management of ursids. In: Hernandez SM, Barron H, Miller EA, et al, editors. Medical management of wildlife species: a guide for practitioners. NJ, USA: Wiley Online Library; 2020. p. 327–41.
66. Hashem BJ. Evaluating the success of an orphaned American black bear (Ursus americanus) rehabilitation program in Virginia. J Wildl Rehabil 2019;39(2):7–12.
67. Beecham JJ, Loeffler IK, Beausoleil RA. Strategies for captive rearing and reintroduction of orphaned bears. J Wildl Rehabil 2016;36(1):7–16.
68. Bowen LE. Natural history and medical management of chiroptera. In: Hernandez SM, Barron H, Miller EA, et al, editors. Medical management of wildlife species: a guide for practitioners. NJ, USA: Wiley Online Library; 2020. p. 353–62.
69. Knight K, van Wick P. Medical and surgical management of deer and relatives. In: Hernandez SM, Barron H, Miller EA, et al, editors. Medical management of wildlife species: a guide for practitioners. NJ, USA: Wiley Online Library; 2020. p. 259–70.

Behavioral Development of Pediatric Exotic Pets and Practical Applications

Marion R. Desmarchelier, DMV, MSc, Dipl. ACZM, Dipl. ECZM (Zoo Health Management), Dipl. ACVB

KEYWORDS

- Behavior • Exotic animals • Development • Epigenetics • Avian • Juvenile
- Hand-rearing • Weaning

KEY POINTS

- Low levels of stress and reduced exposure to methylation agents are required during gametogenesis and the early life stages to maximize adaptability to environmental changes and resilience to stress in adulthood and reduce the risk of behavioral abnormalities.
- Many factors influence the behavioral development and should be carefully taken into consideration when raising or taking care of juveniles: species-appropriate parental care, age and methods of weaning, interspecific and intraspecific social interactions (early handling), environmental enrichment, environmental conditions (temperature, and so forth), nutrition, stress, exposure to drugs, and so forth.
- Combining species-appropriate parent-rearing with appropriately timed human handling is likely to result in individuals better adjusted to life as exotic pets regularly interacting with humans.
- Providing an enriched and safe environment early in life, designed to promote species-specific behaviors, is critical to allow young animals to learn their natural behaviors, such as flying and foraging in birds, and reduce the likelihood of stereotypical behaviors.
- Using operant conditioning with positive reinforcement to train juveniles for daily life behaviors, such as litter training, getting back in their cages, and expressing their needs with appropriate vocalizations for humans, will empower juveniles, reduce inappropriate behaviors (eg, screaming, aggression, and such behaviors), improve the quality of the human-animal bond, and build the foundation of better lifelong welfare.

Department of Clinical Sciences, Faculté de médecine vétérinaire, Université de Montréal, 3200 rue Sicotte, J2S 2M2 Saint-Hyacinthe, Québec, Canada
E-mail address: marion.desmarchelier@umontreal.ca

Vet Clin Exot Anim 27 (2024) 431–448
https://doi.org/10.1016/j.cvex.2023.11.015
1094-9194/24/© 2023 Elsevier Inc. All rights reserved.   vetexotic.theclinics.com

Video content accompanies this article at http://www.vetexotic.theclinics.com.

INTRODUCTION

Raising young animals has always been very challenging at many levels. Every breeder and every owner have observed this and experienced various outcomes throughout the years. Several techniques have been advocated to tame nondomesticated animals and make them mentally and physically healthy pets. For years, separating individuals from their parents and conspecifics as early as at birth/hatching and raising them with humans was believed to be the best way to obtain human-friendly companions. However, science and experience have shown us the severe limitations of this attempt to deny natural biology, as raising animals in an environment that prevents their normal brain development often results in abnormal behaviors affecting the animal's mental health and welfare. The objective of this review is to provide the readers with a summary of the most recent scientific advancements in behavioral development science that can have a significant impact on how we should raise exotic pets. This review is not meant to be exhaustive as the amount of information for each species at each step of development could require its own review article. Instead, the author wishes to provide some information to help deepen the understanding of how the environment we provide in their early life impacts exotic animal health and welfare. The author will also provide some practical applications on how to apply behavioral science while interacting with young animals to reduce the likelihood of inappropriate or problem behaviors and overall improve their well-being.

BEHAVIORAL DEVELOPMENT IN THE POSTGENOMIC ERA
Developmental Plasticity and Epigenetics

Natural selection with random mutations of structural deoxyribonucleic acid (DNA) as the sole agent involved in heritability has been the main paradigm leading behavioral research for years.[1,2] The study of genomics, including one of the largest single investigative projects in modern science, the Human Genome Project, was supposed to revolutionize diagnostics and treatment.[1] As researchers expected between 100,000 and 200,000 genes to compose the genome of our species, a certain disappointment may have occurred as we indeed have between 20,000 and 25,000 genes, just as many as roundworms and less than corn.[1] If the Human Genome Project did not keep its promise to change daily medicine, it did, however, shed a whole new light on how life forms can produce an array of phenotypes with such a low number of genes. Though genetics is undoubtedly involved in behavioral development, many observations could not be fully explained until scientists finally uncovered what had been described by Belyaev, as early as the 1950s, as "on" and "off" switches to genes.[1] Research on developmental plasticity and epigenetics may still be in its infancy but has already opened our scientific minds to the once unthinkable fact that the environment can change our gene expression and that these changes are heritable. The term "epigenetics" was suggested by Waddington in 1942 to refer to all interactions between genes and the environment that bring the phenotype into being.[3] Developmental plasticity represents the process by which a specific genotype can result in a vast array of phenotypes following environmental influences during development.[4] This new paradigm allows us to better comprehend how environmental changes can be rapidly integrated into the epigenome, in a highly adaptive and flexible way, immensely more efficient than random mutations and natural selection could ever be. However, it also proved that phenotypes developed in the early stages of life may affect the individuals for the rest of their lives. For example, all humans are born with the same number of sweat glands but will only activate the number they require during their first 3 years of life.[5] Molecular mechanisms involved in epigenetics are complex and involve DNA methylation (mainly of cytosine), histone hypoacetylation, ribonucleic acid silencing, and other forms of posttranscriptional modification.[1] External factors affecting methylation processes, present in specific food items, drugs, or toxins, for example, have the potential to affect our DNA expression. In 2003, Waterland and Jirtle[6] reported a ground-breaking experiment using mice (*Mus musculus*) carrying the gene **agouti** responsible for turning their fur yellow and also affects their susceptibility to tumors. The parents were fed a diet containing methyl groups (supplemented with extra folic acid, cobalamin, choline, and betaine), commonly found in soy and leafy vegetables, and their offspring born with the agouti gene had brown fur and were no longer susceptible to the same diseases.[6] Their agouti gene had been silenced through methylation.[6] The parents had passed on their DNA and the associated "off" switch.[6] Another striking example is the synthetic estrogen, bisphenol A (BPA), used in plastic and epoxy resins. Over 150 studies showed detrimental effects of BPA, especially with maternal exposure, even to low doses, during gestation.[7] Prenatal exposures resulted in abnormal gain weight, insulin resistance, prostate cancer, and excessive mammary gland later in life.[7] Further human studies led to considering BPA as a toxic substance. Putting an end to the **nature or nurture** debate, this growing body of research reveals the underlying mechanisms affecting the behavioral development of our exotic pets.

Normal Brain and Behavioral Development

As Kolb and Gill wrote so accurately, "The development of the brain reflects more than the simple unfolding of a genetic blueprint but rather reflects a complex dance of genetic and experiential factors that shape the emerging brain. Understanding the dance provides insight into both normal and abnormal development."[8] **Fig. 1** summarizes the main environmental, behavioral, and molecular aspects affecting development. At birth, each of the 100 billion neurons of the human brain has approximately 2500 synapses and will reach 15,000 per neuron by age 2 to 3.[4] The postnatal brain undergoes an impressive combination of neuronal arborization, synaptogenesis, gliogenesis, and myelination.[4] Pruning of synapses occurs to eliminate underused pathways, resulting in about 7 to 8000 synapses per neuron at adult age.[4] For these molecular and cellular processes to result in individuals who are adapted to their environment, performing species-specific behaviors, the early-life environment is critical. Parents should be confronted with an amount of stress that does not compromise their welfare during gametogenesis, gestation, and time during which they care for their offspring. The environment should allow the juveniles to start expressing normal behavior, through play and social interactions when appropriate, creating neurogenesis and synaptogenesis in key brain pathways such as the serotonin and dopamine pathways.[9] There is some evidence that playful social opportunities as juveniles may contribute to the development of the prefrontal cortex and later allow for more flexible behavioral strategies in unexpected situations.[10] Being exposed to stressors, learning what a real environmental danger is, and experiencing an appropriate level of fear are critical to the normal development of the hypothalamic-pituitary-adrenal (HPA) axis and the norepinephrine pathways for a functional response to stress in adulthood.[9] Though interacting positively with the human species may not be part of the genetic programming of nondomestic animals, flexibility of the epigenome can be taken advantage of to integrate human beings as part of the normal environment of the juvenile. Interactions should be timed based on each species' normal developmental stages and literature-based knowledge and should be as positive as possible if the goal is to

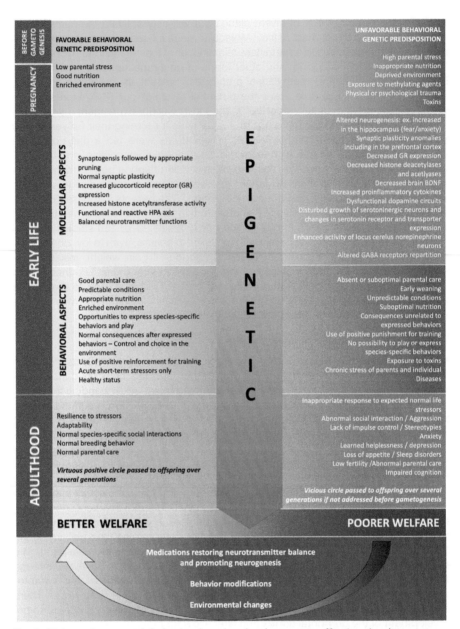

Fig. 1. Main environmental, behavioral, and molecular aspects affecting development.

produce pets who will thrive in human company. The reward system involves the cortico-basal ganglia-thalamo-cortical (CBTC) loop and is essential to individual fitness, motivating the animal to engage in behaviors increasing their likelihood of survival and reproduction, triggering positive emotions.[11] Using operant conditioning techniques with positive reinforcement will not only allow for rewarding interactions but will also allow the stimulation of specific chosen behaviors and the empowerment of juveniles by giving them control over their environment. From normal behavioral development should arise mentally and physically healthy animals, displaying species-appropriate breeding behavior, passing on their epigenome, and therefore improving the welfare of the next generation.

Effects of Early-life Stressors on Behavioral Development

Although encountering and learning to manage expected minor stressors is a normal part of development, undergoing chronic stress and major environmental disruptions or, conversely, being raised in a barred environment can challenge the resilience and flexibility of the individual. **Fig. 1** presents several mechanisms involved in abnormal behavioral development. Early-life abnormal or excessive stressors including an unpredictable environment induce a modulation of the neuroendocrine and sympathetic systems, leading to inflammation, oxidative stress, and neurobiological abnormalities throughout the brain's major pathways.[9,12] Maternal separation in rodents is one of the best research models used to induce early-life stress to mimic childhood trauma and negligence in humans. Sadly, this research model reflects the reality of many exotic pets undergoing premature separation from their parents. Abnormal epigenetic changes in the serotonin and dopamine receptors and transporters are observed with chronic stress, predisposing juveniles to anxiety, depression, and compulsive behaviors later in life.[9] Another pathway affected by maternal care during the first week of life of young rats is the gamma-aminobutyric acid (GABA) system with permanently affected GABA A/central benzodiazepine receptors possibly affecting fear response and predisposing to anxiety disorders.[13] Abnormalities of the rat prefrontal cortex development have been reported following a variety of early-life stressors.[8] Research also demonstrates that an appropriate environment should allow for behaviors to be meaningful to the animals. Providing young Mongolian gerbils (*Meriones unguiculatus*) with substrate to dig did not reduce the occurrence of stereotypic digging. However, providing access to an artificial burrow did reduce the stereotypic behavior.[14] This is essential to comprehend as we often see supposedly enriched environments that are not emulating any normal behaviors, such as a large enclosure to allow for physical exercise without including any motivation for the animal to use it purposefully. The lack of cohesion between the individual behavior and the associated consequence, using inconsistent punishment, for example, can lead to severe dysfunction of the CBTC loop, manifested by learned helplessness, depression, and compulsive/stereotypic behaviors. Early-life stress in juveniles carries consequences in adulthood with apoptosis of mature neurons, activation of immune responses, and reduction of neurotrophic factors, thus causing psychiatric disorders as well as cognitive dysfunction.[9]

Recent scientific advances of the postgenomic era show us that gene expression with relevance for behavior occurs within powerful environmental contexts, especially in the critical stages of early life.[15] These findings have a lot of practical applications on how to take care of juvenile exotic animals.

DEVELOPMENTAL MILESTONE OF THE BEHAVIOR OF EXOTIC PET SPECIES

To understand how and when our environmental intervention acts on our exotic pets, we need to be able to discern their normal developmental stages. Each species has evolved very different adaptative strategies to allow for optimal behavioral development from birth or hatching to adulthood. In mammals, we generally recognize 4 major stages including the neonatal stage (birth to eye opening), transition stage (open their eyes, start exploring in the nest, and interact with littermates), weaning stage (start to nibble on solid foods, more active, play, key socialization period), and adolescence (start to get more independence from parents, explore the environment, lasts until sexual maturity). **Table 1** summarizes these stages in some exotic pet species. In many species, the mother will nurse and groom the newborns, keeping them warm, during the neonatal period. They grow very rapidly during this time and are protected mainly by their mother. Even in species born with their eyes open (precocial species such as long-tailed chinchillas and guinea pigs), the first weeks of life still involve a lot of physical maternal care. Psittacine species also follow a similar pattern of behavioral development with major variations in the duration of each period in different species: neonate/hatching, neophyte/nestling, and fledgling stages. Hatchling parrots are altricial with closed eyes and very little down feathers. Very early on, they can stand straight and vocalize when hungry, leading to feeding by their parents, thereby starting the feedback loop of meaningfully interacting with their environment.[16] They will gain weight very rapidly and grow their feathers, as parents regurgitate food for them and protect them from any intruder approaching the nest (Video 1).[17] Neonate behaviors are contextually related: snuggling before sleeping, pumping before eating, and wiggling before defecating (Video 1).[16] As they open their eyes and enter the nestling/neophyte phase, they start exploring the nest and interacting with their parents and clutch mates (Video 1). Neophytes require an environment providing both stimulation and comfort, large enough for practicing wing flapping, climbing, and hiding, allowing for muscle development for future flying and landing behaviors (Video 1).[16,17] Their ears open and they discover their sound environment and intraspecific and interspecific vocalizations through various social interactions. They develop their beak and tongue fine motor skills while preening and eating various food items with different structures and consistencies (Video 1).[16] The fledgling stage is a key step in chick development. They continue to practice movements leading to their eventual first flight (Video 1). They approach the hole of the nest and start discovering the outside environment (Video 1). They gain significant muscular strength during this phase.[17] Once they have fledged, juvenile parrots start a new exploration phase. New vocalizations such as contact calls will be heard.[16] However, they still rely on their parents' protection, even more distant than before, and seek protection from the nest when frightened.[16] They start socializing with other individuals, learning about flock dynamics, and advancing their communication skills. They then start to forage for their own food and, for most species, go through a very progressive phase of weaning (Video 1). A few exceptions include kakapos (*Strigops habroptila*) and some other parrot species, as they can exhibit a more rapid phase of weaning, especially when resources are scarce.[18] It is important though to understand that there are a lot of possible individual variations in this timeline, even within juveniles of the same clutch. Juvenile of most parrot species will take years to reach sexual maturity and their parents can remain an important influence for them for prolonged periods of time.

Table 1
Developmental stages of various mammalian exotic pet species[4]

Phases	Rabbits	Ferrets	Rats	Chinchillas	Guinea Pigs	Degus
Neonatal stage	0–2 wk	0–2 wk	0–12 d	0–3 wk (born eyes open)	0–3 wk (born eyes open)	0–3 wk (born eyes open or eyes open soon after birth)
Transition stage	2–3 wk	2–4 wk	12–18 d			
Weaning stage	3–8 wk	4–8 wk	18–28 d	3–6 wk	3–6 wk	3–6 wk
Adolescence	8–12 wk	8–16 wk	28 d to 5–6 wk	6–24 wk	6–16 wk	6–16 wk

Hatchling reptiles are the opposite; they are mainly precocial and will focus on developing survival skills very early in life, such as reaching water (for turtles), hiding from predators, and seeking shelter. They rapidly begin to hunt for food. Many species are solitary outside of breeding, so socialization may be limited to occasional encounters during subadult and adult stages in the wild. Female crocodilians guard their nests, actively help hatchlings reach water, and defend them from predators during their early lives. Gila monsters (*Heloderma suspectum*), some *Boidae* species, geckos, and agamids guard their eggs. Some species, such as the diamond python (*Python spilotes*), can provide heat to the eggs.[19] A few viviparous female snakes will provide protection to their offspring (eg, boa constrictors [*Boa constrictor*], garter snakes [*Thamnophis sirtalis*], green anacondas [*Eunectes murinus*]).

During normal development in a natural environmental, changes are expected to happen and lead to normal brain development, building adaptability and resilience. When bred in captivity, exotic animals may experience either a lack of normal brain stimulation, abnormally stressful conditions, or inconsistent responses to their behaviors, which can all affect normal behavioral development.

IMPACT OF SELECTED ENVIRONMENTAL FACTORS ON BRAIN DEVELOPMENT
Environmental Conditions During Incubation and Early Life

Environmental variations, including those experienced by birds and reptiles during incubation, can significantly affect the behavioral phenotype of juveniles.[20,21] Though meant to be adaptive, inappropriate conditions such as those possibly encountered in captive settings may result in suboptimal phenotypes.[20] Temperature is one of the most important factors that has been studied. In rats (*Rattus norvegicus*), when given the opportunity, females will make their nest at 86 to 93°F (30–34°C), far from the usual laboratory cage temperatures.[22] Nest temperature has been shown to affect maternal care and pup adrenal gland size in rats.[22] In another study, ducklings incubated at the lowest temperature displayed more proactive behaviors than those incubated at the 2 higher temperatures.[21] In skinks, individuals incubated at a higher temperature were more explorative and demonstrated a larger behavioral repertoire compared to lizards incubated at a lower temperature.[23] Another factor that could influence behavioral development in captivity is lighting. Constant lighting during the perinatal period in rats induced anxietylike behaviors that were retained in adulthood.[24] Artificial switch from diurnal to nocturnal activities has been associated with anxiety and depression-like behaviors in rodents.[25] Comfort, with appropriate substrate and shelter, is also critical in many species. Disruption and limitation of litter supply at an early age in domestic chicks increased severe feather picking, feather damage, and fearfulness.[26] Finally, adequate nutrition, in quality and quantity, is also key to normal brain development, cognitive function, and decreased risk of emotional and behavioral problems in all studied species.[27,28] Links between food, gut microbiome, neurodevelopment, and abnormal behaviors have been established in many species.[29–31] Providing the same quality and variety of food available in the wild to many nondomestic species can be very challenging and could be affecting the behavior development of many psittacines and reptiles. More research may be needed in this area.

Parental Care versus Hand-rearing

There is a whole body of evidence showing the importance of parental care in behavioral development in species where it is part of their biology. Maternal separation is used as a model to induce severe early-life stress in research. Physiologic effects of early maternal separation have been detailed previously. Studies on the behavioral effects of early maternal separation are numerous and all demonstrate how the brain and stress response cannot develop normally when parental care is significantly different from the species' natural biology.[32] Many examples in rodents show that lower levels of maternal care lead to difference in stress reactivity throughout life and affect behavioral and emotional responses.[33] Normal attachment and social behaviors are conditioned by appropriate early social interactions, mainly provided by the mother in altricial mammals in the first weeks of life.[34] Social learning was affected in adult rats that had received lower levels of maternal attention.[35] Stereotypic behaviors and self-mutilations have been documented in relation to early-life stress and maternal deprivation in rodents and many other species.[36] Exotic pet mammals are rarely hand raised, but parents could experience some excessive stress under inappropriate environmental conditions and early weaning or impaired maternal care could participate in neurobiological impairment leading to some of the observed abnormal repetitive behaviors (eg, fur chewing in chinchillas (*Chinchilla lanigera*), corner digging and bar chewing in gerbils, barbering in mice, and so forth).[36–38] Exotic pet birds have historically been hand-reared, if not from hatching, from a much younger age than their wild counterparts, mainly with the goal of producing tame individuals, enjoying human contact and with less fear of what constitutes a captive environment.[39] Unfortunately, after decades of hand-raising parrots, experimental and epidemiologic evidence points toward a different outcome of hand-rearing chicks. Several studies have been comparing the behavioral development of hand-raised versus parent-raised captive parrots. A study on over 100 African gray parrots (*Psittacus erithacus*) showed that hand-raised parrots were more aggressive toward humans than parent-reared birds.[40] Hand-raised parrot chicks that were less than 5 weeks old when removed from their nest developed stereotypies more often than the chicks that stayed longer with their parents.[40] Feather-picking behavior appears to be much less prevalent in parent-raised birds (1.3%) versus hand-raised birds (around 17%) in another study, but confounding variables were considerable (eg, parent-raised birds are more often used as breeding birds than as house pets).[41] A study on 122 peach-faced lovebirds (*Agapornis roseicollis* Vieillot) showed that hand-raised birds were 5 times more at risk to develop feather picking than parent-raised ones.[42] Parental stress, even before hatching, has been associated with severe feather picking and anxiety in chicken (*Gallus gallus domesticus*).[26] Several studies suggest that sexual imprinting occurs in parrots.[39] Myers and colleagues demonstrated that hand-raised cockatiels (*Nymphicus hollandicus*) had less reproductive success than those that were parent-raised because of a combination of abnormal sexual and nesting behaviors.[43] Hand-rearing of orange-winged Amazon parrots (*Amazonica amazonica*) alters juvenile social preferences and vocalizations between 3 and 12 months of age.[39] Hand-raised juvenile Amazons also showed a strong preference for social contact with humans and reduced preference for conspecifics.[39] Hand-raising pet parrots may, therefore, have consequences on later reproductive behaviors, though more studies are needed in this area.[39] Parent-raised birds were shown to have a delayed onset of neophobia, as measured by latency to approach a novel object (6 months vs before 4.5 months of age), but both parent-raised and hand-raised birds were similar at 12 months of age.[44] This study concluded that the differences of exposure to novel objects in the environment at a young age may have influenced the behavior independently of the breeding method.[39,44] This is not to be confused with the sudden fearfulness and generalized anxiety exhibited by some hand-raised parrots at the age where they would normally become independent from their parents, which may be more related to the abnormal development of their HPA axis, as well as their GABA, serotonin, and dopamine pathways.[39] In Williams'[45] study on large parrot species, hand-reared birds exhibited increased incidences of stereotypic behaviors, more learned vocalizations, and inter-acted less with enrichment than parent-reared birds. The lower level of interaction with enrichment is particularly concerning as this could indicate important neurotransmitter dysfunctions preventing the bird from benefiting from an enriched environment if pro-vided later in life. In reptiles, effects of maternal stress are likely underestimated. Glucocorticoid-mediated maternal effects have been shown to be stronger in mam-mals and viviparous squamate reptiles than oviparous species.[46] However, though studies are lacking about long-term effects on reptile behavior development directly linked to parental care, the effects of social environment have been studied in reptiles and other species.

Early Social Environment with Conspecifics

Many exotic pet species give birth to multiple offsprings who would spend weeks to months in very close relationship under natural circumstances. Interactions with clutch or littermates are a part of their normal behavioral development. Keeping individuals in appropriate social groups, as mentioned by Brandão & Mayer,[47] is key to their welfare and normal social development. Keeping social animals as singletons can lead to chronic stress as it denies them the opportunity to display a range of natural behaviors such as play, allogrooming, and group vigilance.[48] Studies across species have shown that social isolation, especially in early life, can lead to cognitive impairments and mental health issues.[49] In rabbits (*Oryctolagus cuniculus*), for example, keeping juve-niles in mixed-sex groups between 6 and 11 weeks of age decreased the frequency of stereotypic behaviors.[50] Keeping growing rabbits as pairs decreased their fear levels and allowed them to express a wider range of behaviors.[51] Play deprivation has been demonstrated in rats, even without complete social isolation, showing how important this complex behavior is for periadolescent rats.[52] On the other hand, keep-ing solitary animals (ie, golden hamster [*Mesocricetus auratus*]) in groups may be stressful and result in aggression.[53] But group-housed hamsters in enriched environ-ments appear to prefer company.[53] Many rodents are kept in unisex groups to decrease the potential of reproduction and aggression. However, there are very few species living in unisex groups in the wild and more studies are needed to understand the impact of this type of grouping.[53] Single or pair housing of adolescent Amazon par-rots that had been parent-raised for their first 6 months was compared in an experi-mental controlled environment.[54] Results were striking: no pair-housed bird developed any stereotypies, versus 57% of singly housed birds; pair-housed birds used their enrichment more, screamed less, preened more, spent less time being inac-tive, climbed, walked, and flew more, and were less fearful of unfamiliar handlers.[52] There was no difference in interaction with familiar handlers.[54] Another study on zoo-housed parrots also showed that solo-housed birds preened less and display more stereotypic behaviors.[45] In reptiles, few studies have been published and envi-ronmental confounding variables are difficult to examine independently of social hous-ing. Early social isolation affected the behaviors regrouped to represent boldness and sociability traits of young garter snakes, with sex-dependent effects.[55] Hatchling veiled chameleons (*Chamaeleo calyptratus*) raised in isolation fled more and curled up into a ball more during social interactions and had lower performance in a foraging task.[56] They also interestingly expressed different colors than those raised in groups.[56] Viperine water snakes *(Natrix maura)* incubated from eggs without physical contact with other eggs were less social than those from clustered eggs: they were more active, aggregated less, and did not physically get in contact with others as often as the other group.[57] Another study in a social lizard species, the tree skink (*Egernia strio-lata*), found evidence of an impact of social environment on behavioral development but also documented some negative impact for 1 of the 2 lizards that were paired during development.[58] The authors also highlighted the fact that lack of social interaction and the nature of social interactions are factors of potential impact and divergence across behavioral development.[58] Tree skinks appeared to cope well in social isolation, which could be explained by possible social variations in wild rearing conditions.[58] Though it may seem intuitive to follow natural rearing conditions to improve individual welfare, this may be an oversimplification of what is actually observed under captive conditions. More research is also required in this area.

Early Human Handling

An important question when raising animals intended to live close to humans throughout their lives is: how much human interaction should we provide, when, and how should we do it? There are only partial answers to these key questions in the current literature. What have been well documented are the effects of early handling of rats, consisting of transferring all pups together in another cage and then back after a few minutes.[59] Repeating this procedure every day for the first 21 days of life resulted in decreased HPA responsivity to stress throughout adulthood.[59] In a study with orange-winged Amazon parrots, chicks were temporarily removed from the nest box and handled at various times during the nestling period.[60] Parent-reared birds that had been handled exhibited approximately equal preference for human and conspecific companionship.[60] Handled birds showed willingness to approach and be picked up by the handler, indifference to dorsal contact, cooperation during intravenous blood withdrawal, acceptance of food from the handler, willingness to sit on the handler's arm, and lack of an increase in respiration rate in the presence of the handler.[60]

The investigators suggest that "neonatal handling may enable captive parrots to react in a more physiologically benign manner to the potential stress of human presence, intrusion, or contact" and "appears to enhance the ability of parrots to adapt to exigencies of the captive environment."[60] Chicks handled a little later appeared to be tamer than those handled earlier.[60] Collette and colleagues repeated these results with all indicators of tameness being increased in handled birds.[61] However, they noted that some chicks resisted being handled, mostly associated with parental defensive behavior toward the handler.[61] Cramton[62] studied the effects of handler empathy on parrot tameness and showed that though no significant differences in tameness could be detected between low-empathy or high-empathy handlers, chicks handled by low-empathy handlers experienced significantly more stress. This shows that there are a very large number of environmental factors that can individually affect a young parrot's experience during early handling and that more research is required to better comprehend the impact and timing of handling during early life.

Environmental Enrichment

Effects of environmental enrichment are challenging to analyze and summarize as there are an infinite number of ways to provide enrichment to growing animals, whether it be a different substrate, a place to hide or to dig, social opportunities, food enrichment, and so forth. In some studies, enrichment provided could lead to aggression between individuals if they were to fight for access to enrichment, which is obviously not the intended goal.[50] Rabbits provided wood sticks for enrichment would show more aggression but resulted in less skin wounds and less stereotypic behaviors.[50] However, when appropriately designed, several studies have shown that environmental enrichment can actually reverse some of the adverse effects of maternal deprivation and reduce anxietylike behaviors in adulthood.[63,64] There is an extensive body of literature on the positive effects on the brain and neurodevelopment of enrichment in laboratory rodents. Enriched environments with physical, sensory, and stimulatory additions can optimize the birds' development.[65] Enriched environments also have the potential to enhance immune function through the application of mild stressors that promote adaptability.[65] An experimental study in orange-winged Amazon parrots revealed that juvenile parrots raised in barred cages developed significantly more stereotypic behaviors than parrots raised in enriched cages.[66] Onset of stereotypic behavior, as well as rate and magnitude, also increased between the 2 groups.[66] Another study using the same species showed that the effects of enrichment were similar but highly variable between individuals.[67] Enrichment also reduced the fear response to novel objects and increased the motivation to explore and interact with those objects in young Amazons and reduced fear of unfamiliar handlers.[68] A critical review on behavioral effects of enrichment in psittacines has been published.[69] They observed that documented types of enrichment involve foraging and physical modifications, while enrichment based on sensorial stimuli was lacking.[69] The investigators concluded that "In addition to being biologically relevant, enrichment should include opportunities to solve challenges and exert control on the environment."[69] Behavioral complexity of reptilian and amphibian species makes enrichment necessary to encourage natural behaviors and welfare in captivity.[70] However, there is a lack of knowledge on the effects of environmental enrichment on reptilian and amphibian behavioral development.[70] Finally, though this article mainly focuses on exotic animals kept as pets, it is worth noting that environmental enrichment is critical when breeding individuals from endangered species intended to be reintroduced in the wild.[71] Captive breeding programs need to provide growing animals with all opportunities to learn predator avoidance, foraging, normal social interaction, habitat selection, as well as exercise for physical fitness.[71]

Pain and Medications

Though painful elective procedures are not common in juvenile exotic pets, it is important for practitioners to be aware that an extensive amount of literature has documented the long-term consequences of neonatal inflammation and pain in many species, from rodents to humans. These include abnormal pain sensitivity, fear, anxiety, abnormal response of the HPA axis to stress, alterations in spatial cognition, social behavior, and reproductive development. All these can be observed throughout the individual's life and even impact the next generation.[72,73] In addition, many drugs administered very early in life can impact the developing brain. This has been demonstrated with almost all tested anesthetic drugs (including ketamine, midazolam, isoflurane, sevoflurane, and other such drugs) shown to induce dose-dependent and duration-dependent neurologic impairments, assumed to be related to anesthetic-induced neuronal inhibition.[74]

In summary, almost every sensorial, social, or physiologic event in early life will shape the developing brain, sometimes with long-term consequences. More research is needed to better understand some of the effects associated with raising nondomestic animals in human-controlled environments, particularly regarding the way humans and animals interact together.

PRACTICAL RECOMMENDATIONS FOR DEVELOPING EXOTIC PETS

Behavioral issues reported in exotic pets include a variety of presentations ranging from abnormal repetitive behaviors, excessive vocalizations, food begging, aggression, house soiling, and so forth. Each of these presentations must be considered in

Box 1
Recommendations to promote behavioral health in developing exotic pets[16,27,34,47,48,53,54,75,76]

- Carefully consider the choice of owning a nondomestic animal as a pet.

- Breed behaviorally healthy and human-conditioned animals in low-stress but enriched environments, before and during pregnancy.

- Incubate eggs under conditions resembling natural ones:
  - Keep reptile eggs close to each other to allow communication.
  - Allow parents to incubate avian eggs in species-appropriate nests.
  - Use cameras to monitor eggs and chicks without disturbing parents.

- Allow parental behavior to be expressed with minimal disruption:
  - Interactions between humans and juveniles could occur when parents allow these to happen without any major stress noted.

- Provide a low-stress, enriched, and predictable environment for the parents to raise their juveniles when species-appropriate:
  - Provide opportunity to dig and hide for burrowing animals.
  - Promote species-specific behaviors including flying and foraging behaviors in psittacine birds.

- Provide an environment that empowers developing animals to the greatest extent possible and promotes species-appropriate behaviors:
  - Physical environment allows motor skill and emotional development
  - Juveniles need to experience the consequences of their behaviors.

- Provide species-appropriate nutrition, in quality, quantity, variety, colors, consistency, and taste.

- Do not perform any physical alterations resulting in the prevention of learning specific behaviors:
  - Do not clip feathers in developing birds.

- Train juveniles using operant conditioning with positive reinforcement as early as possible.

- All forms of punishment should be avoided as much as possible.

- Promote appropriate social interactions:
  - Keep litter and clutch mates together as biologically appropriate, promoting learning social behaviors and play.
  - Monitor social interactions and adjust the environment as needed.
  - Consider individual variations as some species may be solitary in the wild but enjoy intraspecific interaction in captivity, and the opposite may also be true.
  - Keep parrots in pairs or in larger groups allowing pairing if separated from their parents after weaning.

- Allow some minor stress to be experienced, but avoid any major stressor during gametogenesis, pregnancy/incubation, and early development:
  - Avoid predator presence or smell in a prey environment.
  - Avoid unnecessary medical interventions.

- Train with operant conditioning with positive reinforcement for basic behaviors:
  - Litter training/house training
  - Moving from a point to another
  - Recall behavior

- Provide species-appropriate medical care without excessive early intervention:
  - Promote biomedical training from an early age.
  - Habituate animals to be gently handled in a towel.

- Regularly assess the individual behavior and welfare, and adjust the environment accordingly:
  - Owners should be educated about their pet's body language and biological needs.

- Individuals presenting with dysfunction of their stress and emotional response system (severe stereotypies, generalized anxiety, and so forth) may benefit from environmental changes, behavior modification training, and drugs promoting neurogenesis in the serotonin and dopamine pathways.

the context of the unique physical, biological, and physiologic environment of each patient. Behavior being the result of such complex interactions, including during development as the author just demonstrated in this article, it is and should remain, as well expressed by Dr Susan Friedman, the "study of one."[16] However, based on the current literature, some recommendations could be made to try to prevent behavior problems from occurring and to improve animal welfare and the human-animal bond. These may have to be reviewed as we keep learning more about the behavioral development in exotic pet species. **Box 1** summarizes the most important recommendations to support our exotic animal behavioral health.

SUMMARY

As our knowledge in epigenetic and brain-environment interactions progresses, our understanding on how we can adjust our captive breeding conditions of exotic pets keeps expanding. To develop resilient, flexible, and adaptive stress (HPA axis, norepinephrine) and emotional (serotonin, dopamine, GABA) responses, growing individuals need to be conceived from mentally healthy parents, under normal environmental conditions during incubation or pregnancy, and grow in a physically and intellectually challenging environment, surrounded by an appropriate social group, positively learning to interact with this environment. Though more research is needed, current evidence suggests that some common practices may have a negative impact on animal health and welfare, such as premature weaning, hand-raising, or keeping animals in environments that prevent them from displaying natural behaviors, such as flying in birds. Many studies are now showing how alternative ways of raising exotic animals, for example, by providing both parental care and well-timed human interactions, could decrease behavioral and mental health issues encountered in some of our patients. Empowering growing animals to control their environment, making their behaviors meaningful, will likely help them adjust better to long-term life as pets. With adequate positive training from early age, juvenile exotic pets become easier to handle and may seek human contact, which will improve their welfare, the human-animal bond, and ultimately their health.

CLINICS CARE POINTS

- Breed behaviorally healthy and human-conditioned animals in low-stress but enriched environments, before and during pregnancy.
- Allow parental behavior to be expressed with minimal disruption in a low-stress, enriched and predictable environment.
- Provide an environment that empowers developing animals and promotes species-appropriate behaviors.
- Do not perform any physical alterations resulting in prevention of learning specific behaviors (ex. feather clipping).
- Train juveniles using operant conditioning with positive reinforcement as early as possible without disrupting normal intraspecific interactions.
- Promote appropriate social interactions.
- Individuals presenting with dysfunction of their stress and emotional response system (severe stereotypies, generalized anxiety, etc.) may benefit from environmental changes, behavior modification training, and drugs promoting neurogenesis in the serotonin and dopamine pathways.

DISCLOSURE

I have no commercial or financial conflict of interest.

SUPPLEMENTARY DATA

Supplementary data related to this article can be found online at https://doi.org/10.1016/j.cvex.2023.11.015.

REFERENCES

1. LaFreniere P, MacDonald K. A post-genomic view of behavioral development and adaptation to the environment. Dev Rev 2013;33(2):89–109.
2. Dugatkin LA. The silver fox domestication experiment. Evol Educ Outreach 2018; 11(1):16.
3. Deichmann U. Epigenetics: The origins and evolution of a fashionable topic. Dev Biol 2016;416(1):249–54.
4. van Dyck LI, Morrow EM. Genetic control of postnatal human brain growth. Curr Opin Neurol 2017;30(1):114–24.
5. Stevens LM, Landis SC. Developmental interactions between sweat glands and the sympathetic neurons which innervate them: Effects of delayed innervation on neurotransmitter plasticity and gland maturation. Dev Biol 1988;130(2): 703–20.
6. Waterland RA, Jirtle RL. Transposable Elements: Targets for Early Nutritional Effects on Epigenetic Gene Regulation. Mol Cell Biol 2003;23(15):5293–300.
7. Chemical & Engineering News: Government & Policy - Bisphenol A On Trial. Accessed July 31, 2023. https://pubsapp.acs.org/cen/government/85/8516gov2.html.
8. Kolb B, Gibb R. Brain Plasticity and Behaviour in the Developing Brain. J Can Acad Child Adolesc Psychiatry 2011;20(4):265–76.
9. Lee SH, Jung EM. Adverse effects of early-life stress: focus on the rodent neuroendocrine system. Neural Regen Res. 2024;19(2):336-341.
10. Siviy SM. A Brain Motivated to Play: Insights into the Neurobiology of Playfulness. Behaviour 2016;153(6–7):819–44.
11. Schultz W. Neuronal Reward and Decision Signals: From Theories to Data. Physiol Rev 2015;95(3):853–951.
12. Rosenblum LA, Andrews MW. Influences of environmental demand on maternal behavior and infant development. Acta Paediatr Oslo Nor 1994;397:57–63, 1992 Suppl.
13. Meaney MJ. Maternal Care, Gene Expression, and the Transmission of Individual Differences in Stress Reactivity Across Generations. Annu Rev Neurosci 2001; 24(1):1161–92.
14. Wiedenmayer C. Causation of the ontogenetic development of stereotypic digging in gerbils. Anim Behav 1997;53(3):461–70.
15. Rende R. Behavioral resilience in the post-genomic era: emerging models linking genes with environment. Front Hum Neurosci 2012;6:50.
16. Linden PG, Luescher AU. Behavioral Development of Psittacine Companions: Neonates, Neophytes, and Fledglings. In: Luescher A, editor. *Manual of parrot behavior.* John Wiley & Sons, Ltd; 2006. p. 93–111. https://doi.org/10.1002/9780470344651.ch11.
17. Harcourt-Brown N. Development of the skeleton and feathers of dusky parrots (*Pionus fuscus*) in relation to their behaviour. Vet Rec 2004;154(2):42–8.

18. Powlesland RG, Lloyd BD, Best HA, et al. Breeding biology of the Kakapo *Strigops habroptilus* on Stewart Island, New Zealand. Ibis 1992;134(4):361–73.

19. Harlow P, Grigg G. Shivering Thermogenesis in a Brooding Diamond Python, Python spilotes spilotes. Copeia 1984;1984(4):959–65.

20. Hope SF, Kennamer RA, Moore IT, et al. Incubation temperature influences the behavioral traits of a young precocial bird. J Exp Zool Part Ecol Integr Physiol 2018;329(4–5):191–202.

21. While GM, Noble DWA, Uller T, et al. Patterns of developmental plasticity in response to incubation temperature in reptiles. J Exp Zool Part Ecol Integr Physiol 2018;329(4–5):162–76.

22. Jans JE, Woodside BC. Nest temperature: effects on maternal behavior, pup development, and interactions with handling. Dev Psychobiol 1990;23(6):519–34.

23. de Jong M, Phillips BL, Llewelyn J, et al. Effects of developmental environment on animal personality in a tropical skink. Behav Ecol Sociobiol 2022;76(10):137.

24. Roman E, Karlsson O. Increased anxiety-like behavior but no cognitive impairments in adult rats exposed to constant light conditions during perinatal development. Ups J Med Sci 2013;118(4):222–7.

25. Bilu C, Zimmet P, Vishnevskia-Dai V, et al. Diurnality, Type 2 Diabetes, and Depressive-Like Behavior. J Biol Rhythms 2019;34(1):69–83.

26. Haas EN de, Bolhuis JE, Kemp B, et al. Parents and Early Life Environment Affect Behavioral Development of Laying Hen Chickens. PLoS One 2014;9(3):e90577.

27. Black M, Dubowitz H. Failure-to-Thrive: Lessons from Animal Models and Developing Countries. J Dev Behav Pediatr 1991;12(4):259.

28. Ajmone-Cat MA, De Simone R, Tartaglione AM, et al. Critical Role of Maternal Selenium Nutrition in Neurodevelopment: Effects on Offspring Behavior and Neuroinflammatory Profile. Nutrients 2022;14(9):1850.

29. Warner BB. The contribution of the gut microbiome to neurodevelopment and neuropsychiatric disorders. Pediatr Res 2019;85(2):216–24.

30. Hartman S, Sayler K, Belsky J. Prenatal stress enhances postnatal plasticity: The role of microbiota. Dev Psychobiol 2019;61(5):729–38.

31. Sachser N, Zimmermann TD, Hennessy MB, et al. Sensitive phases in the development of rodent social behavior. Curr Opin Behav Sci 2020;36:63–70.

32. Czerwinski VH, Smith BP, Hynd PI, et al. The influence of maternal care on stress-related behaviors in domestic dogs: What can we learn from the rodent literature? J Vet Behav 2016;14:52–9.

33. Caldji C, Diorio J, Meaney MJ. Variations in maternal care in infancy regulate the development of stress reactivity. Biol Psychiatr 2000;48(12):1164–74.

34. Packard K, Opendak M. Rodent models of early adversity: Impacts on developing social behavior circuitry and clinical implications. Front Behav Neurosci. 2022;16 https://www.frontiersin.org/articles/10.3389/fnbeh.2022.918862. Accessed August 11, 2023.

35. Lindeyer CM, Meaney MJ, Reader SM. Early maternal care predicts reliance on social learning about food in adult rats. Dev Psychobiol 2013;55(2):168–75.

36. Latham NR, Mason GJ. Maternal deprivation and the development of stereotypic behaviour. Appl Anim Behav Sci 2008;110(1–2):84–108.

37. Vergneau-Grosset C, Ruel H. Abnormal Repetitive Behaviors and Self-Mutilations in Small Mammals. Vet Clin Exot Anim Pract 2021;24(1):87–102.

38. Waiblinger E, König B. Housing and husbandry conditions affect stereotypic behaviour in laboratory gerbils. ALTEX; 2007.

39. Fox R, Hand-Rearing. Behavioral Impacts and Implications for Captive Parrot Welfare. In: Luescher A, editor. *Manual of parrot behavior.* John Wiley & Sons, Ltd; 2006. p. 83–91. https://doi.org/10.1002/9780470344651.ch10.

40. Schmid R, Doherr MG, Steiger A. The influence of the breeding method on the behaviour of adult African grey parrots (*Psittacus erithacus*). Appl Anim Behav Sci 2006;98(3):293–307.

41. Costa P, Macchi E, Tomassone L, et al. Feather picking in pet parrots: sensitive species, risk factor and ethological evidence. Ital J Anim Sci 2016;15(3):473–80.

42. Ebisawa K, Kusuda S, Nakayama S, et al. Effects of rearing methods on feather-damaging behavior and corticosterone metabolite excretion in the peach-faced lovebird (*Agapornis roseicollis* Vieillot). J Vet Behav 2022;54:28–35.

43. Myers SA, Millam JR, Roudybush TE, et al. Reproductive Success of Hand-Reared vs. Parent-Reared Cockatiels (*Nymphicus hollandicus*). The Auk 1988; 105(3):536–42.

44. Fox RA, Millam JR. The effect of early environment on neophobia in orange-winged Amazon parrots (*Amazona amazonica*). Appl Anim Behav Sci 2004; 89(1–2):117–29.

45. Williams I, Hoppitt W, Grant R. The effect of auditory enrichment, rearing method and social environment on the behavior of zoo-housed psittacines (Aves: Psitta-ciformes); implications for welfare. Appl Anim Behav Sci 2017;186:85–92.

46. MacLeod KJ, While GM, Uller T. Viviparous mothers impose stronger glucocorticoid-mediated maternal stress effects on their offspring than oviparous mothers. Ecol Evol 2021;11(23):17238–59.

47. Brandão J, Mayer J. Behavior of Rodents with an Emphasis on Enrichment. J Exot Pet Med 2011;20(4):256–69.

48. McBride EA. Small prey species' behaviour and welfare: implications for veteri-nary professionals. J Small Anim Pract 2017;58(8):423–36.

49. Cacioppo JT, Hawkley LC. Perceived social isolation and cognition. Trends Cog-nit Sci 2009;13(10):447–54.

50. Bozicovich TFM, Moura ASAMT, Fernandes S, et al. Effect of environmental enrichment and composition of the social group on the behavior, welfare, and relative brain weight of growing rabbits. Appl Anim Behav Sci 2016;182:72–9.

51. Trocino A, Majolini D, Tazzoli M, et al. Housing of growing rabbits in individual, bicellular and collective cages: fear level and behavioural patterns. Animal 2013;7(4):633–9.

52. Holloway KS, Suter RB. Play deprivation without social isolation: Housing con-trols. Dev Psychobiol 2004;44(1):58–67.

53. Sørensen DB, Krohn T, Hansen HN, et al. An ethological approach to housing re-quirements of golden hamsters, Mongolian gerbils and fat sand rats in the labo-ratory—A review. Appl Anim Behav Sci 2005;94(3):181–95.

54. Meehan CL, Garner JP, Mench JA. Isosexual pair housing improves the welfare of young Amazon parrots. Appl Anim Behav Sci 2003;81(1):73–88.

55. Skinner M, Brown S, Kumpan LT, et al. Snake personality: Differential effects of development and social experience. Behav Ecol Sociobiol 2022;76(10):135.

56. Ballen C, Shine R, Olsson M. Effects of early social isolation on the behaviour and performance of juvenile lizards, Chamaeleo calyptratus. Anim Behav 2014; 88:1–6.

57. Aubret F, Bignon F, Kok PJR, et al. Only child syndrome in snakes: Eggs incu-bated alone produce asocial individuals. Sci Rep 2016;6(1):35752.

58. Riley JL, Noble DWA, Byrne RW, et al. Early social environment influences the behaviour of a family-living lizard. R Soc Open Sci 2017;4(5):161082.

59. Meaney MJ, Diorio J, Francis D, et al. Early environmental regulation of forebrain glucocorticoid receptor gene expression: implications for adrenocortical responses to stress. Dev Neurosci 1996;18(1–2):49–72.

60. Aengus WL, Millam JR. Taming parent-reared orange-winged Amazon parrots by neonatal handling. Zoo Biol 1999;18(3):177–87.

61. Collette JC, Millam JR, Klasing KC, et al. Neonatal handling of Amazon parrots alters the stress response and immune function. Appl Anim Behav Sci 2000; 66(4):335–49.

62. Cramton B, Handler. Attitude and Chick Development. In: Luescher A, editor. Manual of parrot behavior. John Wiley & Sons, Ltd; 2006. p. 113–31.

63. Ciucci F, Putignano E, Baroncelli L, et al. Insulin-Like Growth Factor 1 (IGF-1) Mediates the Effects of Enriched Environment (EE) on Visual Cortical Development. PLoS One 2007;2(5):e475.

64. Baldini S, Restani L, Baroncelli L, et al. Enriched Early Life Experiences Reduce Adult Anxiety-Like Behavior in Rats: A Role for Insulin-Like Growth Factor 1. J Neurosci 2013;33(28):11715–23.

65. Campbell DLM, de Haas EN, Lee C. A review of environmental enrichment for laying hens during rearing in relation to their behavioral and physiological development. Poultry Sci 2019;98(1):9–28.

66. Meehan CL, Garner JP, Mench JA. Environmental enrichment and development of cage stereotypy in Orange-winged Amazon parrots (Amazona amazonica). Dev Psychobiol 2004;44(4):209–18.

67. Cussen VA, Mench JA. The Relationship between Personality Dimensions and Resiliency to Environmental Stress in Orange-Winged Amazon Parrots (Amazona amazonica), as Indicated by the Development of Abnormal Behaviors. PLoS One 2015;10(6):e0126170.

68. Meehan CL, Mench JA. Environmental enrichment affects the fear and exploratory responses to novelty of young Amazon parrots. Appl Anim Behav Sci 2002;79(1):75–88.

69. Rodríguez-López R. Environmental enrichment for parrot species: Are we squawking up the wrong tree? Appl Anim Behav Sci 2016;180:1–10.

70. Burghardt GM. Environmental enrichment and cognitive complexity in reptiles and amphibians: Concepts, review, and implications for captive populations. Appl Anim Behav Sci 2013;147(3):286–98.

71. Reading RP, Miller B, Shepherdson D. The Value of Enrichment to Reintroduction Success. Zoo Biol 2013;32(3):332–41.

72. Adcock SJJ. Early Life Painful Procedures: Long-Term Consequences and Implications for Farm Animal Welfare. Front Anim Sci. 2021;2 https://www.frontiersin. org/articles/10.3389/fanim.2021.759522. Accessed July 24, 2023.

73. McGrath PJ, Stevens BJ, Walker SM, et al. Oxford textbook of paediatric pain. OUP Oxford; 2013.

74. Istaphanous GK, Loepke AW. General anesthetics and the developing brain. Curr Opin Anesthesiol 2009;22(3):368.

75. Daugette KF, Hoppes S, Tizard I, et al. Positive Reinforcement Training Facilitates the Voluntary Participation of Laboratory Macaws With Veterinary Procedures. J Avian Med Surg 2012;26(4):248–54.

76. Friedman Sg, Martin S and Brinker B. Behavior Analysis and Parrot Learning, In: Luescher A, editor. Manual of parrot behavior, 2006, John Wiley & Sons, Ltd, 147–163.

77. Pignon C, Mayer J, Pigs Guinea. In: Quesenberry K, Orcutt CJ, Mans C and Carpenter JW. Ferrets, rabbits, and Rodents - Clinical Medicine and Surgery, 4th edition, 2021, W.B. Saunders, 270–297.
78. Jekl VDE, Degus. In: Quesenberry K, Orcutt CJ, Mans C, Carpenter JW. Ferrets, rabbits, and Rodents - Clinical Medicine and Surgery, 4th edition, 2021, W.B. Saunders, 323–333.
79. Mans C and Donnelly TM. Chinchillas, In: Quesenberry K, Orcutt CJ, Mans C, Carpenter JW. Ferrets, rabbits, and Rodents - Clinical Medicine and Surgery, 4th edition, 2021, W.B. Saunders, 298–322.
80. Frohlich J, Rats and Mice, In: Quesenberry K, Orcutt CJ, Mans C, Carpenter JW. Ferrets, rabbits, and Rodents - Clinical Medicine and Surgery, 4th edition, 2021, W.B. Saunders, 345–367.
81. Fisher PG. Chapter 4 - Ferret behavior. In: Bays TB, Lightfoot T, Mayer J, editors. Exotic pet behavior. W.B. Saunders; 2006. p. 163–205.
82. Bays TB. Chapter 5 - Guinea pig behavior. In: Bays TB, Lightfoot T, Mayer J, editors. Exotic pet behavior. W.B. Saunders; 2006. p. 207–38.
83. Evans EI. Chapter 6 - Small rodent behavior: mice, rats, gerbils, and hamsters. In: Bays TB, Lightfoot T, Mayer J, editors. Exotic pet behavior. W.B. Saunders; 2006. p. 239–61.
84. Bays TB. Chapter 1 - Rabbit behavior. In: Bays TB, Lightfoot T, Mayer J, editors. Exotic pet behavior. W.B. Saunders; 2006. p. 1–49.

Nutritional Considerations for Juvenile Exotic Companion Animals

Amanda Ardente, DVM, PhD[a],*, Barbara Toddes, MS[b],
Rhiannon L. Schultz, MA[c]

KEYWORDS

- Small mammal • Reptile • Avian • Nutrition • Juvenile • Pediatric • Exotic pet

KEY POINTS

- Natural history, feeding strategy, energy requirement, digestive physiology and diet digestibility, and key nutrients of concern are all necessary factors to consider when determining an appropriate diet for pediatric exotic species.
- Small exotic companion mammals range from strict carnivores to specialist omnivores to herbivores, so understanding natural history and dietary needs is necessary to promote appropriate growth and gastrointestinal health.
- Particularly for captive reptiles, husbandry practices, including lighting, humidity, temperature, and substrate, work in concert with diet to ensure optimal health.
- Bird owners must closely monitor body weight and offer food for enrichment and/or training only after the complete feed portion of the diet is consumed.

INTRODUCTION

Pediatric exotic companion animal nutrition is a broad topic, spanning small mammals, reptiles, and birds. As with any animal, it is important to provide these species with appropriate diets while growing, to set them up for a healthy life in adulthood. Little research has been done focusing on the juvenile life stages of these species because they are largely adopted by clients as young adults. The information that does exist has been compiled by wildlife rehabilitators, commercial breeders, and/ or exotic captive breeding programs, such as those that exist in zoologic facilities. Husbandry practices are also closely tied to the health and wellness of juvenile exotics and directly influence the diet provided and/or consumed. Although discussion of husbandry and behavioral wellness is beyond the scope of this article, species-specific

[a] Ardente Veterinary Nutrition LLC, 399 Southeast 90th Street, Ocala, FL 34480, USA;
[b] Philadelphia Zoo, 3400 West Girard Avenue, Philadelphia, PA 19104, USA; [c] Animal Welfare Expertise Ltd, Littleton Manor, Winchester, SO22 6QU, UK
* Corresponding author.
E-mail address: amanda@ardentevetnutrition.com

Vet Clin Exot Anim 27 (2024) 449–463
https://doi.org/10.1016/j.cvex.2023.11.016
1094-9194/24/© 2023 Elsevier Inc. All rights reserved.

considerations may be discussed in later sections if strongly relevant to an animal's nutritional health.

Natural history, feeding strategy, energy requirement, digestive physiology and diet digestibility, and key nutrients of concern are all necessary factors to consider when determining an appropriate diet for pediatric exotic species. In terms of energy, the basal metabolic requirement (BMR) must be met, and to support growth, a surplus of energy, with sufficient protein, calcium, and vitamin D are necessary. The use of a commercial complete feed is generally recommended as the base diet for all species to ensure energy requirements and micronutrient needs are met. Many of the products on the market have been formulated for specific species' nutrient recommendations.

Of the 86.9 million households in the US owning pets, approximately 37% have exotic pets.[1] Of these client-owned exotics, species variability is vast. This article, therefore, cannot discuss all aspects of pediatric nutrition for each nondomestic species kept as a pet. Nevertheless, we will attempt to summarize important species-specific diet considerations during the juvenile life stage for some of the most commonly encountered exotic pets in veterinary practice.

CONSIDERATIONS FOR SMALL MAMMALS

Rabbits (*Oryctolagus cuniculus*), guinea pigs (*Cavia porcellus*), and chinchillas (*Chinchilla* spp) are herbivorous hindgut fermenters with a large cecum to accommodate microbial fermentation, synthesis of B-vitamins and amino acids, and nutrient recycling by cecotrophy. Rabbits are born altricial and should not be adopted before 12 weeks of age. Instead, rabbits should be adopted postweaning with well-formed stool. Guinea pigs and chinchillas, however, are born precocial. Guinea pigs nurse until ~4 weeks of age, whereas chinchillas nurse for 6 to 8 weeks. Chinchillas can start consuming semisolid/solid food as early as 1 week, and guinea pigs as early as 2 weeks. Guinea pigs can be purchased/adopted the earliest, as soon as 2 to 4 weeks of age, or once greater than 250 g body weight, and chinchillas at 10 weeks of age.[2–4]

Neonatal hand-rearing is beyond the scope of this article, so the discussion regarding juvenile nutrition will start postweaning. Generally, these species are not considered fully grown until 12 to 15 months or as soon as 9 months for some large breed rabbits.[2–4] Growing rabbits require 2 to 3 times the energy required for a healthy adult at maintenance, calculated as $\sim 100 \times$ (body weight kg)$^{0.75}$.[4,5] Smaller breeds and colder environmental temperatures increase the energy requirement to approximately 3 times maintenance.[2,4] For guinea pigs, healthy adults weighing 400 to 600g require 136 kcal metabolizable energy (ME)/$BW_{kg}^{0.75}$ but growing guinea pigs should be provided $\sim 3,000$ kcal ME/kg of diet.[3,4] No equation has been suggested for chinchillas but their energetic needs are likely comparable.

Rabbits and guinea pigs are diurnal species but chinchillas are crepuscular and, therefore, should be fed a large portion of their diet in the evening.[6] Diets primarily consist of a species-specific commercial pellet formulated with grass hay, and grass hay (eg, orchard, timothy, Bermuda) fed *ad libitum*. Some feeding recommendations include leguminous hay (eg, alfalfa) but high protein and calcium concentrations may facilitate rapid growth, which is likely not ideal for pet owners, and predispose future development of calcium-based uroliths.[5–9] The inclusion of *ad libitum* hay in the diet is necessary to ensure adequate dry matter (DM) intake, with appropriately long fibrous strands to support dental, gastrointestinal, and microbial health.[10] Related key nutrients of concern for these growing, herbivorous, hind-gut fermenters are protein and essential amino acids, fiber, minerals and vitamins, specifically calcium and vitamin D3, and, for guinea pigs, vitamin C.

The protein requirement of growing rabbits is 15% to 16% DM and is slightly greater for guinea pigs and chinchillas at 18% to 20%.[4,5,7] Essential amino acid requirements can be met with a high-quality protein source and appropriate cecotrophy.[4,10,11] Concerning fiber, feeding a total daily amount and appropriate forms (short vs long fibers) from an early age will establish optimal gut and dental health for adulthood. Insufficient fiber can lead to gastrointestinal tract dysfunction (eg, functional ileus), resulting in abdominal discomfort, scant feces, anorexia, and death. Commercial pellets should contain 10% to 16% fiber DM for guinea pigs and as much as 20% to 25% fiber DM for rabbits.[5,8] Pellets supply short fiber strands, whereas leguminous hays supply long fiber strands necessary for long-term gut health.[4,5] It is important to note, however, that high-protein, high-calcium legume hays should not be fed long term due to the risk of obesity and development of calcium-based urolithiasis; therefore, a gradual transition to grass hay as animals reach adulthood is recommended to prevent these health problems.[4]

Mineral requirements rely on relative concentrations and interactions. If a high-quality, plant-based commercial pellet and hay are fed, all mineral requirements should be met and balanced. Requiring additional consideration are calcium and phosphorus because of their role in bone growth. The recommended calcium-to-phosphorous ratio (Ca:P) for growth is approximately 1.5 to 2. Dietary deficiency of these minerals, or a low Ca:P, can lead to nutritional secondary hyperparathyroidism, or metabolic bone disease (MBD), characterized by fibrous osteodystrophy and osteomalacia; however, excess dietary calcium can cause mineral imbalances/deficiencies, tissue mineralization, and calcium-based urolithiasis. Oversupplementation should therefore be avoided, and particularly once animals have reached sexual maturity, ensure grass hay (not leguminous hay) is provided.[3,5,7,9]

Vitamin requirements are again generally met by a high-quality diet and appropriate cecotrophy, except vitamin C for guinea pigs. Vitamin C, or ascorbic acid, is an essential nutrient for guinea pigs because guinea pigs lack L-gulonolactone oxidase, which synthesizes ascorbic acid from glucose in vivo. This nutrient must therefore be provided by the diet to avoid deficiency symptoms, such as scurvy. Complete feeds formulated for guinea pigs are generally fortified with a shelf-stable vitamin C; however, pellet formulation, feed storage temperature and humidity, length of storage time, and exposure to air can all cause rapid oxidation of ascorbic acid. Supplementation is therefore recommended. Aqueous solutions of vitamin C added to drinking water lose potency rapidly, so, instead, options include (1) crushing a vitamin C tablet and adding it to feed or providing as a chewable tablet, (2) adding an aqueous supplement to a small amount of water that is rapidly, voluntarily consumed; or (3) providing produce rich in ascorbic acid (eg, bell peppers, tomatoes, and kale).[7] During growth, the recommended dietary vitamin C required to prevent deficiency symptoms is 30 mg/kg daily.[3,6,7]

Any changes made to the diet of rabbits, guinea pigs, or chinchillas, should be done gradually, allowing time for new diet item acceptance and proper shifts in the hindgut microbial population. If leguminous hay was fed early in the animal's life, for example, the transition to providing grass hay only should begin before full growth is reached (~10 months for guinea pigs and small-to-medium rabbits; ~7 months for large breed rabbits) and take 2 to 4 weeks to complete, ensuring the grass hay is being well-consumed. Ensure sufficient water is provided using a preferred method. For guinea pigs, water is most commonly offered via a cage-side bottle drinker but for rabbits, consumption may be optimized when offered water from a bowl.[5,12] Daily appetite, body weight, body condition, fecal production (frequency and consistency), and cecotrophic behavior should be closely monitored by clients and if any concerns, reported to the veterinarian immediately to avoid a rapid decline in health.

Domestic ferrets (*Mustela furo*) are born altricial and weaned by 6 to 8 weeks. Kits should be offered soft, moist foods as early as 3 weeks of age until about 14 weeks when ferrets are ~90% fully grown.[4,13] As obligate carnivores, the gastrointestinal tract is simple, transit time rapid (3–4 hours), and metabolic rate high; therefore, ferrets should be provided food at least 3 times/day and/or free choice to prevent fasting for more than 3 hours.[4,13,14] The diet should provide sufficient calories for growth, approximating 1.5 to 3 times adult maintenance of 200 to 300 kcal ME/kg of body weight daily, and contain 35% protein and 20% or greater fat "as fed" to support growth.[4,13,15,16] Appropriate diet items range from whole prey, to fresh or freeze-dried complete meat products, to dry kibble. Commercial dry kibble should be of high quality and formulated for ferrets, containing animal-based ingredients (vs plant) and supplying plenty of protein with minimal carbohydrates/fiber. If it is not possible to obtain ferret-specific feed, a premium kitten or all-life-stage cat food can be considered. Early on, dry kibble should be moistened with water or, if growth rate is slow, goat milk has successfully been used to boost caloric intake.[17] Vitamin E deficiency has been reported in growing kits fed diets high in polyunsaturated fatty acids but low in vitamin E. Clinical symptoms include lethargy, vocalizing when handled, reluctance to move, and death. Firm subcutaneous swellings indicating steatitis and fatty liver degeneration are key postmortem findings.[14,18] This condition, however, would be avoided if high-quality, varied diets were provided, as is recommended for juvenile ferrets.

Specialist omnivores, such as 4-toed hedgehogs (*Atelerix albiventris*; insectivorous) and sugar gliders (*Petaurus breviceps*; gummivorous), are popular exotic pets. For both species, obesity and MBD are the most commonly encountered nutritional disorders. Juveniles must therefore be provided sufficient but not excessive energy for growth and appropriate protein, fat, and minerals. Additionally, husbandry practices must support thermoregulation, which impacts diet digestibility and nutrient absorption, and encourage activity while in captivity.

Neonatal hedgehogs, or hoglets, are born altricial, weaned between 4 and 6 weeks, begin eating solid food as early as 3 weeks of age, and can be acquired by owners as early as 8 weeks.[19] Hoglets grow rapidly in their first few months of life; however, growth rates and related energy requirements have not been established.[20–22] Hedgehogs are crepuscular and should be fed in the evening. The diet should comprise a high-quality commercial insectivore diet supplemented with gut-loaded insects (eg, mealworms, crickets, and Dubia roaches), providing 30% to 50% protein and 10% to 20% fat relative to DM basis.[19,20,23] Hedgehogs likely have a greater requirement for fiber, in the form of chitin, due to the ingestion of insect exoskeletons.[19,24] The energy required for growth has not been reported. Hedgehog adult maintenance energy requirements vary with species, body mass, and ambient temperature. To ensure growth is appropriate, therefore, simply monitor body weight, body condition, and diet consumption, to ensure growth rate is not excessive, and encourage exercise/activity to mitigate the onset of obesity.[19,20] Ensuring complete feed consumption and that insects are gut-loaded and/or dusted with a calcium supplement is necessary for MBD prevention. In hoglets aged younger than 4 weeks, hindlimb paresis/paralysis has responded to thiamine supplementation, indicating a deficiency possibly due to a gastrointestinal disturbance limiting nutrient absorption.[2] If kept well-fed and warm (70°F–80°F; 21°C–27°C) year-round, hedgehogs will not hibernate, which will help avoid nutritional diseases in captivity.[20,23]

Sugar gliders are marsupials, with neonates nursing in the pouch until 70 days of age. At ~130 days, young are weaned and moved into the nest.[14,25] At 200 days of age, juveniles are considered subadults and sexual maturity occurs by 8 to 12 months for females and 12 to 15 months for males.[14] The natural diet of sugar gliders primarily consists of saps, gums, nectar, and insects/arachnids.[14] In captivity, diets should include high-quality complete feed, fruit, vegetables, and insects (eg, mealworms, crickets, and Dubia roaches).[14,24] Commercial diets marketed for sugar gliders are available but few studies have verified their "complete" nature for the species. Alternatively, a premium dry complete feed formulated for omnivores or a high-protein supplement specifically formulated for sugar gliders may be used to satisfy the species' protein requirement.[26,27] These items, however, may provide other nutrients in excess or cause their dilution and result in undesirably low concentrations; therefore, ideally if such products are used, the complete diet should be reviewed by a nutritionist to ensure nutrient-balance.[27] Diets offering excessive produce, particularly those with a low calcium-to-phosphorus ratio (**Table 1**), should be avoided due to inadequate protein and calcium, predisposing the joeys to MBD and dental disease.[14]

To support growth, one study reported an average intake of 24 to 35 kcal/d for sugar gliders weighing 96 g.[26] Body mass, activity level, and ambient temperature all affect the species' energy needs. Therefore, the proper amount of energy and nutrients can be supplied by offering 1-part (by weight) commercial feed to 1-part produce (as 75% fruits, 25% vegetables), and, as the sugar glider reaches adulthood, shift the ratio to 1-part commercial diet to 2-parts produce to help mitigate obesity.[24] Fruit sugars, such as nectar or sap (eg, maple syrup, honey, and artificial nectar products), and gum arabic are often recommended but their digestibility requires further investigation.[14] These diet items could be offered on a weekly basis as enrichment but should not be a base component of the daily diet.

Sugar gliders are nocturnal and should be fed in the evening to optimize feeding behaviors and diet consumption and provided with adequate dietary vitamin D_3 to support bone growth. Hind limb paresis/paralysis caused by MBD is a significant concern and tends to occur when fed an excessive amount of unsupplemented insects or produce with an inverse Ca:P. Insects should be gut-loaded or dusted with a calcium supplement, and depending on the consumption of complete feed, one that also includes

Table 1
Examples of fruits that can be fed to sugar gliders and their respective calcium-to-phosphorous ratios, classified as inadequate (<1:1), marginal (~1:1), or adequate (>1:1)

Calcium-To-Phosphorous Ratio (Ca:P)	Example Fruits
< 1:1	Grapes
	Bananas
	Apples
	Pears
	Watermelon
~ 1:1	Cantaloupe
	Honeydew
	Strawberries
	Raspberries
	Pineapple
> 1:1	Blueberries
	Citrus (orange and grapefruit)
	Figs
	Mango
	Flower blossoms (roses and hibiscus)

vitamin D3. The diet should contain at least 1% calcium, 0.5% phosphorous, 1 to 2:1 Ca:P, and 1500 IU/kg vitamin D3 on a DM basis.[14] The total amount of insects, especially high-fat species such as mealworms and wax worms, fed should also be closely controlled to maintain desired body weight and nutrient balance. Further, browse for perching should be offered daily from an early age as juveniles are growing, to encourage chewing (supporting dental health) and jumping (encouraging activity).[25]

CONSIDERATIONS FOR REPTILE SPECIES

For captive reptiles, husbandry practices, including proper lighting, humidity, temperature, and substrate, work in concert with the diet to optimize health.[28,29] For herbivorous reptiles, poor husbandry practices are exacerbated by insufficient dietary minerals provided under human care. Cultivated vegetation typically fed to these captive herbivores lacks sufficient calcium and vitamin A, making them more susceptible to nutritional MBD than insectivorous reptiles.[29] Advanced MBD often results in skeletal deformities, soft, rubber-like jaw structure, and easily fractured limbs but earlier stages of the disease are less obvious and often more treatable.[30] Dusting vegetation with a mineral supplement is recommended; however, the specific minerals required can vary by species, age, and sex. Most commonly, supplementation of calcium and vitamin D_3 is key for the prevention of MBD. This is also true for insectivorous reptiles, where insects can be supplemented before feeding. Dusting, or lightly coating insects, is one method of supplementation; however, the timing of application is key. Many insects groom themselves and move around the enclosure before the reptile has a chance to consume them, so insects should be dusted immediately before feeding to minimize supplement loss. Preferably, insects can be "gut loaded" by being fed a diet hyperdosed with minerals and vitamins so that the reptile is consuming an enriched, or fortified, diet item.

In addition to dietary supplementation, providing appropriate ultraviolet B (UVB) light is essential, particularly for juvenile reptiles, to ensure proper calcium absorption and metabolism through the conversion of dehydrocholesterol in the skin to vitamin D.[31] UVB requirements vary by species, so it is essential to review species-specific requirements when making recommendations for husbandry plans. Veiled chameleons (Chamaeleo calyptratus), for example, must meet their calcium requirements from both their diet and UVB exposure for vitamin D synthesis,[28] whereas the nocturnal crested gecko (Correlophus ciliates) may obtain the required vitamin D from diet alone and may not have a substantial UVB light requirement.[32]

Obesity is a common issue in reptiles under human care and can usually be linked to inappropriate diet and/or lack of physical activity.[30] Hypovitaminosis A due to insufficient nutritional vitamin content or absorption is also often suspected in reptiles but can be difficult to diagnose without treatment with vitamin A supplementation or beta-carotene for confirmation.[30] Other considerations that are pivotal to the care of juvenile reptile nutrition are temperature, humidity, and available space because these aspects influence feeding behaviors and/or digestion.[31,33]

Central bearded dragons (Pogona vitticeps) are popular pets and are usually purchased at the juvenile stage. Wild juvenile bearded dragons consume approximately a 50:50 ratio of animal matter to vegetation, increasing vegetation consumption to 90% as they mature into adults.[34] Cricket sizes no larger than the width of the reptile's head and gut-loaded with preformed vitamin A are recommended for juvenile bearded dragons and should be fed alongside an assortment of high-fiber produce (eg, dark leafy greens, carrots, and squashes).[34,35] Vegetables should be dusted with a phosphorus-free vitamin D_3 supplement at least 2 to 4 times per month.[34,36] A diet consisting of more than 50% insects, even a variety of insect species, is not suitable for bearded dragons at any life stage and may contribute to a greater risk of hypercholesterolemia.[34,37] Many reptile keepers observe a hesitancy to eat, or a total reduction in diet consumption, as bearded dragons are transitioned toward the vegetation-based adult diet. This can be alarming and often cause keepers to revert to an insect-heavy diet, which can lead to severe health issues over time. One way to potentially mitigate this response is to advise owners of this natural diet shift well in advance and make a slow, gradual transition. It may be helpful to provide insects on top of or mixed into the vegetation portion of the diet because some bearded dragons will continue to feed on available vegetation once stimulated to feed by the movement of the offered insect(s). Suggested feeding schedules for bearded dragons at different life stages include 2 to 3 times daily for hatchlings, twice daily for juveniles, and once daily for adults.[34] Feeding should take place during the morning, or just before the warmest part of the day, to aid in appropriate digestion.[33] It should also be noted that the presence of fruit in the diet has been significantly associated with dental disease in bearded dragons and should therefore be fed rarely or not at all.[36,38]

Geckos are a common reptile pet for both new and experienced keepers. Some of the most commonly kept gecko species are leopard geckos (*Eublepharis macularius*) and crested geckos, both of which are often considered "beginner" species for reptile-keeping novices. Gecko dietary requirements vary significantly by species as wild geckos are widely distributed throughout a range of habitats. For instance, leopard geckos are primarily insectivorous at all life stages.[31] Live, moving prey is often used to stimulate reliable feeding,[31] so gut-loading and/or dusting is of particular importance. Crested geckos, however, are a tropical arboreal species, which are both insect-eaters and fruit-eaters. Juvenile crested geckos can be more easily housed together than adults, so it is key to provide ample feeding space to ensure each individual can access their appropriate diet. Although commonly practiced in adults, checking the oral calcium sacs (ie, pouch-like structures located on the oral palate) of juvenile crested geckos may not provide sufficient assessment of diet calcium availability because it does not account for different life stage requirements (eg, growth and breeding). Fortunately, various complete diets are commercially available for crested geckos, and these diets seem to be sufficient for all life stages.

Common green iguanas (*Iguana iguana*) are herbivorous at all life stages, including as juveniles,[39] and should be fed a variety of dark leafy greens, tropical fruits, and flowers. A common mistake made is providing a large proportion of lettuces, which are not nutritionally dense enough to represent the bulk of the animal's diet.[39] Research has demonstrated that hatchlings require at least 22.5% protein for appropriate growth[40–42] and iguanas, similar to other herbivorous reptiles, can readily develop MBD from a Ca:P that deviates too far from 2:1.[43] Some foods can also contribute to thyroid issues (eg, Bok choy, kale, turnips, chard, rutabaga, and *Brassica* flowers) and should be fed sparingly.[39,44] Other foods may be too high in tannins and should also be avoided or fed rarely. These include bananas, grapes, and carrots.[39] Frozen-thawed vegetables should be avoided in iguana diets as the phytothiaminases present in such foods have been linked to the development of thiamine deficiency.[30,45] Commercial diets are available for iguanas but it should be noted that these diets may not provide the required moisture and should be fed with water available at all times.[39,41]

Snakes are a popular pet reptile due to the availability of docile species that are readily available from pet stores and breeders. These include the commonly kept corn snake (*Pantherophis guttatus*), royal "ball" python (*Python regius*), and rosy boa (*Lichanura trivirgata*).[46] Each of these species has a unique life history and preferred wild diet items but as juveniles kept in captivity, they have similar dietary recommendations. Because snakes are carnivores and have a relatively simple digestive system, highly digestible whole-prey items should be provided.[44] Typically, frozen-thawed pinkie mice are an appropriate starter food item for juvenile snakes but prey should increase in size as body length and head/jaw width increase. Live prey feeding is not usually necessary or recommended because it can pose a significant risk of injury to the snake, especially to inexperienced juveniles.[46] Euthanized or frozen-thawed food items should be offered several times first to determine the receptiveness of individual snakes. Increasing surface temperature of the thawed food item directly before feeding often encourages pitted snakes (ie, those containing pit organs used for heat sensing), such as pythons and boas, to pursue dead prey. However, the use of a microwave oven or scalding water to increase surface temperature of prey items is not recommended because this can lead to "hot spots" in the prey item that can damage the snake's sensitive oral and digestive anatomy.[44] Anorexia in captive snakes is commonly reported with hypothermia and/or parasite infection being typical causes.[46] It is also important to note that some species, such as ball pythons, may experience seasonal shifts in feeding behavior, and that not all reluctance to eat is a sign of illness in snakes.[44]

In the United States, there are regulations against the purchase of turtles and tortoises with a shell less than 4 inches in diameter (eg, the 1975 "4-inch rule" of the US Food and Drug Administration) but smaller animals are still commonly available to purchase from private dealers and breeders. Often turtles and tortoises are purchased in the juvenile stage, especially for larger, fast-growing tortoise species such as aldabra (*Aldabrachelys gigantea*), sulcata (*Centrochelys sulcata*), and leopard tortoises (*Stigmochelys pardalis*), whereas others, such as many of the small-to-medium-sized tortoises and semiaquatic turtles, Russian tortoises (*Testudo horsfieldii*), Indian star tortoises (*Geochelone elegans*), and box turtles (*Terrapene* spp), are often acquired later in developmental stage because it takes longer for them to meet the 4-inch rule. Important nutritional considerations for juvenile turtles and tortoises are similar to those for other reptiles, with special care needed to ensure proper diet calcium, protein, fiber, thiamine, and vitamin A contents and ratios are met.[29,30,47] For herbivorous turtles and tortoises, high-fiber vegetation should constitute most of the diet, with various complete diets commercially available but sometimes avoided due to apparent palatability issues. Some vegetation such as spinach, cabbage, and beet greens are known to contain high levels of oxalate that binds calcium and thus should be fed rarely or avoided entirely.[48] Aquatic and semiaquatic turtles consume both plant and animal matter. These species are susceptible to thiamine deficiency if fed frozen fish thawed slowly, hastening enzymatic breakdown of thiamine, or fish known to have naturally higher concentrations of thiaminase (eg, common feeder fish, goldfish, and fathead minnows).[30] As with other reptiles, MBD is of primary concern, so adequate UVB lighting and appropriate diet Ca:P are paramount.

CONSIDERATIONS FOR AVIAN SPECIES

The juvenile stage for birds extends from fledging to reproductive maturity and varies in length depending on species. Precocial birds such as backyard chickens have a short juvenile stage (~20 weeks), whereas sexual maturity in large parrots may not occur until 6 years of age. This section will discuss common dietary needs of juvenile birds as well as associated issues and diseases in 4 orders commonly kept as pets.

Backyard chickens have become very popular, and the National Animal Health Monitoring system is planning a Backyard Animal Keeping 2024 Study.[49] Commercial feeds for production chickens can be problematic for juvenile pet birds. These feeds are designed to produce a 2 kg broiler from 3.4 kg of feed in less than 40 days.[50] This rapid growth can promote skeletal deformities such as tibial dyschondroplasia and angular bone deformities.[51] Additionally, chicks and growing birds that consume layer feeds can develop osteomalacia and renal insufficiency because chicks do not use the additional calcium in these feeds, resulting in an inverse Ca:P.[52,53] Use of a grower ration designed for backyard flocks will help prevent diet-related health conditions. Although not the only company with quality products for backyard birds, Purina Mills provides an excellent online guide to help consumers select the best food for life stage and region of the country. Parasitic infections are another common issue for growing backyard chickens. These birds typically ingest parasite eggs through contaminated feed or water or by direct consumption of parasite-carrying snails, earthworms, or other insects (intermediate hosts). Large roundworms (*Ascaridia galli*) pose the most significant risk. Although the ingestion of insects and earthworms can be a parasite source, most flock infections are from food and bedding soiled with fecal material of infected chickens. Good hygiene practices, including the removal of old food and maintaining clean and dry bedding, will help reduce parasite infestation.[54]

Ducks, geese, and swans are frequently kept as pets and are sometimes combined with chickens and, as with chickens, need to be maintained on feeds appropriate for juvenile growth. The majority of domestic ducks are descended from either mallard (*Anas platyrhynchos*) or Muscovy duck (*Cairina moschata*).[55] The Pekin is a commercial mallard type duck and is popular due to its fast growth. As with chickens, commercial ducks have been selectively bred to grow extremely fast. Pekin ducks can reach a 2 kg body weight in 60 days.[56] The most common issue associated with diet in juvenile pet ducks, geese, and swans is a condition called "angel wing." Angel wing (AW) presents as one or both wings twisting unnaturally outward.[57] The causes of AW may be varied and can include genetic aspects as well as toxin exposure[58]; however, excessive growth associated with a high-protein diet, or insufficient calcium and phosphorus intake, have also been linked to development of AW. As with chickens, it is important for their long-term health to transition these birds from a starter diet to a maintenance diet, and not directly to a breeder diet (**Table 2**).

Exercise is also an important consideration in the avoidance of skeletal deformities. Shredded greens can be scatter fed to promote foraging. The particle size of the greens should be increased as the birds grow. Additionally, mealworms can be added as a scatter feed beginning at 2 weeks of age. Approximately 5 mealworms per bird is enough to promote excitement and foraging. Both greens and mealworms add little to the diet's nutrient profile, so the amount offered should be limited and instead used as a means of promoting exercise and activity.

Pigeons and doves are kept as pets, often in large mixed species and breed colonies. Pigeons and doves are both Columbiformes with a crop that serves as a reservoir for ingested food. Although pigeons are commonly known as scavengers, doves are more discerning and have a wide range of species-specific diets. Pigeons kept as

Table 2
A simple diet progression, used by the Philadelphia Zoo, credited with the avoidance of excessive growth and skeletal deformities in collection waterfowl

Age	Diet Phase
Week 1–2	Appropriate commercial waterfowl starter diet
Week 3–5	2-parts commercial starter diet: 1-part commercial maintenance diet
Week 6–12	1-part commercial starter diet: 2-parts commercial maintenance diet
Week 13-breeding	Commercial maintenance diet

pets or in captive flocks have physical or behavioral attributes that make them desirable. These birds have been bred specifically for these attributes.

Crop stasis is likely the most feared digestive issue in Columbiformes. Crop stasis in juvenile birds is associated with environmental contaminants, such as lead,[59] viruses,[60,61] and pathogenic bacterial or fungus infections.[61] Hyperkeratosis is associated with vitamin A deficiency in many species of birds and is a common finding in association with candidiasis and crop stasis.[62] Vitamin A deficiency may also interfere with normal growth by altering the proliferation and maturation of cells of the intestinal mucosa.[63]

Flocks of pigeons and doves maintained on a commercial food appropriate for life stage and activity level, will stave off diet-related issues when fed properly. Companies, such as Mazuri Exotic Animal Nutrition, have developed feeding systems (ie, Nutritiblend Feeding System, Mazuri Exotic Animal Nutrition, St. Louis, MO, USA) for mixed species/breed flocks. Use of a commercially available feeding system that provides complete and balanced nutrition is a superior approach to nutrient supplementation. Excess vitamin A, as well as deficiency, can cause hyperkeratosis, as can deficiencies in biotin or zinc, affecting feather quality and beak and nail growth. Furthermore, nutrients work in conjunction with each other (ie, vitamin A supplementation without adequate vitamin E will have little effect), so supplementing just one nutrient at a time may have undesired effects on others.[63]

Psittacines are popular pets. Generally, pet psittacines can be grouped into 3 broad categories: small (<100 g such as parrotlets, budgerigars, lovebirds, cockatiels, and small conures), medium (110–140 g such as quaker and Senegal parrots, mini macaws, lorikeets, and many conures), and large (>150 g). In the United States, pet juvenile psittacines are captive-bred. Small psittacines are typically parent-reared, whereas medium and large birds are often hand-reared. Psittacines are classified as folivores; however, many species consume a variety of plant parts. Subclassifications include granivores (grain or seed-based diet: budgerigars and cockatiels), frugivores (fruit-based diet: macaws), and nectarivores (nectar-based diet: lorikeets and lories). Additionally, within the category of granivores, smaller birds select grass seeds, whereas larger birds add higher protein seeds from shrubs and trees.[64]

Crop stasis develops when the bird is a chick and can persist in juveniles, leading to death. The most common nutritional cause of crop stasis is tube feeding in chicks.[65] Other nutritional issues common in psittacines are gout, which is associated with energy intake and amino acid imbalance, obesity, and conversely, malnutrition. The best way to avoid nutritional issues in juvenile birds is to offer a nutritionally complete diet, using a pellet size appropriate for the size of the bird, and a feeding plan to ensure the needs of the owner and bird are both met.

For growing juveniles, the BMR can be calculated as $78 \times (BW_{kg}^{0.75})$. All energy needed to meet BMR should be provided using a nutritionally complete commercial biscuit or pellet. Seeds and nuts should be avoided for this base portion of the diet because birds tend to sort, only eating preferred items, which will lead to amino acid imbalances and other nutrient deficiencies.[64,66,67] Pet psittacines need twice the calculated BMR to sustain growth; however, the energy provided to support growth must be reduced as the bird approaches adult weight. Individually housed adult birds only require 1.2 to 1.4 times BMR; therefore, owners need to reduce the energy allowance above BMR to mitigate the development of obesity.

A simple feeding plan successfully used by the Philadelphia Zoo is as follows:

1. Calculate BMR $78 \times (BW_{kg}^{0.75})$ using the Atwater factors of 4 kcal/g protein, 9 kcal/g fat, and 4 kcal/g carbohydrate.[68]

2. Provide BMR as a commercial, species-appropriate, pellet or biscuit (or nectar, for appropriate species).
3. Provide 85% of the energy allotment above BMR as appropriate enrichment foods, avoiding seeds and nuts.
4. Allow 15% of the energy allotment above BMR for training/bonding foods. It is within this portion of the diet that seeds and nuts can be appropriate. If no training/bonding is taking place, incorporate this portion of the allotted energy into enrichment.

Owners should regularly monitor the body weight of their bird and only offer enrichment and training allotments after the commercial portion of the diet is consumed. The amount of commercial feed needed to meet a caged bird's BMR is visually less than expected.

SUMMARY

Veterinary involvement early in the life of exotic companion animals can help ensure proper nutrition is provided from the outset, to support growth and establish a strong foundation for healthy transition into adulthood. Unfortunately, limited research has been performed on the energy and nutrient requirements of pediatric exotic pets. Decisions must be made based on what is known about growth across species: supplying sufficient energy, meeting calcium and vitamin D3 requirements, and providing appropriate husbandry to optimize diet intake and metabolism. Further, an understanding of species-specific natural history will help address other important diet considerations, such as satisfying a rabbit's fiber needs, supplementing a juvenile bearded dragon with calcium, and encouraging a parrot to consume its complete feed. Exotic pediatric pets should have weekly body weight measurements, ideally at home with an appropriate scale, with concurrent body condition assessment, quantification/qualification of diet offered versus consumed, and observation of fecal output. If any concerns are noted, immediate veterinary intervention should be encouraged to thwart a rapid decline in health.

CLINICS CARE POINTS

- Nutritional secondary hyperparathyroidism, gastrointestinal stasis, and vitamin deficiencies are the most common nutritional diseases of juvenile small exotic mammals. Energy intake and the development of obesity in adulthood are directly affected by the nutrition received in the juvenile life stage.

- Changes made to the diet of rabbits, guinea pigs, or chinchillas, should be done gradually, allowing time for new diet item acceptance and proper shifts in the hindgut microbial population.

- Nutritional MBD is a significant risk for juvenile reptiles but can be prevented through appropriate nutrition and UV lighting.

- Many whole food items available for reptiles have an inappropriate Ca:P, and thus pure calcium supplementation may be necessary, especially for herbivorous species.

- For avian species, it is important to transition animals from a starter diet to a maintenance diet and not move directly to a breeder diet.

- A successful juvenile avian diet is based on the consumption of an appropriate commercial diet.

DISCLOSURE

Dr A. Ardente is the founder and owner of a for-profit nutrition consulting company (Ardente Veterinary Nutrition, LLC). R.L. Schultz is the Project Manager for a for-profit animal welfare consultancy (Animal Welfare Expertise). B. Toddes has no conflicts of interest.

REFERENCES

1. American Pet Products Association. Pet industry market size & ownership statistics. American Pet Products Association; 2023. Available at:.
2. National Research Council Subcommittee on Laboratory Animal Nutrition. Nutrient requirements of rabbits. 2nd revised edition. Washington DC: National Academies Press; 1977.
3. National Research Council Subcommittee on Laboratory Animal Nutrition. Nutrient requirements of Guinea pigs. 4th revised edition. Washington DC: National Academies Press; 1995.
4. Carpenter JW, Wolf KN, Kolmstetter C. Chapter 70: Feeding Small Pet Mammals. In: Hand MS, Thatcher CD, Remillard RL, et al, editors. Small animal clinical nutrition. 5th edition. Mark Morris Institute; 2010. p. 1215–36.
5. Smith SM. Gastrointestinal physiology and nutrition of rabbits. In: Quesenberry KE, Orcutt CJ, Mans C, et al, editors. Ferrets, rabbits, and rodents clinical medicine surgery. 4th edition. Elsevier; 2009. p. 1–12.
6. Donnelly T, Brown CJ. Guinea pig and chinchilla care and husbandry. Vet Clinics Exotic Anim Pract 2004;7:351–73.
7. Pignon C, Mayer J. Chapter 4: guinea pigs. In: Quesenberry KE, Orcutt CJ, Mans C, et al, editors. Ferrets, rabbits, and rodents. Elsevier; 2020. p. 270–97.
8. Oglesbee BL, Lord B. Gastrointestinal diseases of rabbits. ferrets, rabbits, and rodents. Elsevier; 2020. p. 174–87.
9. Edell AS, Vella DG, Sheen JC, et al. Retrospective analysis of risk factors, clinical features, and prognostic indicators for urolithiasis in guinea pigs: 158 cases (2009-2019). J Amer Vet Med Assoc 2022;260(S2):S95–100.
10. Ayers LS, Typpo JT, Krause GF. Isoleucine requirement of young growing male guinea pigs. J Nutr 1987;117(6):1098–101.
11. Typpo JT, Anderson HL, Krause GF, et al. The lysine requirement of young growing male guinea pigs. J Nutr 1985;115(5):579–87.
12. Balsiger A, Clauss M, Liesegang A, et al. Guinea pig (*Cavia porcellus*) drinking preferences: do nipple drinkers compensate for behaviourally deficient diets? J Anim Physiol Anim Nutr 2017;101(5):1046–56.
13. Powers LV, Perpinan D. Basic anatomy, physiology, and husbandry of ferrets. In: Quesenberry KE, Orcutt CJ, Mans C, et al, editors. Ferrets, rabbits, and rodents clinical medicine surgery. 4th edition. Elsevier; 2021. p. 1–12.
14. Johnson-Delaney C. Sugar gliders. In: Quesenberry KE, Orcutt CJ, Mans C, et al, editors. Ferrets, rabbits, and rodents clinical medicine surgery. 4th edition. Elsevier; 2021. p. 385–400.
15. Bell JA. Ferret nutrition. Vet Clin North Am Exot Anim Pract 1999;2(1):169–92.
16. Fox JG, Bell JA, Broome R. Growth and reproduction. In: Fox JG, Marini RP, editors. Biology and diseases of the ferret. 3rd edition. John Wiley & Sons; 2014. p. 187–209.
17. Morton EL, Mathis C. Ferrets: a complete pet owner's manual. Barron's Educational Series Inc.; 1985.

18. McLain DE, Thomas JA, Fox JG. Nutrition. In: Fox JG, editor. Biology and diseases of the ferret. Lea & Febiger; 1988. p. 135–52.

19. Doss GA, Carpenter JW. African pygmy hedgehogs. In: Quesenberry KE, Orcutt CJ, Mans C, et al, editors. Ferrets, rabbits, and rodents clinical medicine surgery. 4th edition. Elsevier; 2021. p. 401–15.

20. Bexton S. Hedgehogs. In: BSAVA manual of wildlife casualties. BSAVA Library; 2016. p. 117–36.

21. Bunnell T. Growth rate in early and late litters of the European hedgehog (*Erinaceus europaeus*). Lutra 2009;52(1):15–22.

22. Ivey E, Carpenter JW. African hedgehogs. In: Quesenberry KE, Carpenter JW, editors. Ferrets, rabbits, and rodents: clinical medicine and surgery. 3rd edition. Saunders-Elsevier; 2012. p. 411–28.

23. Hoefer HL. Hedgehogs Veterinary Clinics of North America: Small Animal Practice 1994;24(1):113–20.

24. Dierenfeld ES. Feeding behavior and nutrition of the sugar glider (*Petaurus breviceps*). Vet Clin Exot Anim Pract 2009;12(2):209–15.

25. Barnes M. Ch 9: Sugar gliders. In: Gage LJ, editor. Hand-rearing wild and domestic mammals. Blackwell Pub; 2002. p. 55–62.

26. Dierenfeld ES, Thomas D, Ives R. Comparison of commonly used diets on intake, digestion, growth, and health in captive sugar gliders (*Petaurus breviceps*). J Exot Pet Med 2006;15(3):218–24.

27. Dierenfeld ES, Whitehouse-Tedd KM. Evaluation of three popular diets fed to pet sugar gliders (*Petaurus breviceps*): Intake, digestion and nutrient balance. J Anim Physiol Anim Nutr 2018;102:e193–208.

28. Hoby S, Wenker C, Robert N, et al. Nutritional metabolic bone disease in juvenile veiled chameleons (*Chamaeleo calyptratus*) and its prevention. J Nutr 2010; 140(11):1923–31.

29. Fledelius B, Jørgensen GW, Jensen HE, et al. Influence of the calcium content of the diet offered to leopard tortoises (*Geochelone pardalis*). Vet Rec 2005;156(26): 831–5.

30. Mans C, Braun J. Update on common nutritional disorders of captive reptiles. Veterinary Clinics: Exotic Animal Practice 2014;17(3):369–95.

31. Oonincx D, van Leeuwen J. Evidence-based reptile housing and nutrition. Veterinary Clinics: Exot Anim Prac. 2017;20(3):885–98.

32. Kubiak M. In: *Handbook of exotic pet medicine*. Hoboken, NJ, USA: John Wiley & Sons; 2020.

33. Divers SJ, Stahl SJ, editors. Mader's reptile and amphibian medicine and surgery. Elsevier Health Sciences; 2018.

34. Raiti P. Husbandry, diseases, and veterinary care of the bearded dragon (*Pogona vitticeps*). J Herpetol Med Surg 2012;22(3–4):117–31.

35. Stahl SJ. General husbandry and captive propagation of bearded dragons, *Pogona vitticeps*. Bulletin of the Association of Reptilian and Amphibian Veterinarians 1999;9(4):12–7.

36. Barboza T, Bercier M. An Update on Companion Inland Bearded Dragon (Pogona vitticeps) Nutrition. Vet Clin North Am Exot Anim Pract 2024;27(1):71–84.

37. Schilliger L, Lemberger K, Chai N, et al. Atherosclerosis associated with pericardial effusion in a central bearded dragon (*Pogona vitticeps*). J Vet Diagn Invest 2010;22(5):789–92.

38. Mott R, Pellett S, Hedley J. Prevalence and risk factors for dental disease in captive Central bearded dragons (*Pogona vitticeps*) in the United Kingdom. J Exot Pet Med 2021;36:1–7.

39. Bogoslavsky B. Iguana nutrition. Iguana Times 2000;8(4):17–20.
40. Donoghue S. Growth of juvenile green iguanas (*Iguana iguana*) fed four diets. J Nutr 1994;124:2626S–9S.
41. Donoghue S, Vidal J, Kronfeld D. Growth and morphometrics of green iguanas (*Iguana iguana*) fed four levels of dietary protein. J Nutr 1998;128(12):2587S–9S.
42. Allen ME, Oftedal OT. Nutrition in captivity. *husbandry and veterinary management of the green iguana*. Krieger Publishing Company; 2003. p. 47–74.
43. Frye FF. The importance of calcium in relation to phosphorus, especially in folivorous reptiles. Proc Nutr Soc 1997;56(3):1105–17.
44. Maslanka MT, Frye FL, Henry BA, et al. Nutritional Considerations. In: Health and welfare of captive reptiles. Springer International Publishing; 2023. p. 447–85.
45. Calvert I. Nutritional problems. In: Girling SJ, Raiti P, editors. BSAVA manual of reptiles. British Small Animal Veterinary Association; 2004. p. 289–308.
46. Mitchell MA. Snake care and husbandry. Veterinary Clinics: Exotic Animal Practice 2004;7(2):421–46.
47. Rawski M, Mans C, Kierończyk B, et al. Freshwater turtle nutrition–a review of scientific and practical knowledge. Ann Anim Sci 2018;18(1):17–37.
48. Donoghue S. Nutrition in reptile medicine and surgery. 2nd edition. Saunders-Elsevier; 2006. p. 251–98.
49. USDA APHIS. (2023). Retrieved July 6, 2023, from https://www.aphis.usda.gov/aphis/ourfocus/animalhealth/monitoring-and-surveillance/nahms/nahms_smallscale_studies.
50. Siegel PB, Wolford JH. A review of some results of selection for juvenile body weight in chickens. J Poult Sci 2003;40(2):81–91.
51. Waldenstedt L. Nutritional factors of importance for optimal leg health in broilers: A review. Anml Feed Sci Tech 2006;126(3–4):291–307.
52. Barber, DL (n.d.). Basic guide for the backyard chicken flock. Retrieved July 14, 2023, from https://journals.flvc.org/edis/article/download/118543/116467/.
53. Henry ME, Ryals JM, Halbritter A, Barber DL. Raising Backyard Chickens for Eggs. 2019. https://edis.ifas.ufl.edu/publication/an239.
54. Butcher GD, Miles RD. Intestinal Parasites in Backyard Chicken Flocks. 2021.
55. Makram A, Galal A, El-Attar AH. Effect of natural versus artificial incubation on embryonic development of pekin, muscovy and sudani (*Egyptian Muscovy*) ducks crosses. J Genetic and Environmental Resources Conservation 2021; 9(2):51–9.
56. Chen X, Shafer D, Sifri M, et al. Centennial review: history and husbandry recommendations for raising pekin ducks in research or commercial production. Poultry Sci 2021;100(8):101241.
57. Arican M, Parlak K, Yalcin M. Angel wings syndrom in swans (Cygnus cygnus and cygnus atratus). Kafkas Üniversitesi Veteriner Fakültesi Dergisi 2019;25(6):873–7.
58. Zhu X, Shao B, Guo Y, et al. Incidence rate of angel wing and its effect on wing bone development and serum biochemical parameters in geese. Poult Sci 2021; 100(11):101450.
59. Boyer IJ, Cory-Slechta DA, DiStefano V. Lead induction of crop dysfunction in pigeons through a direct action on neural or smooth muscle components of crop tissue. J Pharmacol Exp The 1985;234(3):607–15.
60. Rahimi Sardo E, Talazadeh F, Jafari RA, et al. Phylogenetic analysis of pigeon adenovirus 1 in clinical specimens of domestic pigeons (*Columba livia domestica*) in Iran. Vet Res Forum: An International Quarterly Journal 2023;14(6): 329–34.

61. Rubbenstroth D, Peus E, Schramm E, et al. Identification of a novel clade of group a rotaviruses in fatally diseased domestic pigeons in europe. Transboundary and Emerging Diseases 2019;66(1):552–61.
62. Talazadeh F, Ghorbanpoor M, Masoudinezhad M. Phylogenetic analysis of pathogenic Candida spp. in domestic pigeons. Vet Res Forum 2023;14:8.
63. Harrison GJ, McDonald D. Nutritional considerations section II. Clin Avian Med 2006;108–40.
64. Koutsos EA, Matson KD, Klasing KC. Nutrition of birds in the order psittaciformes: a review. J Avian Med Surg 2001;15(4):257–75.
65. Romagnano A. Psittacine incubation and pediatrics. veterinary clinics. Exotic Animal Practice 2012;15(2):163–82.
66. Cummings AM, Hess LR, Spielvogel CF, et al. An evaluation of three diet conversion methods in psittacine birds converting from seed-based diets to pelleted diets. J Avian Med Surg 2022;36(2):145–52.
67. Ullrey DE, Allen ME, Baer DJ. Formulated diets versus seed mixtures for psittacines. J Nutr 1991;121:S193–205.
68. Atwater WO. Farmer's Bulletin no. 142: Principles of nutrition and nutritive value of food, Special Collections. USDA National Agricultural Library; 1910. p. 1–48.

Moving?

Make sure your subscription moves with you!

To notify us of your new address, find your **Clinics Account Number** (located on your mailing label above your name), and contact customer service at:

Email: journalscustomerservice-usa@elsevier.com

800-654-2452 (subscribers in the U.S. & Canada)
314-447-8871 (subscribers outside of the U.S. & Canada)

Fax number: 314-447-8029

Elsevier Health Sciences Division
Subscription Customer Service
3251 Riverport Lane
Maryland Heights, MO 63043

*To ensure uninterrupted delivery of your subscription, please notify us at least 4 weeks in advance of move.

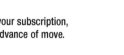

Printed and bound by CPI Group (UK) Ltd, Croydon, CR0 4YY

03/10/2024

01040468-0014